T0146067

ABORTION ACROSS BORDERS

ABORTION ACROSS BORDERS

Transnational Travel and Access to Abortion Services

EDITED BY Christabelle Sethna & Gayle Davis

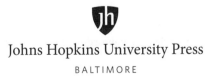

Johns Hopkins University Press

BALTIMORE

Johns Hopkins University Press
2715 North Charles Street
Baltimore, Maryland 21218-4363
www.press.jhu.edu

Library of Congress Cataloging-in-Publication Data

Names: Sethna, Christabelle, editor. | Davis, Gayle, editor.
Title: Abortion across borders : transnational travel and access to abortion services /
    [edited by] Christabelle Sethna and Gayle Davis.
Description: Baltimore, Maryland : Johns Hopkins University Press, 2019. |
    Includes bibliographical references and index.
Identifiers: LCCN 2018020740 | ISBN 9781421427294 (hardcover : alk. paper) |
    ISBN 142142729X (hardcover : alk. paper) | ISBN 9781421427300 (electronic) |
    ISBN 1421427303 (electronic)
Subjects: | MESH: Abortion, Induced—history | Medical Tourism—history |
    Abortion, Legal—legislation & jurisprudence | Health Policy | Women's Rights |
    Internationality | History, 20th Century
Classification: LCC HQ767 | NLM WA 11.1 | DDC 362.1988/8—dc23
LC record available at https://lccn.loc.gov/2018020740

A catalog record for this book is available from the British Library.

*Special discounts are available for bulk purchases of this book. For more information,
please contact Special Sales at 410-516-6936 or specialsales@press.jhu.edu.*

Johns Hopkins University Press uses environmentally friendly book materials,
including recycled text paper that is composed of at least 30 percent post-consumer
waste, whenever possible.

CONTENTS

The idea for this edited volume took root over lunch in a café in Edinburgh, Scotland, a number of years ago. The editors would like to thank the contributors for their enthusiasm and most of all for their patience as this volume shape-shifted over time. Angela Chnapko kindly steered the manuscript in the direction of Robin W. Coleman at Johns Hopkins University Press. We are grateful to Robin for believing in the book, to his colleagues Adelene Jane Sapal, Sahara Clement, and Juliana McCarthy, and to copyeditor Nicole Wayland for all their efforts. The remarkable personal and professional dedication of Senior Production Editor Debby Bors to preparing this manuscript for publication is deeply appreciated.

This volume owes much to the Social Sciences and Humanities Research Council of Canada and the research assistants hired, notably young and dedicated feminists Erin Jex and Julie Vautour. A special note of gratitude is extended to Agata Ignaciuk and Jesse Olszynko-Gryn, whose fabulous research skills are matched by their good cheer; to Catelynne Sahadath for her ability to unearth with lightning speed any reference requested; to Jessica Campbell for investing significant effort into our index; and to Steven Devine for his impressive technical skills and unstinting support.

Gayle wishes to thank Roger Davidson, University of Edinburgh; Lesley Hall, Wellcome Library, London; and Sally Sheldon, University of Kent, for encouraging and improving her research on women's reproductive health. Christabelle acknowledges Denis Prud'homme and Geneviève Rail for their understanding. Marion Doull has been invaluable throughout. And Ruth Roach Pierson continues to inspire.

ABORTION ACROSS BORDERS

Introduction

CHRISTABELLE SETHNA

A TELEVISION JOURNALIST asked American president-elect Donald Trump in November 2016 what would happen if *Roe v. Wade*, the 1973 Supreme Court decision protecting abortion rights in the United States of America (USA), were overturned. Trump ventured that, as individual states would then determine whether to provide abortion services, women without access to them would "have to go to another state."[1] Across the Atlantic a year later, Ailbhe Smyth, a spokeswoman for the group Coalition to Repeal the Eighth Amendment in the Republic of Ireland (hereafter Ireland), expressed concern about Brexit, the decision made by the United Kingdom (UK) in a June 2016 referendum to leave the European Union (EU). She alleged that Irish women traveling to the UK to access abortion services could end up having later-term abortions because of potential delays at the border, saying: "If the UK decides limitations on the kinds of services people from other jurisdictions can access, then there are so many questions up in the air."[2]

Despite the controversial status of abortion, safe, legal abortion is recognized as an essential medical service for women in many parts of the world.[3] If access to abortion services is unavailable or hindered by legal and extralegal obstacles, women are compelled to carry their pregnancies to term, seek an illegal abortion, or self-induce.[4] A lesser-known option, to which Trump and Smyth refer in their comments, is travel undertaken across domestic and international borders to access surgical or medical abortion services.[5]

This is the first edited volume to provide a strong focus specifically on the transnational aspects of travel, in the broadest sense of the word, for abortion services in the past and present. It emerges out of growing academic attention paid to the nexus of reproductive healthcare, mobility, and globalization. While there are many definitions of globalization, it is generally understood as the liberalization of economic markets all over the globe and the rapid movement of people, goods, and services but also networks, ideas, and ideologies that cross borders. Cross-border mobility has been accelerated by the explosion of transportation systems and telecommunications technologies since the 1990s. The periodization of globalization is imprecise; it varies greatly, with some supposing that globalization is ages old, or a more recent iteration of colonialism, or a verifiable new historical epoch dating back to the late twentieth century. For some, globalization has had a positive effect by creating more economic opportunities, but others are convinced that it has widened the gap between rich and poor. Feminist scholars, too, are divided on whether globalization has been bad for women, with some claiming that it has deepened economic inequality, especially in the Global South, while others contend that it has created more job opportunities for women and has spurred the growth of transnational feminist activist networks addressing women's rights.[6] However, in the past several years a growing focus on national security, especially in countries pursuing the populist politics of white nationalism, has intensified international border "thickening." Border zones have been militarized and extensive checks have been placed on cross-border mobility, upending the original potent promise of globalization.[7]

Transnational travel for abortion services remains a noteworthy example of cross-border mobility in search of reproductive healthcare. Chapters in this volume cover North America, the UK, Western Europe, Eastern Europe, Australia, and New Zealand. It is but a small snapshot of transnational abortion travel because there are substantial swathes of the world it does not include, namely Africa, the Middle East, Asia, and Latin America, categorized roughly as the Global South despite many individual exceptions. In any case, reproductive matters are not necessarily generalizable by geographical region; the Global South encompasses countries that have some of the world's most liberal *and* some of the most restrictive abortion laws, leading in the latter instance to the world's first "abortion refugee" to be granted asylum.[8] Additionally, the American government's intermittent deployment of the Ronald Reagan–era Mexico City Policy, commonly known as the "Global Gag Rule," which forbids any overseas organization that provides abortions or counseling about abortion from receiving American foreign aid, even if abortion were legal in the country in which it operates, has since the 1980s decimated reproductive health services in regions with already high rates of conflict, poverty, and maternal and infant mortality.[9] Close attention needs to be paid to the role of cross-border travel for abortion services in these regions, especially given the enmeshed histories of migration, colonial dominance, and globalization in relation to the Global North. In this light, Gail Pheterson and Yamila Azize have found that many laws determining abortion provision in the Caribbean are holdovers of "colonial jurisprudence." They argue that "travel between countries is a constant feature of life in most of the region," with women compelled to travel to other Caribbean islands, or to one side of an island from another, in order to access abortion services anonymously.[10]

Laws and policies concerning abortion remain a moving target. In global terms, Russia was the first country to legalize abortion in 1920, and although this trend was liable to reversals, legalization was also seen in Eastern European countries by the 1950s. Sweden legalized abortion in the 1930s, and Japan in the 1940s, largely for eugenic reasons. A general trend toward the legalization or liberalization of abortion laws and policies in the Global North since the 1960s is apparent, with Malta, the Vatican, Ireland, and Northern Ireland among the longtime holdouts. After the fall of the Berlin Wall in 1989, some Eastern European countries—Poland in particular—introduced serious constraints on legal abortion.[11] In a 2018 referendum in Ireland, a sizeable majority of the populace voted to repeal the Eighth Amendment. The amendment gave equal constitutional protection to a pregnant woman and her fetus, amounting to a virtual ban on legal abortion on Irish soil. In the USA it is speculated that a more conservative Supreme Court might overturn *Roe v. Wade*, emboldening many states to gut access to abortion services even further.[12] This volume is not, however, about abortion legislation or abortion policies per se in the regions it covers but about the historical and contemporary ebb and flow of interconnected local and global mobilities, and the ways in which they shape and are shaped by legal and extralegal obstacles to abortion services, even in countries that supposedly have liberal abortion laws.

Travel for abortion services is implicated heavily in the politics of reproductive rights, choice, and justice but is understudied.[13] When entire works are devoted to the study of abortion, abortion travel is mostly absent, or referred to only in a piecemeal fashion. Even in the case of the USA, where all politics are said to be reproductive politics, abortion remains central to federal and state decision-making in many contexts, and there is ample evidence of the need for many women to travel from one state to another due to state-imposed restrictions on access.[14]

Travel for abortion services inside and outside the USA has been necessary both before and after *Roe v. Wade*. Linda Greenhouse and Reva B. Siegal, in *Before Roe v. Wade: Voices That Shaped the Abortion Debate before the Supreme Court's Ruling,* reprint detailed instructions from the Society for Humane Abortion about traveling from San Francisco to Tokyo to access abortion providers, while Johanna Schoen's *Abortion after Roe* gives a fleeting nod to women's travel for abortion services in the pre–*Roe v. Wade* era. Katha Pollitt's *Pro: Reclaiming Abortion Rights* mentions abortion travel as a historical fact and as a factor that continues to place American women at risk of later-term abortions. Carol Sanger, in *About Abortion: Terminating Pregnancy in Twenty-First-Century America,* briefly acknowledges the importance of traveling for abortion services in the past, given that individual states have been "hacking away at the abortion right in every way they can." More awareness of the ongoing travel of doctors and patients in order to provide or access a patchwork system of abortion services is present throughout Carole Joffe's *Dispatches from the Abortion Wars: The Costs of Fanaticism to Doctors, Patients, and the Rest of Us.* And although her book is neither about abortion nor abortion travel exclusively, Jennifer Nelson's *More Than Medicine: A History of the Feminist Women's Health Movement* raises the issue of travel for abortion services, linking together feminist activism and abortion referral services established in the state of Washington. Each of these texts finds that socioeconomic and racial inequality factor greatly into women's ability to access an abortion or not.[15]

Particularly useful to this volume is strong academic interest in the "mobility turn" and the consequent examination of the movement of people, goods, and services between, through, and across space, time, and place. Mobility can be embodied, practiced, or represented.[16] For example, for a woman to access abortion services, she might travel to an abortion provider by car, train, ferry, bus, or plane. However, the prospect of medical (as opposed to surgical) abortion may mean that the same woman living in a healthcare jurisdiction where abortion is illegal, or otherwise difficult to access, may not have to leave it at all. She might swallow a combination of mifepristone and misoprostol, abortion-inducing drugs most effective in the first trimester of pregnancy, that she purchased online from a feminist activist group in another country and that was delivered to her home by the postal service.[17]

Cross-border exchanges of various kinds factor crucially into a wide range of mobilities that are directly or tangentially associated with access to abortion services. Thus, while travel for abortion services is most closely associated with the embodied cross-border travel of women seeking pregnancy termination through surgical (and sometimes medical) abortion, this volume allows that it must also be understood more fluidly to include: fluctuations in laws and policies; variable roles of individuals, organizations, and agencies on the local, national, and international scene; the random flow of ideas, media, and communications networks; haphazard professional and nonprofessional medical care; irregular transportation and accommodation; changes to geographical, political, economic, and jurisdictional boundaries; oscillations between prochoice and anti-abortion activism; variations in medical protocols for abortion; the merry-go-round of private and public sector abortion provision; and personal experiences of succeeding or failing to access abortion services, whether legal or illegal, away from one's community.

Originally, the term "abortion tourism" was used to signal women's physical travel across international borders to access abortion services. Now, it is often employed to describe the phenomenon of women's travel across international and domestic borders for the purposes of pregnancy termination, but it is sometimes seen as pejorative or is considered to have anti-abortion connotations, and the usefulness of the term itself is contested.[18] Travel for abortion services is sometimes considered a subset of "medical tourism," which is said to be one of the most salient commercial outcomes of globalization.[19] Like globalization, medical tourism is difficult to define. Scholars disagree over its scope (is it distinct from "health tourism"?), reach (does it involve international *and* domestic border crossings?), emergence (can it be dated to the 1990s?), and connection to holiday-making (are vacation packages part of the recuperation process?). The terminology itself warrants scrutiny, with some arguing in favor of expressions like "medical travel."[20] Generally, it is agreed that medical tourism is a billion-dollar transnational global industry linking patients with medical services outside one's designated healthcare jurisdiction to destination hubs all over the world.[21] Most of the travel for medical services is regional, and it often involves close geographical neighbors.[22] Although it is uncertain as to who counts as a medical tourist, the growth of medical tourism since the 1990s has been exponential, attracting "patients without borders."[23] The literature on medical tourism is sizeable, and it raises fascinating and challenging logistical, legal, and ethical questions. However, among its current weaknesses, the literature often fails to explore women's involvement in medical tourism and, particularly, the travel of women for medical services, including abortion services. Travel for abortion services—which is considered unique to (cisgendered) women but can also involve queer, gender nonconforming individuals, and transmen—is often given short shrift by scholars.[24]

Research in medical tourism can be found in health studies, women's and gender studies, geography, law, bioethics, sociology, medical anthropology, and urban, tourism, and migration studies. Yet when scholars in these fields acknowledge the influence of gender, concerted attention to travel to access abortion services is largely absent. Well-received edited collections related to medical tourism continue to illustrate just how little space is taken up by travel for abortion services. In *Fieldwork in Tourism: Methods, Issues and Reflections*, edited by C. Michael Hall, contributors Audrey Bochaton and Bertrand Lefebvre discuss the flow of medical tourists to India and Thailand for various medical procedures, yet they do not refer to abortion.[25] Medical tourism guides sometimes make note of travel for abortion services; in *Medical Tourism: A Reference Handbook*, by Kathy S. Stolley and Stephanie Watson, abortion merits only two brief references in relation to "reproductive tourism" and "illegal procedures."[26] One of the best-known edited collections on medical tourism and its various permutations is *Medical Tourism: The Ethics, Regulation, and Marketing of Health Mobility*, edited once again by C. Michael Hall. Here there are scattered mentions of travel for fertility and abortion services, but with little to no elaboration.[27] Raywat Deonandan's chapter on fertility tourism to India in *Bon voyage: Essais sur le tourisme medical/Travelling Well: Essays in Medical Tourism*, coedited by Ron Labonté et al., briefly tackles abortion tourism and wonders about the possibility that women from countries in which abortion (or other stigmatized medical services) were illegal may be prosecuted upon returning home.[28] A helpful edited collection by I. Glenn Cohen, *The Globalization of Health Care: Legal and Ethical Issues*, raises various concerns over cross-border travel including, at times, travel for abortion or fertility services.[29] Abortion travel makes a brief appearance in a chapter by Tamra Lysaght and Douglas Sipp in *Bodies across Borders: The Global Circulation of Body Parts, Medical Tourists and Professionals*, coedited by Bronwyn Parry et al., positioning it within the category of "morally contestable activities."[30]

There are several reasons for this lacuna. It may be because scholarship on medical tourism is more interested in niche markets for medical services and tends to portray the "medical tourist" as a generic figure unmoored from identity variables (aside from nationality) such as gender, race, class, and sexuality.[31] Or, despite its commonality, abortion remains a stigmatized medical service even when it is legal, and more so in some countries as opposed to others. Still, travel for abortion services is rarely included, even in research on travel to access other stigmatized medical procedures, such as organ transplants and doctor-assisted suicide.[32] Moreover, and crucially for this volume, the vast majority of medical tourism research, aside from some interest in health tourism, is focused overtly on the present. Yet a historical perspective reveals that women have traveled to and fro in considerable numbers for abortion services in Eastern Europe, Japan, Britain, Mexico, the UK, Canada, and the USA since at least the 1960s, predating the rise of medical tourism in the 1990s.[33]

Another possible reason why travel for abortion services is generally ignored may be that when attention is concentrated on women's travel for medical services, it is limited to, and most closely associated with, fertility services. These fertility services are said to be accessed most often by white, middle-class, Western, heterosexual, and, increasingly, gay individuals and couples, although these demographics have been challenged as all too stereotypical.[34] The intention here is to (re)produce a much-wanted child, a goal promoted as benefiting the creation of stable and loving families, and befitting to women for whom motherhood is still considered foundational in many societies. Moreover, as reproductive technologies have been harnessed to globalization and commercialization, scholarship on fertility services has boomed, with travel for abortion services left behind in its shadow. Abortion travel is not included in "medical travels" involving access to gametes (as well as other body parts), although this type of mobility is said to be "illustrative of a new globalized and neoliberal bioeconomy in which people's desperation, hopes, and longing for health, reproduction, and normality fuel the transactions and travels that take place."[35] Conversely, the divide between travel for abortion services and travel for fertility services is challenged, as evidenced by attempts by Guido Pennings and

I. Glenn Cohen to unite the two under terms such as "reproductive tourism" and "circumvention tourism," respectively.[36]

Regardless, the omission in the literature is odd given that individuals who cross borders for many kinds of medical services encounter very similar legal and extralegal obstacles in their healthcare jurisdictions as do women seeking abortion services. These obstacles, which can run from laws or policies prohibiting or restricting the required medical service to unavailable or untrained medical personnel, inadequate hospitals or clinic facilities, travel distance to the medical provider, scarce transportation, high costs, a lack of insurance coverage, long wait lists, and social stigma, raise the issue of the social privilege of those who travel. Medical tourism tends to be associated with neoliberal freedoms, autonomy, and choice on the part of patients who are economically stable enough to contemplate traveling to another health jurisdiction and paying the attendant costs. However, travel to access medical services, among them abortion services, is often a response to inequality of access at the local level, reinforcing or exacerbating discrimination by gender, race, class, sexuality, age, and region.

The dance between privilege and inequality is a prevalent theme in the work of scholars who have staked a claim to the importance of studying travel for abortion services at a domestic level, especially when a country is large in size, some regions are sparsely populated, transportation over long distances is unavailable or unaffordable, and the provision of abortion services is determined greatly by individual healthcare jurisdiction. Pollitt would agree, for she states: "If a teenage girl shows up at a Swedish hospital twenty weeks pregnant and frantic, ways can be found to quietly help her. Moreover, should a German woman be denied a second-trimester abortion, she can probably get to the Netherlands, and a French one to London, more easily than a woman [from the USA] in the Mountain States or the Rio Grande Valley or much of the Deep South can travel to the nearest clinic hundreds of miles away."[37]

Christabelle Sethna and Marion Doull have studied the travel of women to abortion clinics in Canada, revealing the "spatial disparities" between the underserved Atlantic provinces and coastal, rural, and northern areas of the country, as well as urban areas that are well serviced in regard to abortion provision. They found that women who travel are most likely to be young and economically underprivileged.[38] Angel Foster et al. show that women in the Canadian Atlantic province of New Brunswick continue to have a great deal of difficulty accessing abortion services. Stymied by wait times, out-of-pocket expenses, the travel required due to multiple visits to hospitals, and some physicians' refusal to refer patients for abortions, some women leave the province to have costly abortions in neighboring Nova Scotia.[39] Stanley K. Henshaw and Lawrence B. Finer show convincing evidence of large geographical gaps in the provision of abortion services in the USA. They highlight the negative impact of the distance to abortion providers as one of the main extralegal obstacles to access that is especially detrimental to low-income women.[40] In research on the tightening legal restrictions on abortion that have resulted in the closure of many American abortion clinics, Lisa Pruitt and Marta R. Vanegas argue that the women who are hit hardest are those living the farthest from urban centers. According to the authors, the assumption of "urbanormativity" underlies judicial decisions that do not take into consideration the burdens imposed by the long distances one needs to traverse to reach an abortion provider.[41] Medical abortion may be a game changer for some women who live far from an abortion provider. However, as long as access to medical abortion is regulated by strict protocols and remains under the control of medical professionals, it may not be easily accessible, especially when doctors and pharmacists raise the issue of conscientious objection.[42]

The main exception to the sparseness of the literature on travel to access abortion services is the enormous amount of research that continues to proliferate on Ireland and Northern Ireland, where religiously based pro-life sentiments run high. Women from both regions travel to Britain or the Netherlands in the thousands for pregnancy termination every year. Their travel has spawned a wealth of reports from nongovernmental organizations, personal accounts, edited collections, books, journal articles, chapters in books, blogs, and documentaries, all dealing in some fashion with abortion travel. Notably, in a first-time special issue of *Signs: Journal of Women in Culture and Society* on gender and medical tourism in 2011, Annette B. Ramírez de Arellano comments in a few sentences on American women's abortion travel to Cuba before Fidel Castro took power, allowing for the euphemistic "Havana weekend" that included "a standard package including airfare, medical care, and hotel accommodations." Such instances of "crossing borders to get health care," she remarks, have gone from "cottage industry" to "a worldwide phenomenon involving large-scale medical complexes that specialize in combining healing and hospitality."[43] However, in this special issue, Mary Gilmartin and Allen White's coauthored contribution on Ireland is the only one to deal squarely with travel, mobility, and abortion services.[44]

In Ireland, the life of the fetus has been protected by the Irish Constitution, but a number of court rulings in the 1980s and 1990s secured the right of Irish women to receive abortion counseling that includes information about accessing abortion services overseas and to travel abroad for an abortion. Several of these rulings have been based on instances of "crisis pregnancies" that are the result of rape, threaten the woman's life, or are complicated by abnormalities in fetal development.[45] In Northern Ireland, where a pro-life lobby is also powerful, access to abortion services is likewise severely restricted. It has resulted in the annual travel of an estimated 1,000 Northern Irish women to the mainland UK for abortion services. The costs of travel and accommodation are compounded by the fact that abortions on Northern Irish women were not covered by the UK's National Health Service, although this policy was reversed in mid-2017.[46] Stories about the hardships of travel to access abortion services abroad figured prominently in the buildup to the 2018 Irish referendum on the Eighth Amendment, which also saw Irish expatriates travel back to their home country to cast their vote. The referendum result has opened the door somewhat to the liberalization of abortion provision in Ireland and has also placed pressure on the Northern Irish government to reform its own abortion laws.[47]

Despite obvious points of connection between medical tourism and abortion tourism, the two are a contentious fit. Much of the Irish literature uses the term "travel" rather than tourism, signaling the right of Irish women to travel abroad for abortion services. Some scholars, such as those contributing to a 2016 special issue of the *Columbia Journal of Gender and Law*, prefer to use "abortion travel" specifically "to avoid the consumerist and individualist connotations" of abortion tourism or even medical tourism.[48] While acknowledging that travel to abortion services may be experienced as an act of liberation, it is generally portrayed as a punitive and stigmatizing form of "banishment," or as a "diaspora," and women who travel for these purposes have been compared to "exiles," "refugees," "trans-status subjects," and "accidental tourists."[49] Difficulties in accessing abortion services can be prolonged even after women return home, because they may be unable to receive appropriate and nonjudgmental postabortion medical attention.[50] Finally, irrespective of terminology, the literature points to the hypocritical stance of governments that actively block access to abortion services. In so doing, they effectively download the procedure onto other healthcare jurisdictions and, in the process, encourage cross-border traffic in abortion services.

This volume's strengths are that it showcases the phenomenon of transnational travel for abortion services in addition to and apart from the travel of Irish women, who receive the lion's share of notice in this regard. Furthermore, it illustrates that women have traveled for abortion services years before Irish women began traveling in large numbers for abortion services, and well before medical tourism was recognized as one of the major commercial outcomes of globalization. This concentration on abortion travel in the past and present is rare. As well, placing abortion travel in the context of medical tourism makes this volume all the more valuable to the immense amount of scholarship in this area.

What is apparent throughout this volume is that travel for abortion services, like medical tourism itself, is best examined using a transnational lens. *Abortion in the New Europe: A Comparative Handbook*, coedited by Bill Rolston and Anna Eggert, is an excellent older text that surveys abortion laws and abortion services in 19 European countries, including the former Soviet Union. Because of a strong historical focus, there are several references to women traveling to neighboring countries for abortion services once their abortion laws were liberalized.[51] A more recent coedited volume, *A Fragmented Landscape: Abortion Governance and Protest Logics in Europe*, courtesy of Silvia De Zordo, Joanna Mishtal, and Lorena Anton, can be viewed as an update of Rolston and Eggert's work, post–Soviet Union. It tackles the impact of public and private protest in contemporary Europe for and against abortion provision. The coeditors declare in part that an "uneven [abortion rights] policy landscape" in the EU combined with the rise of religiously fueled anti-abortion sentiment has compelled some women to travel for abortion services.[52]

Sandra Coliver, the general editor of *The Right to Know: Human Rights and Access to Reproductive Health Information*, looks at reproductive rights from a human rights perspective. Aside from Coliver's own chapter on Ireland, various chapters mention travel from other countries for abortion services (from Algeria to Tunisia; from Malawi to South Africa and Zambia; and from Poland to the Ukraine, Germany, and the Netherlands) and stress the financial difficulties of doing so.[53] Rebecca J. Cook, Joanna N. Erdman, and Bernard M. Dickens, coeditors of *Abortion Law in Transnational Perspective: Cases and Controversies*, illustrate that while there is a global trend toward the decriminalization of abortion, policies operate to deny access to abortion services in practice, even when these services are legal. Although this particular collection does not tackle women's travel for abortion services, it is valuable for establishing the value of seeing international patterns in abortion access and affirming that domestic abortion laws are deeply influenced by international and regional events.[54] A much-needed volume coedited by Shannon Stettner et al., *Transcending Borders: Abortion in the Past and Present*, takes a multidisciplinary approach to the experiences of women seeking abortion services in Global North and Global South nations. It allows that national boundaries are artificial constructs and upholds the value of the transnational in researching and writing about abortion. It highlights the significance of reproductive justice, asking just which reproductive choices are structurally possible for women when considering the functions of time, space, geography, and culture. This volume also includes a chapter by Joanna Mishtal on the roles played by the Catholic Church and healthcare providers in relation to the travel of Irish women abroad.[55]

Currently, a noticeable rollback of reproductive rights in many parts of the world has coincided with a jump in anti-globalization sentiment, the spread of populism, and an emphasis on securing national borders against racialized immigrants, migrants, and refugees. These developments mean that the present volume makes a timely appearance.[56] Chapters are organized generally in chronological order to give readers a sense of sequential developments in the different regions spotlighted. They are sectioned into three parts—"Flight Risks," "Domestic Transgressions," and "Democratic Transitions"—which are constructed largely around the following arguments: (1) legal and extralegal obstacles to abortion services in a specific healthcare jurisdiction must always be viewed through a transnational lens; (2) abortion services do not have to be illegal in order to be inaccessible; (3) domestic and international travel to access abortion services cannot be viewed as two distinct trends because they are profoundly interrelated responses to the existence of legal and extralegal obstacles to abortion services at local levels; (4) uneven access to abortion services in local healthcare jurisdictions reinforces or exacerbates discrimination by gender, race, class, sexuality, age, and region; and (5) by making gender in relation to other identity variables central, travel to access abortion services can enrich research on medical tourism. Chapter authors approach these themes from historical and contemporary perspectives, apply a range of disciplinary frameworks, and use a variety of terminologies to depict travel for abortion services. At appropriate points, each chapter cross-references others across the entire volume to reinforce its overall coherence and enrich its regional and thematic associations. Nevertheless, this volume's multidisciplinary nature, the variety of regions and time periods it covers, the local specifics involved, and the range of writing styles mean that each chapter is necessarily distinctive in its approach to travel for abortion services transnationally.

Part I, "Flight Risks," deals with the rich and largely untold history of women traveling for abortion services across international borders in the 1960s and 1970s, as well as the fallout of these journeys. Made possible by flight paths that also serviced a booming international tourist industry, they permitted scores of women to take flight when they found themselves hemmed in by their home countries' abortion legislation. Significantly, a focus on this earlier period contradicts and retemporalizes the popular understanding of medical tourism as a phenomenon dating to the 1990s. Lena Lennerhed introduces readers to Sherri Finkbine, a pregnant American wife and mother who flew to Sweden in the early 1960s for an abortion after discovering that she had taken a drug, thalidomide, that damages fetal development. By analyzing the Swedish debate surrounding Finkbine's abortion, Lennerhed lays the groundwork for a discussion that links together eugenics, disability, and Sweden's abortion laws. Christabelle Sethna writes about the geopolitical and biopolitical transnational dimensions of the Abortion Law Reform Association (ALRA)'s campaign strategy in Britain, its defense of the 1967 British Abortion Act, and its response to the travel of nonresident women to Britain after the act's passage. The new law, which had no residency requirements, attracted women primarily from Western Europe—and, to a lesser extent, Canada and the USA—to seek abortions in Britain's private sector. Their travel raised the uncomfortable prospect of profiteering from abortion and underlined the porous nature of international borders in an increasingly globalizing world. Hayley Brown zeroes in on the facilitation of travel of New Zealand women to Australia for abortion services. She believes that this kind of travel has been ignored by historians who focus far more on experiences of male bonding between the two countries. Particularly notable is the involvement of New Zealand feminist activists, who, unable to prevent the passage of restrictive abortion laws, invested their energy into alliances with their Australian counterparts to ensure that New Zealand women were able to access abortion services in the Australian cities of Melbourne and Sydney.

Abortion is often vilified as a transgression committed against motherhood or fetal personhood, but the chapters in part II, "Domestic Transgressions," lean toward illustrating how federal, state, and provincial governments have transgressed against women—especially if they are socially, racially, or economically marginalized—when it comes to accessing abortion services, and even when abortion laws have been liberalized. This part provides ample evidence of abortion travel as contained within national boundaries, giving pause to those who assume that medical tourism occurs only across international borders. Gayle Davis, Jane O'Neill, Clare Parker, and Sally Sheldon examine the initial implementation of the British Abortion Act (1967), which is often portrayed as having sat at the vanguard of a wave of liberalizing legislation across Western nations but in fact "medicalized" the abortion decision-making process, thereby leaving women dependent on the medical profession's sympathy and goodwill. The result was a profound geographic variability in abortion provision across Britain and the need for domestic abortion travel to access private and charitable services when resident women were denied a free National Health Service abortion. The authors map abortion provision and travel networks in the early years of the act and explore the tensions that constrained provision in certain parts of the country and propelled women elsewhere. Mary Gilmartin and Sinéad Kennedy insist on exploring the wider background of voluntary and involuntary "reproductive mobility" in Ireland rather than focusing on abortion alone. They argue that Ireland has historically regulated and disciplined women's fertility on the whole and has constructed some women's mobility as more problematic than that of others. Throughout, the authors showcase the ways in which different generations of reproductive rights activists have incorporated powerful symbols of reproductive mobility into their protest campaigns.

As abortion is regulated in Australia by state governments, Barbara Baird examines the state-by-state ebb and flow of the provision of abortion services in a country that is vast in size, with a population that is concentrated mainly in cities. Baird is careful to underline the importance of local-global connections, including the impact of pro-life support, legal precedents, and neoliberal policies in the structuring of abortion access. Baird is cognizant of the difficulties Indigenous women and women in rural and remote areas in Australia face, noting that since the liberalization of abortion laws, intrastate travel signals the greatest geographical disadvantage Australian women seeking abortions face. Lori Brown emphasizes the ongoing assault against abortion services in Texas, USA. Proudly pro-gun and pro-life, the Texas legislature has forced several abortion clinics to shut down, extending the distance one must travel to an abortion provider. Most at risk are women without medical insurance, poor women, and young Hispanic and Latina women. In Canada, Cathrine Chambers, Colleen MacQuarrie, and Jo-Ann Mac-Donald turn their gaze toward the country's smallest province, Prince Edward Island (PEI). Promoted as a magical tourist attraction and the home of storybook heroine Anne of Green Gables, this resolutely pro-life island in the Atlantic has, up until recently, compelled PEI women to seek abortion services off island. The coauthors assert that the tedious pathways to abortion services heighten PEI women's sense of geographical isolation and personal shame, and confirm that mobility is a privilege unavailable to many.

The final part, "Democratic Transitions," refers to major shifts in governance ranging from fascism, socialism, and communism toward democracy. However, democratic governments are not necessarily women- or abortion-friendly. In fact, abortion services can become a point of contention in democratic societies, even though they may have been liberally available earlier in more politically illiberal regimes. Restricting access to abortion services can also be an indication of a decline in the status of women. Agata Ignaciuk tracks the journeys of Spanish women to London in search of an abortion during the final years of General Francisco Franco's dictatorial regime. The criminalization of abortion, alongside other laws that, for example, placed women under the control of their fathers and husbands, reinforced the government's strong ties to the Catholic Church. Ignaciuk finds that a successful campaign to legalize contraception after Franco's death led feminist activists to mobilize against illegal abortions, circulate information about abortion clinics abroad in the Spanish press, and enable women's travel to Britain for abortions. Anna Bogic provides an alternative angle on travel by taking into consideration multiple meanings of language translation. She focuses on the translation into Serbian of the popular American feminist text *Our Bodies, Ourselves* and illustrates how the 1992 version traveled linguistically and culturally in a postsocialist, pronatalist regime. Bogic contends that a series of international encounters between American and Eastern European women both before and after Serbia's transition to democracy advanced the travel of ideas about abortion at local and global levels.

Ewelina Ciaputa examines changes to Poland's abortion laws over decades, tracing their impact on the domestic illegal abortion underground, and Polish women's abortion tourism to neighboring countries. Ciaputa finds that the resurgence of the Catholic Church in postcommunist Poland has fueled the growth of illegal abortion and abortion tourism because of its influence on the government's attempts to restrict legal abortion. These attempts have been resisted by feminist activists inside and outside Poland who have rallied to help Polish women access abortion services. In the volume's final and most contemporaneous chapter, Niklas Barke speculates what the result of the UK's 2016 democratic referendum on membership in the EU and the 2018 Irish referendum on the repeal of the Eighth Amendment might mean for nonresident women who seek abortion services in Britain. Barke suggests that EU policies that guarantee the freedom of movement of EU citizens cannot always be taken for granted, and neither can political stability in democratic societies. Anticipating the obstacles to freedom of movement that nonresident women might face under a "soft Brexit" or a "hard Brexit" departure from the EU, Barke outlines several complications that could arise in relation to the travel of women from Ireland and Northern Ireland, constituting the largest contingent of women traveling to Britain for abortion services.

In sum, this volume shines a scholarly light on the neglected phenomenon of transnational travel for abortion services across a variety of regions and time periods. Travel for abortion services in the past and present across domestic and international borders must be understood as fluid and wide ranging. It poses a challenge to any notion of a genderless medical tourism while giving pause to the perception that reproductive rights, choice, and justice are something that all women everywhere can attain freely and equally.

Notes

1. Emily Crockett, "Trump on 60 Minutes: If *Roe v. Wade* is Overturned, Women Will 'Have to Go to Another State,'" *Vox*, November 14, 2016, https://www.vox.com/policy-and-politics/2016/11/13/13618556/trump-60-minutes-roe-v-wade-abortion.

2. Mary Minihan, "Brexit 'May Lead to Later Abortions for Irish Women,'" *Irish Times*, August 12, 2017, https://www.irishtimes.com/news/social-affairs/brexit-may-lead-to-later-abortions-for-irish-women-1.3183960.

3. David A. Grimes et al., "Unsafe Abortion: The Preventable Pandemic," *Lancet* 368, no. 9550 (2006): 1908–19.

4. For more information on obstacles, see Ernestina Coast et al., "Trajectories of Women's Abortion-Related Care: A Conceptual Framework," *Social Science and Medicine* 200, no. 1 (2018): 199–210.

5. Christabelle Sethna, "All Aboard? Canadian Women's Abortion Tourism, 1960–1980," in *Gender, Health and Popular Culture*, ed. Cheryl Krasnick Warsh (Waterloo: Wilfred Laurier University Press, 2011), 89–108.

6. For example, see Kevin H. O'Rourke and Jeffrey G. Williamson, *Globalization and History: The Evolution of a Nineteenth-Century Atlantic Economy* (Cambridge, MA: MIT Press, 1999); Ulrich Beck, *What Is Globalization?*, trans. Patrick Camiller (Cambridge: Polity Press, 2009 [1997]); and Valentine M. Moghadam, *Globalizing Women: Transnational Feminist Networks* (Baltimore: Johns Hopkins University Press, 2005).

7. For example, see Gilberto Rosas, "Diffused Exceptionality and 'Immigrant' Social Struggles during the 'War on Terror,'" *Cultural Dynamics* 18, no. 3 (2006): 335–49.

8. Marge Berer, "Abortion Law and Policy Around the World: In Search of Decriminalization," *Health and Human Rights Journal* 19, no. 1 (June 2017): 13–27. See also Lara M. Knudsen, *Reproductive Rights in a Global Context* (Nashville: Vanderbilt University Press, 2006), and Amnesty International, *Body Politics: A Primer on Criminalization of Sexuality and Reproduction* (London: Amnesty International, 2018). María Teresa Rivera from El Salvador was jailed after a miscarriage and later granted asylum in Sweden in 2017. See Jorge Rivas, "I Am the World's First Abortion Refugee," *SPLINTER*, July 31, 2017, https://splinternews.com/i-am-the-worlds-first-abortion-refugee-1797403271.

9. Sarah Hawkes and Kent Buse, "Trumped Again: Reinstating the Global Gag Rule," *British Medical Journal* (online), 356, no. 1 (February 7, 2017), https://search.proquest.com/openview/998211dod3a7e22736f250841d2a9f79/1?pq-origsite=gscholar&cbl=2043523.

10. Gail Pheterson and Yamila Azize, "Abortion Practice in the Northeast Caribbean: 'Just Write Down Stomach Pain,'" *Reproductive Health Matters* 13, no. 26 (2005): 44–53. See also Caroline Levander and Walter Mignolo, "Introduction: The Global South and World Dis/Order," *Global South* 5, no. 1 (Spring 2011): 1–11.

11. Carole Joffe, "Abortion and Medicine: A Sociopolitical History," in *Management of Unintended and Abnormal Pregnancy: Comprehensive Abortion Care*, ed. Maureen Paul et al. (Chichester, UK: Wiley-Blackwell, 2009), 1–9; Lena Lennerhed, "Troubled Women: Abortion and Psychiatry in Sweden in the 1940s and 1950s," in *Transcending Borders: Abortion in the Past and Present*, ed. Shannon Stettner et al. (London: Palgrave Macmillan, 2017), 89–100; and Tiana Norgren, *Abortion before Birth Control: The Politics of Reproduction in Postwar Japan* (Princeton, NJ: Princeton University Press, 2001).

12. See Henry McDonald, Emma Graham-Harrison, and Sinead Baker, "Ireland Votes by Landslide to Legalise Abortion," *Guardian*, May 26, 2018, https://www.theguardian.com/world/2018/may/26/ireland-votes-by-landslide-to-legalise-abortion, and Reva Siegal, "The End of Abortion," *New York Times*, June 28, 2017, https://www.nytimes.com/2018/06/28/opinion/abortion-kennedy-supreme-court-trump.html?action=click&pgtype=Homepage&clickSource=story-heading&module=opinion-c-col-right-region&region=opinion-c-col-right-region&WT.nav=opinion-c-col-right-region.

13. See Jane Kirby, *Fired Up about Reproductive Rights* (Toronto: Between the Lines, 2017); Erica Millar, *Happy Abortions: Our Bodies in the Era of Choice* (London: Zed Books, 2017); and Loretta J. Ross and Rickie Solinger, *Reproductive Justice: An Introduction* (Oakland: University of California Press, 2017).

14. Laura Briggs, *How All Politics Became Reproductive Politics: From Welfare Reform to Foreclosure to Trump* (Oakland: University of California Press, 2017); Jonathan M. Bearak, Kristen Lagasse Burke, and Rachel K. Jones, "Disparities and Change over Time in Distance Women Would Need to Travel to Have an Abortion in the USA: A Spatial Analysis," *Lancet* 2, no. 11 (November 2017): e493-e500; and Gretchen E. Ely et al., "Where Are They from and How Far Must They Go? Examining Location and Travel Distance in US Abortion Fund Patients," *International Journal of Sexual Health* 29, no. 4 (May 2017): 1–12.

15. Linda Greenhouse and Reva B. Siegal, *Before Roe v. Wade: Voices That Shaped the Abortion Debate before the Supreme Court's Ruling* (New York: Kaplan Publishing, 2010), 8–11; Johanna Schoen, *Abortion after Roe* (Chapel Hill: University of North Carolina Press, 2015); Katha Pollitt, *Pro: Reclaiming Abortion Rights* (New York: Picador, 2014), 6, 39, 41–42, 94, 184, 194; Carol Sanger, *About Abortion: Terminating Pregnancy in Twenty-First-Century America* (Cambridge, MA: Harvard University Press, 2017), xi; Carole Joffe, *Dispatches from the Abortion Wars: The Costs of Fanaticism to Doctors, Patients, and the Rest of Us* (Boston: Beacon Press, 2010); and Jennifer Nelson, *More than Medicine: A History of the Feminist Women's Health Movement* (New York: New York University Press, 2015), 57–89.

16. Saskia Sassen, *Globalization and Its Discontents: Essays on the New Mobility of People and Money* (New York: New Press, 1999); Tim Cresswell, *On the Move: Mobility in the Modern Western World* (New York: Routledge, 2006); and Mary Gilmartin and Allen White, "Interrogating Medical Tourism: Ireland, Abortion, and Mobility Rights," *Signs* 36, no. 2 (Winter 2011): 275–80.

17. "Buy Abortion Pills, Mifepristone Online, Misoprostol Online," Women on Web, accessed October 20, 2017, https://www.womenonweb.org/en/page/3074/buy-abortion-pills-mifepristone-online-misoprostol-online. See also Michelle Oberman, *Her Body, Our Laws: On the Front Lines of the Abortion War, from El Salvador to Oklahoma* (Boston: Beason Press, 2018), 7–10.

18. Christabelle Sethna and Marion Doull, "Accidental Tourists: Canadian Women, Abortion Tourism and Travel," *Women's Studies: An Interdisciplinary Journal* 41, no. 4 (2012): 458.

19. Sethna and Doull, "Accidental Tourists," 457–75.

20. John Connell advocates for the use of the term "medical travel" to describe cross-border movement for the purposes of medical care. See John Connell, "Contemporary Medical Tourism: Conceptualisation, Culture and Commodification," *Tourism Management* 34, no. 1 (2013): 7–10.

21. John Connell, "Medical Tourism: Sea, Sun, Sand and . . . Surgery," *Tourism Management* 27, no. 6 (December 2006): 1093–1100; Bapu P. George, Tony L. Henthorne, and Alvin J. Williams, "Determinants of Satisfaction and Dissatisfaction among Preventative and Curative Medical Tourists: A Comparative Analysis," *International Journal of Behavioural and Healthcare Research* 2, no. 1 (2010): 5–19; Rory Johnston et al., "What is Known about the Effects of Medical Tourism in Destination and Departure Countries? A Scoping Review," *International Journal for Equity in Health* 9, no. 24 (2010): 1–13; and Simon Hudson and Xiang Li, "Domestic Medical Tourism: A Neglected Dimension of Medical Tourism Research," *Journal of Hospitality Marketing and Management* 21, no. 3 (December 2012): 227–46.

22. John Connell, "Reducing the Scale? From Global Images to Border Crossings in Medical Tourism," *Global Networks* 16, no. 4 (2016): 531–50.

23. Nathan Cortez, "Patients without Borders: The Emerging Global Market for Patients and the Evolution of Modern Health Care," *Indiana Law Journal* 83, no. 1 (2008): 71–132; Andrea Whittaker, Lenore Manderson, and Elizabeth Cartwright, "Patients without Borders: Understanding Medical Travel," *Medical Anthropology* 29, no. 4 (2010): 336–43; and Valerie Crooks, Meghann Ormond, and Ki Nam Jin, "Reflections on 'Medical Tourism' from the 2016 Global Healthcare Policy and Management Forum," *BMC Proceedings* 11, Suppl. 8 (2017): 6.

24. Jason Behrmann and Elise Smith, "Top 7 Issues in Medical Tourism: Challenges, Knowledge Gaps, and Future Directions for Research and Policy Development," *Global Journal of Health Science* 2, no. 2 (October 2010): 80–90. Far more research on the contraceptive and abortion needs of queer, gender nonconforming individuals, and transmen also needs to be done. See Lauren M. Porsch, Ila Dayananda, and Gillian Dean, "An Exploratory Study of Transgender New Yorkers' Use of Sexual Health Services and Interest in Receiving Services at Planned Parenthood of New York City," *Transgender Health* 1, no. 1 (2016): 231–37.

25. Audrey Bochaton and Bertrand Lefebvre, "Interviewing Elites: Perspectives from the Medical Tourism Sector in India and Thailand," in *Fieldwork in Tourism: Methods, Issues and Reflections*, ed. C. Michael Hall (New York: Routledge, 2011), 70–80.

26. Kathy S. Stolley and Stephanie Watson, *Medical Tourism: A Reference Handbook* (Santa Barbara, CA: ABC-CLIO, 2012), 7, 60.

27. C. Michael Hall, ed., *Medical Tourism: The Ethics, Regulation, and Marketing of Health Mobility* (London: Routledge, 2013).

28. Raywat Deonandan, "An Introduction to the Ethical Dimensions of Reproductive Medical Tourism," in Ron Labonté et al., *Bon voyage: Essais sur le tourisme medical / Travelling Well: Essays in Medical Tourism* in Collection d'études transdisciplinaires en santé des populations / Transdisciplinary Studies in Population Health Studies 4, no. 1 (2013): 151–77, https://www.researchgate.net/publication/235443103_Travelling_Well_Essays_in_Medical_Tourism

_2012_Collection_d%27etudes_Transdisciplinary_transdisciplinaires_en
_Studies_in_Population_sante_des_populations_Health_Series_Vol_41.

29. I. Glenn Cohen, ed., *The Globalization of Health Care: Legal and Ethical Issues* (Oxford: Oxford University Press, 2013).

30. Tamra Lysaght and Douglas Sipp, "Dislodging the Direct-to-Consumer Marketing of Stem Cell–Based Interventions from Medical Tourism," in *Bodies across Borders: The Global Circulation of Body Parts, Medical Tourists and Professionals*, ed. Bronwyn Parry et al. (London: Routledge, 2015), 212.

31. For example, see Meghann Ormond, "Medical Tourism, Medical Exile: Responding to the Cross-Border Pursuit of Healthcare in Malaysia," in *Real Tourism: Practice, Care and Politics in Contemporary Travel Culture*, ed. Claudio Minca and Tim Oakes (London: Routledge, 2012), 143–61.

32. Leigh Turner, "'Medical Tourism' Initiatives Should Exclude Commercial Organ Transplantation," *Journal of the Royal Society of Medicine* 101, no. 8 (August 2008): 391–94; and Gregory Higginbotham, "Assisted-Suicide Tourism: Is It Tourism?," *Tourismos* 6, no. 2 (2011): 177–85.

33. For example, see Laura Kaplan, *The Story of Jane: The Legendary Underground Abortion Service* (New York: Pantheon Books, 1995); Eleonora Zielińska, "Between Ideology, Politics, and Common Sense: The Discourse of Reproductive Rights in Poland," in *Reproducing Gender: Politics, Publics, and Everyday Life After Socialism*, ed. Susan Gal and Gail Kligman (Princeton, NJ: Princeton University Press, 2000), 23–57; Leslie J. Reagan, "Crossing the Border for Abortions: California Activists, Mexican Clinics, and the Creation of a Feminist Health Agency in the 1960s," *Feminist Studies* 26, no. 2 (Summer 2000): 323–48; Beth Palmer, "'Lonely, Tragic, but Legally Necessary Pilgrimages': Transnational Abortion Travel in the 1970s," *Canadian Historical Review* 92, no. 4 (December 2011): 637–64; and Christabelle Sethna et al., "Choice, Interrupted: Travel and Inequality of Access to Abortion Services since the 1960s," *Labour/Le Travail* 71 (Spring 2013): 29–48.

34. Marcia C. Inhorn, *The New Arab Man: Emergent Masculinities, Technologies, and Islam in the Middle East* (Princeton, NJ: Princeton University Press, 2012); and Amy Speier, *Fertility Holidays: IVF Tourism and the Reproduction of Whiteness* (New York: New York University Press, 2016).

35. Susanne Lundin, Charlotte Kroløkke, Michael N. Petersen, and Elmi Muller, eds., *Global Bodies in Grey Zone: Health, Hope, Biotechnology* (Stellenbosch, South Africa: SUN MeDIA Stellenbosch, 2016), 16. See also Françoise Baylis and Jocelyn Downie, "Introduction," *International Journal of Feminist Approaches to Bioethics* 7, no. 2 (Fall 2014): 1–9. This special issue is confined to commercial surrogacy, egg donations, and sex selection.

36. Guido Pennings, "Legal Harmonization and Reproductive Tourism in Europe," *Human Reproduction* 19, no. 12 (2004): 2689–94; and I. Glenn Cohen, "Medical Outlaws or Medical Refugees? An Examination of Circumvention Tourism," in *Medical Tourism: Understanding the Dynamics of the Global Market for Health Services*, ed. Jill Hodges, Leigh Turner, and Ann Marie Kimball (Santa Barbara, CA: ABC-CLIO, 2012), 207–29.

37. Pollitt, *Pro*, 184.

38. Christabelle Sethna and Marion Doull, "Spatial Disparities and Travel to Freestanding Abortion Clinics in Canada," *International Women's Studies Forum* 38 (May/June 2013): 52–62.

39. Angel Foster et al., "'If I Ever Did Have a Daughter, I Wouldn't Raise Her in New Brunswick': Exploring Women's Experiences Obtaining Abortion Care before and after Policy Reform," *Contraception* 95, no. 5 (2017): 477–84.

40. Stanley K. Henshaw and Lawrence B. Finer, "The Accessibility of Abortion Services in the United States, 2001," *Perspectives on Sexual and Reproductive Health* 35, no. 1 (February 2003): 16–24.

41. Lisa Pruitt and Marta R. Vanegas, "Urbanormativity, Spatial Privilege, and Judicial Blind Spots in Abortion Law," *Berkeley Journal of Gender, Law and Justice* 30, no. 1 (2015): 76–153.

42. Diane Cooper et al., "Medical Abortion: The Possibilities for Introduction in the Public Sector in South Africa," *Reproductive Health Matters* 13, no. 26 (2005): 35–43; and Wendy Chavkin, Liddy Leitman, and Kate Polin, "Conscientious Objection and Refusal to Provide Reproductive Healthcare: A White Paper Examining Prevalence, Health Consequences, and Policy Responses," *International Journal of Gynecology and Obstetrics* 123, Suppl. 3 (2013): S41-S56; and Ronit Y. Stahl and Ezekiel J. Emanuel, "Physicians, Not Conscripts—Conscientious Objection in Health Care," *New England Journal of Medicine* 376, no. 14 (April 2017): 1380–85.

43. Annette B. Ramírez de Arellano, "Medical Tourism in the Caribbean," *Signs* 36, no. 2 (Winter 2011): 289–90.

44. Gilmartin and White, "Interrogating Medical Tourism."

45. For a small sample of research, see Evelyn Mahon, "Abortion Debates in Ireland: An Ongoing Issue," in *Abortion Politics, Women's Movements and the Democratic State: A Comparative Study of State Feminism*, ed. Dorothy MacBride Stetson (Oxford: Oxford University Press, 2001), 157–79; Human Rights Watch, *A State of Isolation: Access to Abortion for Women in Ireland* (New York: Human Rights Watch, 2010); Ruth Fletcher, "Contesting the Cruel Treatment of Abortion-Seeking Women," *Reproductive Health Matters* 22, no. 44 (2014):10–21; Sheelagh McGuinness, "Law, Reproduction, and Disability: Fatally 'Handicapped'?," *Medical Law Review* 21, no. 2 (June 2013): 213–42.

46. Fiona Bloomer and Eileen Fegan, "Critiquing Recent Abortion Law and Policy in Northern Ireland," *Critical Social Policy* 34, no. 1 (August 2013): 109–20. See also Jessica Elgot and Henry McDonald, "Northern Irish Women Win Access to Free Abortions as May Averts Rebellion," *Guardian*, June 29, 2017, https://www.theguardian.com/world/2017/jun/29/rebel-tories-could-back-northern-ireland-abortion-amendment?CMP=Share_iOSApp_Other.

47. Una Mullally, ed., *Repeal the 8th: A Collection of Stories, Essays, Poetry, Art and Photography Emerging from and Inspired by the Movement for Reproductive Rights in Ireland* (London: Unbound, 2018). See also Melissa Davey, "'North is Next': Fresh Fight for Grassroots Power That Beat Ireland Abortion Ban," *Guardian*, June 1, 2018, https://www.theguardian.com/world/2018/jun/02/north-is-next-fresh-fight-for-grassroots-power-that-beat-ireland-abortion-ban.

48. Lisa Kelly and Nicole Tuszynski, "Introduction: Banishing Women: The Law and Politics of Abortion Travel," *Columbia Journal of Gender and Law* 25, no. 1 (2016): 25–26.

49. Kelly and Tuszynski, "Introduction," 26; Ann Rossiter, *Ireland's Hidden Diaspora: The "Abortion Trail" and the Making of a London-Irish Underground, 1980–2000* (London: IASC Publishing, 2009); and Sethna, "All Aboard?," 92–93.

50. Daniel Grossman et al., "Mexican Women Seeking Safe Abortion Services in San Diego, California," *Health Care for Women International* 33, no. 11 (November 2012): 1060–69.

51. Bill Rolston and Anna Eggert, eds., *Abortion in the New Europe: A Comparative Handbook* (Westport, CT: Greenwood Press, 1994).

52. Silvia De Zordo, Joanna Mishtal, and Lorena Anton, eds., *A Fragmented Landscape: Abortion Governance and Protest Logics in Europe* (New York: Berghahn Books, 2017), 1.

53. See Sandra Coliver, *The Right to Know: Human Rights and Access to Reproductive Health Information* (London: Article 19, 1995).

54. Rebecca J. Cook, Joanna N. Erdman, and Bernard M. Dickens, eds., *Abortion Law in Transnational Perspective: Cases and Controversies* (Philadelphia: University of Pennsylvania Press, 2014).

55. Joanna Mishtal, "Quiet Contestations of Irish Abortion Law: Abortion and Politics in Flux?," in Shannon Stettner et al., *Transcending Borders*, 187–202.

56. A recent oral history of the New York–based Clergy Consultation Service, an abortion referral network of volunteers that helped women access abortion services in the 1960s and 1970s, looks to the past to warn about current restrictions on abortion in the USA. See Doris Andrea Dirks and Patricia A. Relf, *To Offer Compassion: A History of the Clergy Consultation Service on Abortion* (Madison, WI: University of Wisconsin Press, 2017). See also Colleen MacQuarrie, Fiona Bloomer, Claire Pierson, and Shannon Stettner (eds.), *Crossing Troubled Waters: Abortion In Ireland, Northern Ireland, and Prince Edward Island* (Charlottetown, PEI: Island Studies Press, 2018).

PART I **FLIGHT RISKS**

[1]

Sherri Finkbine Flew to Sweden

Abortion and Disability in the Early 1960s

LENA LENNERHED

SHERRI FINKBINE flew from the United States of America (USA) to Sweden in August 1962 to obtain an abortion after taking thalidomide and subsequently learning of the risks to the fetus from the drug. After she had undergone a physical examination and received counseling, and after the National Board of Health had deliberated on her case, her application was approved. The operation took place shortly thereafter. It was to become one of the most notorious abortions in Western history. American and European newspapers, television, and radio gave the story day-by-day coverage. Sherri Finkbine became famous.[1] After Finkbine had flown back home, and foreign journalists redirected their attention toward other places and events, within Sweden the spotlight remained firmly on the Finkbine case and its ramifications. Taken in conjunction with the fact that a number of Swedish women had also consumed thalidomide, the Finkbine case resulted in the revision of the Swedish Abortion Act.

At this time, Sweden was seen by many as the epitome of the welfare state, a country based on the principle of equality and characterized by a high standard of living.[2] The foundations for the Swedish welfare state were laid by the Social Democratic Party, which took power in 1932 and was to retain it for more than 40 years. From the 1930s, extensive social reforms were introduced, including the reform of healthcare centers for mothers and children, greater access to contraceptives and abortion, the introduction of a sterilization law, and the teaching of sex education in schools. Swedish women had been able to obtain a legal abortion since 1938 on medical grounds (if the woman was seriously ill), on eugenic grounds (if the woman was carrying a serious inherited disease), on humanitarian grounds (if the woman had become pregnant after rape), and—from 1946—on sociomedical grounds (if the woman's health was predicted to be upset detrimentally by childbirth and caring for a child).[3] In 1963, the year after Finkbine's abortion, fetal defects were added to the Swedish Abortion Act as further grounds for the procedure. Abortion could henceforth be granted "when it can reasonably be assumed that the expected child because of damage during fetal development will suffer severe illness or severe disability."[4]

The aim of this chapter is to analyze the Swedish debate surrounding Finkbine's abortion and to explore its political consequences, as it made a substantial contribution to a revision of Swedish abortion law. Using a variety of primary sources, which include newspaper and television reports, governmental investigations, and parliamentary discussions, three particular aspects of the debate are highlighted: (1) perceptions of women applying for an abortion; (2) conceptions of disability, and of disabled children in particular; and (3) the role of the media, both in the Finkbine case and in the wider public debates on disability and abortion. I show that the media was particularly active in informing the country about Finkbine's abortion and in supporting her case, a significant factor in the move toward abortion law reform. I also show how the concepts of class, race, respectability, and motherhood were crucial factors in bringing about a wider acceptance of abortion.

Thalidomide

Thalidomide was developed in West Germany by Chemie Grünenthal and sold under various names to 46 countries. In total, about 10,000 children were born with deformities caused by thalidomide, most of them in West Germany, where the drug was sold under the name "Contergan" without a prescription. In Britain, as Christabelle Sethna argues in her contribution to this volume, the birth of children affected by thalidomide reinvigorated the Abortion Law Reform Association (ALRA), leading in turn to the passage of the 1967 British Abortion Act, which Gayle Davis et al. analyze in this volume. Thalidomide in Sweden was sold by Astra under the name "Neurosedyn" from January 1959 to December 1961, at which point it was withdrawn. For a while, it was also sold in another form under the name "Noxodyn." The drug was prescribed to a wide selection of patients, including children and pregnant women, for a number of conditions that included insomnia, anxiety, and stress-related headaches. In Astra's advertisements, thalidomide was described as soothing, fast-acting, effective, and with "extremely low toxicity."[5]

The first sporadic warnings were heard in West Germany in 1959 when some linked it to cases of polyneuritis, an inflammation of the nerves, and to phocomelia, a birth defect in which arms and legs are largely lacking and hands and feet are attached near the shoulders and pelvis. Not until a large number of children with such birth defects were born did Chemie Grünenthal withdraw Contergan from the German market, in November 1961. Furthermore, the information was not passed on to companies in other countries that sold the product under license. *Svenska Dagbladet* reported the event in a brief note—"German sedative presumed dangerous during pregnancy"—as did *Dagens Nyheter*, but both these daily newspapers used the drug's German name, Contergan, instead of the Swedish.[6]

Shortly thereafter, the Swedish communist newspaper *Ny Dag* criticized the fact that thalidomide had not yet been withdrawn in Sweden, as it had been in West Germany.[7] Following correspondence with the National Board of Health, Astra distributed a warning letter to Swedish doctors in December 1961, and the agent was withdrawn. No attempt was made to inform the public, and Arthur Engel, director general of the National Board of Health, urged journalists writing about the case to desist, so as not to stir up anxiety.[8]

However, the media's silence was short-lived, broken by an article in the Christian newspaper *Dagen* in February 1962 and by another piece in *Dagens Nyheter* a month later, titled "International Sleeping Pills Scandal. Thousands of Children Deformed. Swedish Investigation."[9] Criticism was directed at the National Board of Health for failing to notify the public. Board representative Karl-Erik Linder responded that it was "normal procedure" to notify doctors by mail. As he explained in *Dagens Nyheter*: "If we had sent out an official notice from the National Board of Health and made a big fuss, we might have caused a panic. There are almost certainly tens of thousands of expectant mothers who no longer know for certain what tranquilizers or other drugs they may have taken. And it's not hard to imagine the consequences of such a terrifying warning."[10] In the magazine *Vecko-Journalen*, journalist Barbro Alving wrote an open letter to the National Board of Health, criticizing it for claiming that the amount of thalidomide on the market was insignificant, thereby trivializing the tragedy.[11] Alving also wrote that it had become clear that information was not passed on from doctors to women. Her conclusion was that the National Board of Health had reduced a matter of human suffering to a matter of procedure.

It has been estimated that about 150 children were born in Sweden with thalidomide-related deformities, and that up to 90 of these children survived, while the others died during or shortly after birth.[12] The story of thalidomide in Sweden brings together the powerful professions of law, medicine, and journalism. It is about care and control, and parents versus authorities, as parents fought to bring their children home as some were institutionalized. It is also about money and disability. As children struggled with the awkward arm and leg prostheses they were expected to use, the issues of liability and compensation were fought over in court. Held in Sweden, the lawyers claimed this to be the world's first thalidomide trial, and it resulted in a 1969 settlement in which the affected children received lifelong financial compensation. Above all, the story of thalidomide is one where an incredibly strong belief in and respect for medicine received a sudden jolt, which led subsequently to a tightening of drug control as well as a change in abortion law.[13]

Sherri Finkbine's Abortion

Unlike the rest of the chapters in this volume, which deal generally with women who travel for abortion services, this chapter homes in on the experience of one specific woman who attracted international attention for her overseas abortion journey. Sherri Finkbine was 29 years old, white, middle class, married to Robert Finkbine, and a mother of four children ranging in age from 1 to 7 years. She had a part-time job as an anchorwoman for a children's television program. During this, her fifth pregnancy, Sherri Finkbine occasionally took tranquillizers that contained the substance thalidomide. It was at about this time that it was discovered that thalidomide could do serious damage to a fetus. In the USA, thalidomide was never licensed, but Robert Finkbine had bought the pills in England while escorting a group of students on a European trip and put them in the couple's medicine cabinet.[14]

Sherri Finkbine applied for an abortion in her home state of Arizona, and her application was approved by several physicians, despite the fact that the state's strict abortion laws permitted abortion only if the woman's life was at risk. In order to warn other pregnant women about the dangers of thalidomide, Sherri Finkbine let herself be interviewed by a local newspaper. Her case gained publicity and a media storm quickly arose, and as a result the physicians felt compelled to rescind their approval. Had these doctors gone through with the abortion, they would, according to the press reports, have risked prosecution and dismissal. Finkbine took her case to court to challenge the decision, but to no avail. According to her own account, her physician then advised her to obtain an abortion in Japan or Sweden, where the laws supposedly were more relaxed. Some doctors attempted to steer pregnant women away from abortions; however, doctors whose hands were tied by abortion laws or abortion provision policies did try to refer women elsewhere for abortion services, as many chapters in this volume make clear, including those by Gayle Davis et al. and Agata Ignaciuk. Finkbine abandoned her plans for Japan because of the long wait for a visa, but Sweden remained a possibility. She was eventually able to have her pregnancy terminated in Stockholm's Karolinska Hospital, where one of the hospital physicians confirmed that the fetus showed the typical thalidomide deformity in both its arms.[15]

Swedish law at that time allowed that abortions could be justified on medical, eugenic, sociomedical, or humanitarian grounds. However, no part of the law allowed the abortion of a fetus that had become ill or damaged during pregnancy. Yet Swedish clinical practice tended to allow abortion in cases of suspected fetal damage—when, for instance, a woman had contracted rubella during the early stages of pregnancy.[16] In such cases, the medical or sociomedical indications were used; it was suggested that a disabled child would endanger the pregnant woman's mental health. It can be argued, therefore, that Sherri Finkbine essentially had her abortion justified on psychiatric grounds, a rationale that Gayle Davis et al. assess in relation to the 1967 British Abortion Act in this volume.

As Finkbine traveled, so too did the news of her abortion. Finkbine's flight to Sweden became the subject of enormous media attention. One of the very first television transmissions from the USA to Europe, via the television satellite Telstar, featured an interview with the Finkbines. They were given celebrity status in Sweden. Viewers of the Swedish news program *Aktuellt* could even watch the airplane land, the door open, and the Finkbines disembark, greeted by camera flashes and a rush of journalists. An on-the-spot airport press conference took place with the tired but composed Finkbines. The Swedish authorities' approval of Sherri Finkbine's abortion made the front pages throughout Europe.[17]

The publicity surrounding her abortion also resulted in a wave of abortion requests from non-Swedish women, strengthening observations made separately by Christabelle Sethna, Agata Ignaciuk, and Anna Bogic in this volume about the function of newspapers, magazines, and manuals in transmitting information about abortion or access to abortion services. However, the National Board of Health, which received 800 letters from American, British, Canadian, and German women between 1962 and 1969, devised a standard reply and warned women against going to Sweden, as did the Swedish Embassy in Washington, DC. Some nonresident women managed, nonetheless, to obtain an abortion in Sweden, including nine American women between 1963 and 1964.[18]

In Sweden, the Finkbines were assisted heavily by the tabloid evening newspaper *Expressen*. While in the country, the couple lived at the home of the newspaper's managing director, and the newspaper's medical reporter assisted Sherri Finkbine in her application for an abortion and in her contacts with the health authorities.[19] In return, the newspaper scooped an internationally acclaimed story. *Expressen* wrote that it was pleased to have the opportunity to publish a series of articles, partly so as to be able to help the Finkbines financially by selling their story to the international press, thus averting the "economic disaster" that threatened them as a result of the cost of their trip to Sweden, and partly in order to give what the newspaper perceived as the "true and positive picture of Swedish attitudes to the abortion question."[20]

For six consecutive days, Sherri Finkbine dominated the front pages of *Expressen*, with headlines such as "Sherri Finkbine Had an Abortion," "My World in Ruins Because of One Brief Telephone Conversation," "I Wish My Situation on No Mother," and "Thank You Sweden, Thank You All Wonderful Swedes."[21] There were, moreover, many evocative photographs of Sherri Finkbine—on the telephone, waiting anxiously with her husband, on the way to the hospital—that culminated in a two-page spread taken directly from the postabortion sickbed. In addition to *Expressen*'s own journalism, Sherri Finkbine contributed five articles herself. "Finkbine" publicity effectively became a serialized abortion novel. Each day added new ingredients to a drama about "how fate struck a happy family" and how an "American tragedy" had reached a happy ending in "humane, down-to-earth" Sweden.[22]

Sherri Finkbine began her series of self-penned articles by recounting the greatest day of her life: the day when her first child was born. She told of the couple's worries over the girl's congenital hip injury, its treatment, and their joy when the girl recovered, as well as their later joy over the arrival of their three additional children. It was hardly a coincidence that maternal love featured so prominently right at the beginning of the series, adding a highly respectable context to proceedings. Sherri Finkbine also stressed that she and her husband were not "brilliant exceptional parents" but a regular family with worries and bills to pay, despite which the children were at the center of their lives. Thalidomide, it was claimed, destroyed "this idyllic existence."[23] With the realization that it was thalidomide that she had taken came deep anxiety and parental agony. She asked: "Could we—we who love kids—give life to a child who would be doomed to suffer throughout its life?"[24]

Sherri Finkbine then gave an account of the events surrounding her Arizona abortion application, the international media coverage that her case acquired, and the resulting trip to Sweden. She noted: "It felt so weird to actually have to flee our own country to get something done which, medically speaking, was unassailable."[25] In the USA, she claimed to have met with condemnation: she was a sinner and what she wanted to do was murder. To counter these religious beliefs, as she perceived them, Finkbine stressed that she too had a God, and that what is right for one person is not necessarily right for another. Once in Sweden, there followed an anxious wait and then huge relief when the abortion procedure was over. In her final article in the series, Sherri Finkbine thanked Sweden, the Swedish people, and the newspaper *Expressen*. She concluded, "Thank you for enabling me to return home to my children as a fully fit and healthy mother."[26] Motherhood and her strong love for her children thus formed the framework around her entire story.

It should be pointed out that Sherri Finkbine's articles were published in *Expressen* in the days after she received the news that her abortion request had been granted. This means that they were not written in order to try to shape public opinion or to influence the National Board of Health's decision. Rather, they were intended as a thank-you to *Expressen* and as an opportunity for Finkbine to offer her own version of events that received international attention and about which so many people had an opinion. Her husband, Robert Finkbine, also wrote about the events in an extensive article titled "Our Case," which appeared in the journal *Industria International* and was published in English by the organization Svenska arbetsgivareföreningen (SAF), the Swedish

Employers' Association.[27] Robert Finkbine was a history teacher, not a business man, and it is not known why SAF decided to publish his article. Just as Sherri Finkbine had done in *Expressen*, Robert Finkbine described the background and events that led to his wife's abortion in Stockholm. Like his wife, Robert Finkbine thanked Sweden and the Swedish people. He also used much of his article to write about the country and the people they had encountered in a way that positioned the couple simultaneously as delighted overseas visitors *and* anxious medical tourists seeking abortion services who were reassured repeatedly by their Swedish contacts. He described a beautiful land with lakes and greenery, walks in Stockholm's Old Town alleyways while awaiting a response on their abortion request, and meetings with slightly formal yet open and friendly Swedes, including the professional and friendly medical staff who, with their broken English, did their best to help the couple. At the hospital, Robert Finkbine relayed, his wife was comforted by a young woman who had had an abortion just a few months earlier after taking thalidomide, and who wanted to give her emotional support and assure her that her decision to seek an abortion was the right one. Robert Finkbine also spoke of "the mother," the wife of the managing director, with whom they stayed in Sweden. She, with tears in her eyes, gave Sherri Finkbine her approval and, when the abortion was granted, apparently said: "I'm so happy for you—it's the only way."[28]

While Robert Finkbine's text was filled with emotion, he also wanted to transmit a picture of Swedish society and explain the larger factors that had made his wife's abortion possible. He remarked, "The national empathy of the Swedish people reached out to Sherri and me, engulfing us in warm waves of understanding, creating the emotional retreat needed so desperately by people on the brink of pain, living on the raw edge of a decision between life and death."[29] Robert Finkbine complimented Sweden with reference to the equality he had witnessed between women and men, the people's open and natural approach to sexuality, and the fact that sex education in schools was mandatory. Illegal abortion, divorce, illegitimate children, and venereal disease existed there too, Robert Finkbine wrote, but in Sweden these were recognized as problems, and, according to him, undogmatic and objective solutions were being sought. Sweden was characterized by an open realism with which Robert Finkbine sympathized and which, according to him, paved the way for his wife to have the abortion denied her in the USA. Of great importance also was the organization of healthcare in the two countries. The American doctors who first approved Sherri Finkbine's abortion risked losing their jobs and medical licenses, while their Swedish counterparts had the state and its institutions fully behind them. Robert Finkbine wrote that as Americans, he and his wife had had negative preconceptions about "socialized medicine" before their trip but that their opinions had been overturned completely while in Sweden. Robert Finkbine did not argue for the introduction of socialized medicine in the USA. He stressed the importance of private enterprise and individual initiatives, but his conclusion was that there was something for Americans to learn from Sweden.

Although Robert Finkbine's article was primarily an attempt to document the journey to his wife's abortion, with the setting and focus he gave it, it joins the ranks of tributes to Sweden, with Marquis Childs's famous book *Sweden: The Middle Way* (1936) being the first and foremost example. Robert Finkbine's image of Sweden, just like Childs's and many other successors, was of an orderly, modern, and progressive welfare state characterized by openness and sensible social solutions. At around the same time, the American magazine *Life* published a story on Sherri Finkbine, accompanied by pictures of a weeping Sherri with her face hidden in her hands, an argumentative and assertive Sherri, and a Sherri with her children. Historian Leslie J. Reagan, who has analyzed this *Life* article, writes: "Finkbine's attributes made her an ideal media representation of the American mother caught in a reproductive dilemma, for she represented the ideal mother and 'every woman.' She was the culture's portrait of the child-centered woman: attractive, white, heterosexual, and a married mother of four."[30]

This portrait of respectable maternity made abortion seem more palatable, as Christabelle Sethna illustrates in her chapter in regard to Britain in this volume. Indeed, the Finkbines also received considerable attention in the press in Australia, a region explored in this volume by Barbara Baird. Historian Clare Parker has argued that the reports on Finkbine and other thalidomide cases pushed the abortion debate in Australia into the public arena and onto the political agenda.[31] Clearly, the Finkbine story is likely to have altered the public perception of abortion, and of women who sought an abortion, in the USA and Australia, as well as in Sweden, and possibly in many other countries besides. In addition to being a wife and mother, Sherri Finkbine had many other attributes. She stood as a successful professional woman with a college education who combined children with a career in television broadcasting. When faced with the cold facts surrounding thalidomide, she insisted on her right to an abortion, both in the USA and in Sweden. She was both articulate and likeable, and she communicated effectively in the interviews she gave and in the articles she wrote. One can hardly get further from the miserable or egotistical and unmotherly female whose image tended to dominate discussions of the abortion issue at this time.[32]

Suzanne Vandeput's "Thalidomide Murder"

In the same year that Sherri Finkbine had her pregnancy terminated in Sweden, Suzanne Vandeput from Liège, Belgium, killed her thalidomide-affected newborn baby.[33] With the support of her husband, mother, sister, and doctor, she gave the child an overdose of sleeping pills. All were charged but acquitted five months later after a highly publicized trial. A key feature of the Vandeput case is the sympathy that the accused received. Several opinion polls at the time showed very strong public support for Vandeput and her actions, as well as for euthanasia and mercy killings more generally.[34] When the accused were released, scenes of joy were played out among the huge crowds that had gathered outside the courthouse.[35]

The case also attracted attention in Sweden, where, similarly, people tended to express their understanding for Vandeput, or "the mother," as she was often called. *Dagens Nyheter* reported the story under the headline "Heartbroken Mother Killed Newborn."[36] The editor in chief, Olof Lagercrantz, wrote that Vandeput had shown courage and acted appropriately, and that it was, therefore, wrong to prosecute her. While respecting human life, Lagercrantz wrote: "Only in a world without love is it possible to value a life without any potential as more holy than everything else."[37] In the intense debate that ensued, while few were quite as charitable as Lagercrantz, it is remarkable that no one appears to have argued for the imprisonment of Suzanne Vandeput.

The philosopher Harald Ofstad shared Lagercrantz's compassion for Vandeput and the child but not his conclusions. According to Ofstad, mercy killing could be morally right: when a person had a fatal disease in combination with severe pain and suffering. However, the Vandeput case was about a disabled child, and Ofstad underlined the importance of not seeing the healthy child as a norm. He argued that "respect for the weak and helpless, for those different, [was] one of the most valuable aspects of our culture."[38] While Pentecostal leader Lewi Pethrus argued that Vandeput's actions should be condemned, he sympathetically declared himself convinced that they arose out of "motherly love." Pethrus added that it was easy to debate the issue from afar and without knowing the facts of the case, and that it was "something completely different to be the mother of a child with no arms."[39] The magazine *Vecko-Journalen* emphasized the Vandeput couple's well-ordered and secure life (considering them "a model family"), their ordinariness ("it could have been any one of us"), and their dream of having a child ("the nursery was ready and waiting"). It accentuated Vandeput's despair when tragedy struck, stating that her act was thought through and that she took responsibility for it. While the article did not expressly support the killing of the child, its thrust was strongly empathetic.[40]

Conversely, Erik Nilsson, editor for the journal *Svensk vanföretidskrift*, published by the disability organization De vanföras väl, declared how "offensive" he found the "applause" for the murder in Liège. Yet he argued that Vandeput had probably acted while in a state of shock, and thus while she should have been sentenced, she should also have been shown mercy.[41] A similar viewpoint was put forward by Hannie Örne, the mother of a little girl disabled by thalidomide. Örne wrote that she, more than anyone else, probably understood the despair that Vandeput had felt. Indeed, Örne wrote a letter to the court in Liège that asked for compassion for a traumatized young woman.[42] At the same time, Örne called for a symbolic sentence in order to maintain a respect for life.

There are several notable similarities between the Finkbine and Vandeput cases. Both involved white, middle class, married women who had taken thalidomide. The women's actions—traveling overseas to procure an abortion or embarking on a "mercy-killing"—received international attention. Their cases appear largely to have aroused sympathy and understanding. When the press wrote about these cases, the dramatic language was similar: "How fate struck a happy family [the Finkbines]" and "A happy couple like any other in Belgium. . . . But then disaster struck [the Vandeputs]."[43] Although Vandeput was slightly younger than Finkbine and did not have the same successful career, the newspapers wrote about and characterized them in strikingly similar ways. It was stressed that they were married, they were mothers, and they were well-adjusted individuals.

It might also be said that the sympathy and support given to Fink-bine and Vandeput was a reflection of contemporary attitudes toward disability. In Sweden—as in the USA—it was customary for children with disabilities to be placed in institutions and for ties between these children and their parents to be broken. The institutionalization of the so-called mentally deficient, crippled, blind, and deaf had started in the 1800s for their protection, care, upbringing, and later education, and this continued to be the approach by the 1960s, though that decade was an era of transition. Institutions were now being subjected to criticism, characterized as old-fashioned and isolated, as a more positive view of disabled children was beginning to emerge.[44] It is reasonable to believe that couples in the 1960s who were expecting or actually had children affected by thalidomide had great difficulty seeing any future for them. They did not appear to imagine that these children could live enjoyable and fulfilling lives. Örne was very much in the minority when attempting to provide an alternative perspective; she described her thalidomide-affected daughter as happy, strong willed, and spirited as her nonaffected siblings.[45]

The Fifth Abortion Indication

That thalidomide severely affected fetuses during pregnancy brought the issue of abortion to the fore in Sweden. The first time a Swedish newspaper raised the matter was in April 1962. However, the angle of the story was significantly different. The front page of the tabloid evening newspaper *Aftonbladet* presented a headline in large black letters that read "Women Using Dangerous Sleeping Pill for Abortion."[46] Inside the newspaper, the message was emphasized further by the headlines, "Doctors (National Board of Health Investigators) Sound the Alarm about a Terrible Rumor: Dangerous Sleeping Pill Used to Cause Abortions. Large Increase in Deformed Children." These were insidious. The National Board of Health had not raised the alarm, but its investigator Jan Winberg was interviewed in the article about an inquiry he had undertaken on the connection between fetal damage and drugs. The newspaper claimed that it understood that "a certain category of women" had regularly taken thalidomide "to dispose of unwanted children." The article did not go into who these women were but nevertheless insisted that the women had no idea that the agent induced severe malformations and used it solely in order to provoke a miscarriage.

"The thought is frightening," announced *Aftonbladet*. "I've heard similar rumors during the inquiry. If they are true, it is terrible," Winberg agreed.[47]

In the *Aftonbladet* article, the focus of the thalidomide debate was, therefore, twisted: from women and newborn children as inadvertent victims of a tragic drug disaster to pregnant women who deliberately tried to get rid of their fetuses. It is unclear why the issue came up at all. At this time, it had not been determined that thalidomide could induce miscarriage. In Winberg's inquiry, which was commissioned by the National Board of Health, there was no information about abortion or miscarriage related to thalidomide.[48] Indeed, the whole *Aftonbladet* article appeared to have been based purely on conjecture: the newspaper "understands" that thalidomide "may have" been used for the purpose of miscarriage. Subsequent debate centered much more on the need for abortion services after the consumption of thalidomide; however, provoking one's own miscarriage has a long tradition in many societies. Women continue to depend on self-induced abortion when access to abortion services is difficult to obtain, as Cathrine Chambers, Colleen MacQuarrie, and Jo-Ann MacDonald find in their study on abortion access in Prince Edward Island, Canada, in this volume.

A few weeks after Sherri Finkbine's abortion took place, *Svenska Dagbladet* published an editorial proposing that the abortion law should be changed, and shortly thereafter the National Board of Health approached the government with a proposal to extend the Swedish Abortion Act with a fifth indication: that abortion should be granted if the fetus were damaged during pregnancy.[49] The background to this proposal was indubitably the events surrounding the use of thalidomide. By that point, 12 applications for abortion had been received from women who had taken thalidomide. Six of these requests had been granted on medical grounds, and three on sociomedical grounds. In one case, the woman had miscarried, and in the remaining two, the applications had been rejected; unfortunately, it is not clear why.

While Swedish abortion legislation did not specifically address the issue of potential fetal defects, the National Board of Health argued that its practice was to allow the woman an abortion in such cases, including rubella or certain parental blood-type combinations or suspected radiation damage. In a single year in the early 1950s, for example, almost 300 pregnant women with rubella had received legal abortions.[50] Children could be born blind, deaf, or with heart problems and intellectual disabilities if their mothers were infected with rubella during pregnancy. However, the National Board of Health declared that it found it unsatisfactory that abortions should be carried out on the basis of indications not specifically designated. It called, therefore, for a revision of the law to include fetal defects explicitly—in effect, to bring the law in line with current clinical practice. It was pointed out that Danish abortion law had been similarly revised in 1956 as a direct result of the numerous cases of rubella.

The National Board of Health's proposal went to the Department of Justice for consultation in 1962.[51] At the same time, the notion of pregnant women deliberately taking thalidomide to cause them to miscarry was raised again, but this time through the possibility of exploiting any potential revision to abortion laws that took fetal defects into account. Brita Rudberg, from the psychiatric clinic in Sahlgrenska Hospital, Gothenburg, criticized the proposal—which would introduce a fetal damage indication to Swedish abortion law—in *Svenska läkartidningen*, a medical journal. She complained that "it would allow the woman in a completely different way than before to decide the fate of the fetus. She can take thalidomide or other teratogenic [causing fetal defects] preparations in order to expose the expected child to the risk of 'severe deformity' and so obtain a legal abortion."[52] Although thalidomide had by now been withdrawn from circulation, women might have some thalidomide pills left over, contended Rudberg, whose sentiments were echoed and supported by other commentators and MPs.

Nonetheless, during this consultation period, the proposal to widen the grounds for abortion to include fetal damage was endorsed by a majority, including the Liberal Party's Women's Federation, the Social Democratic Women's Federation, and several university faculties of medicine. Yet support was by no means unanimous. The Swedish Medical Association declared itself to be opposed to any such revision in the legislation. It claimed that it was not against performing abortions in the case of possible serious fetal defects but felt that the need for this was already covered by the current law. It added that fetal damage could be prevented through more effective drug control and a tightening-up of prescriptions issued to pregnant women. There was, in their view, no medical rationale for the proposed extension to Swedish abortion law.[53] Further arguments against the National Board of Health's proposal included uncertainty in predicting fetal defects and ethical concerns over expanding the law.

In a similar vein, Diakonistyrelsen, an organization that represented deacons, requested a review of the Swedish Abortion Act in order to take it in a more restrictive direction. In its criticism of fetal damage as an indication for abortion, it represented the position of people with disabilities and argued that such an indication could be interpreted as meaning that the community felt it preferable that individuals with disabilities simply did not exist.[54] A similar standpoint was taken by both the Conservative Party's Women's Federation and the disability organization De vanföras väl. The latter argued that "every indication that focuses on the fetus and accepts its extinction for the purpose of relieving suffering hits a group of people in their human dignity and right to exist."[55]

After the government presented its proposal, similar counterarguments were heard from MPs. Conservatives and liberals spoke against the extension of the Abortion Act, as did the social democrat, physician, and chair of the Swedish Association for Sexuality Education (RFSU) Elisabet Sjövall. The suggestion that women would be able to take undue advantage of the abortion law was cited as a problem by many people. Sjövall claimed that it was almost impossible to prove whether a woman had taken a few of the thalidomide pills or not; thus she concluded that the bill would "allow the possibility for any criminal abortion to now be performed legally."[56] A further point of discussion that arose was whether the introduction of a fetal damage indication would represent a fundamental change in abortion law. Many critics of the proposal argued that other indications for abortion were based purely on the woman, allowing abortion if she was raped or ill, whereas a fetal damage indication would allow abortion based on the status of the fetus, which introduced a problematic grading of the value of human life. The government offered the counterargument that the proposal was based on compelling humanitarian reasons and did not involve a new principle, since the existing abortion law's eugenic indication concerned damage to the fetus. It was emphasized that the bill involved no belittlement of the disabled, nor did it pave the way for a gradation of the value of human life.[57]

How are these different attitudes to be interpreted? Eugenic indications were introduced into the abortion and sterilization laws during the 1930s in order to combat the spread of undesirable characteristics in the population. Behind this lay society's desire to raise the population's "quality" by eliminating serious hereditary diseases and to avoid large welfare costs.[58] In the government's 1963 bill, the abortion law's eugenic indication was described as being "colored by" the notion of eradicating diseases but that consideration for the expected child and the parents also played an important role. This is hardly a plausible description of the purpose or application of the eugenic indication during the 1930s, but a practice may have evolved, as confidence in the older eugenics faded, that took greater account of the individual fetus.

To determine if the fifth abortion indication represented a new principle in abortion law is thus problematic, though it is clear that the different sides had an interest in presenting it one way or the other: either as a fundamentally new element in the Abortion Act (conservative MPs, the disability organization De vanföras väl, and individual Christian debaters) or as a legitimization of current practice and an extension of existing law (the government and the newspapers *Dagens Nyheter* and *Svenska Dagbladet*). That is, it was a question of politics.[59]

Conclusion

In the spring of 1963, the proposal to introduce a fetal damage indication became part of Swedish abortion law. This legislative revision, as this chapter has attempted to demonstrate, links directly to abortion travel and the case of Sherri Finkbine, as well as to fetal defects caused by the drug thalidomide more widely. As this volume illustrates, women have historically traveled to many parts of the world to access abortion services and continue to do so today for a variety of reasons and in a variety of contexts. Sherri Finkbine flew to Sweden to have her pregnancy terminated because she had taken thalidomide, and because a termination had ultimately been denied her in her home country, the USA. She arguably represented something new in the history of abortion: a modern, white, middle-class woman who spoke out in favor of abortion. However, her outspokenness was ultimately the catalyst that necessitated her travel.

The events surrounding thalidomide consumption in Sweden resulted in a revised abortion law and a greater understanding of women who wished for an abortion. Yet it was still a concern that some abortion grounds (fetal damage) were weighed more heavily than others (self-determination). And there was still an unsavory element of dividing women into two types. While Sherri Finkbine was depicted by the Swedish press as a good mother and a respectable human being, newspapers such as *Aftonbladet* were issuing warnings about "a certain category of women" who had taken matters into their own hands and used thalidomide to successfully achieve an abortion. Even in parliamentary debates, it was argued that women would duplicitously take advantage of the abortion law by taking, or stating that they had taken, dangerous drugs.

Swedish abortion debates at this time also focused on the controversial subject of disability. During the period of thalidomide consumption, as well as during the earlier outbreak of rubella in the 1950s, women were permitted to have an abortion to alleviate the risk of fetal damage. The birth of a disabled child was generally described as a tragedy, and as a lifetime of suffering for the child as well as the parents. However, the 1960s was a period of transition. Some media representations of children born with injuries caused by thalidomide attempted to contribute to a more positive and optimistic view of disabled children. The 1967 television documentary "Peter och hans kamrater" ("Peter and His Friends") by Maj Ödman spread knowledge about and brought together disabled children and their parents. Reagan notes that the media played a central role during the rubella epidemic in 1960s America;[60] the media occupied an equally active role in Swedish abortion debates, informing the public about thalidomide at a time when the medical establishment hesitated.

The year after the fetal damage indication was incorporated into Swedish law, women's abortion travel was brought to the fore once more. At a 1964 conference titled "Sex and Society," organized by the Liberal Student Union in Stockholm with support from the RFSU, two young women appeared on a darkened stage. Both had had their application for an abortion turned down in Sweden. One was now a single mother, while the other had traveled to communist Poland to obtain an abortion. A few months later, as a result of the conference, Sweden's Office of the Prosecutor-General announced plans to instigate legal proceedings against the many women who had obtained an abortion in Poland—a country whose response to unwanted pregnancy is explored in this volume by Ewelina Ciaputa—and against Hans Nestius, a conference co-organizer, for aiding them. Nestius was brought in for questioning, and his home was searched in an attempt to find names and addresses.[61]

The "Poland Affair," as it became widely known, mobilized the Swedish public. Soon afterward, due to growing support for abortion and anger that women should not be penalized for seeking abortion services, the government decided to grant both the women and Nestius a nolle prosequi. They escaped prosecution. The government then appointed an abortion commission to revise the nation's abortion laws, which culminated in "abortion on demand" from 1975 onward. The Poland Affair thereby provided a second example within just a short period of time that women's abortion travel had wide-ranging political consequences.[62]

Notes

1. Lena Lennerhed, "Sherri Finkbine's Choice: Abortion, Sex-Liberalism and Feminism in Sweden in the 1960s and 1970s," *Women's History Magazine* 73 (Autumn 2013): 13–18. For the wider history of abortion, disability, and the impact of thalidomide, see Leslie J. Reagan, *Dangerous Pregnancies: Mothers, Disabilities, and Abortion in Modern America* (Berkeley: University of California Press, 2010); Trent Stephens and Rock Brynner, *Dark Remedy: The Impact of Thalidomide and Its Revival as a Vital Medicine* (Cambridge, MA: Perseus, 2001): 57–58; and Dagmar Herzog, "Abortion, Christianity, Disability: Western Europe, 1960s-1970s," in *Sexual Revolutions*, ed. Gert Hekma and Alain Giami (Basingstoke, UK: Palgrave Macmillan, 2014), 249–63.

2. Yvonne Hirdman, Jenny Björkman, and Urban Lundberg, *Sveriges historia: 1920–1965* (Stockholm: Norstedts, 2012).

3. Lena Lennerhed, *Kvinnotrubbel: Abort i Sverige 1938–1974* (Uppsala, Sweden: Gidlunds, 2017).

4. *Sweden 1965 års abortkommitté, and Sweden Justitiedepartementet, Abortfrågan: remissyttranden över 1965 års abortkommitté betänkande Rätten till abort (SOU 1971:58)* (Stockholm: Statens offentliga utredningar, 1971), 121.

5. Advertisement for medical products from Astra 1960, uncatalogued, National Library of Sweden. See also Inga-Maj Juhlin, *Rikskuratorn: Omhändertagandet av de neurosedynskadade barnen 1962–1970* (Stockholm: Carlsson, 2012), 10.

6. "German Sedative Presumed Dangerous during Pregnancy," *Svenska Dagbladet*, November 27, 1961; and "German Sedative Presumed Dangerous during Pregnancy," *Dagens Nyheter*, November 27, 1961.

7. *Ny Dag*, December 8, 1961.

8. Nadja Yllner, *Bara en liten vit sömntablett* (Borås, Sweden: Recito, 2007), 62.

9. "International Sleeping Pills Scandal. Thousands of Children Deformed. Swedish Investigation," *Dagens Nyheter*, March 14, 1962. See also Yllner, *Bara en liten*, 83.

10. *Dagens Nyheter*, March 18, 1962. In *Expressen*, March 27, 1962, Linder—together with Åke Liljestrand—explained again: "We feared that more comprehensive measures might create anxiety, which would cause greater damage including potentially serious mental complications in many expectant mothers, who may not even be able to find out what drugs they have used."

11. Barbro Alving, "Open Letter to Director Engel," with response from Engel and further comment by Alving. See Barbro Alving, "Open Letter to Director Engel," *Vecko-Journalen*, March 23, 1962. Later, the German physician Widukind Lenz estimated that five children were born deformed in Sweden as a result of lack of information from the authorities. See Karin Paulsson, *"Dom säger att jag ser mer normal ut med benproteser"*: *om samhällskrav kontra barns behov* (Stockholm: Stockholm University, 1995), 33.

12. The data on the number of children born in Sweden is taken from the National Board of Health's investigator Jan Winberg, "Utredning rörande det eventuella sambandet mellan fosterskador och läkemedel," *Svenska läkartidningen* 61 (1964): 828, but somewhat higher figures have been reported in other contexts.

13. On the impact of thalidomide on Sweden, see Paulsson, *"Dom säger att jag"*; Yllner, *Bara en liten*; Juhlin, *Rikskuratorn*; Erik Ransemar and Halfdan Renling, *"Det idealiska sömnmedlet"*: *En studie i hur neurosedyntragedin publicerades* (Stockholm: Raben and Sjögren, 1970). See also *P3 Radio Documentary*, "Neurosedynkatastrofen," directed by Kristofer Hansson and Frederick Johnsson, broadcasted March 12, 2006, on Sveriges Radio, www.sverigesradio.se.

14. *Expressen*, August 17–22, 1962; Reagan, *Dangerous Pregnancies*, 58–59.

15. See the newspapers *Expressen* and *Aftonbladet*, August 1962.

16. *Kungl.Maj:ts proposition*, no. 100, 1963: 5.

17. "Aktuellt," Swedish Television, August 6, 1962; *Aftonbladet*, August 17, 1962.

18. Mattias Tydén, *Från politik till praktik: De svenska steriliseringslagarna 1935–1975* (Stockholm: Almqvist and Wicksell International, 2002), 338.

19. Åke Ahrsjö (managing director at *Expressen* in 1962) in discussion with the author, May 2007.

20. *Expressen*, August 17, 1962.

21. *Expressen*, August 17, 1962, and August 22, 1962. Even *Dagens Nyheter* reported on the Finkbine case under headings such as "Tears of Joy after Abortion Promise" ("Glädjetårar efter löfte om abort"), August 18, 1962, and "Mrs. Finkbine's Operation! The Foetus is Malformed" ("Fru Finkbines operation! Fostret är missbildat"), August 19, 1962. On August 20, *Dagens Nyheter* reported that the pope had condemned the abortion.

22. Sherri Finkbine, *Expressen*, August 18, 1962; August 22, 1962.

23. Sherri Finkbine, *Expressen*, August 18, 1962; August 22, 1962.

24. Sherri Finkbine, *Expressen*, August 19, 1962.

25. Sherri Finkbine, *Expressen*, August 21, 1962.

26. Sherri Finkbine, *Expressen*, August 22, 1962.

27. Sherri Finkbine, *Expressen*, August 22, 1962.

28. Robert Finkbine, "Our Case," *Industria: International Extra: For and about Swedish Industry* (1962): 132.

29. Finkbine, "Our Case," 132.

30. Reagan, *Dangerous Pregnancies*, 86.

31. Clare Parker, "From Immorality to Public Health: Thalidomide and the Debate for Legal Abortion in Australia," *Social History of Medicine* 25, no. 4 (2012): 863–80.

32. Lena Lennerhed, *Historier om ett brott: Illegala aborter i Sverige på 1900-talet* (Stockholm: Atlas, 2008), chapter 5.

33. *Dagens Nyheter* called the Vandeputs case "Thalidomide Murder" on the newspaper's front page: "Belgiskt rättsdrama om neurosedynmord ["Belgian Thalidomide Murder Courtroom Drama"]," *Dagens Nyheter*, August 21, 1962.

34. Richard Oulahan, "Euthanasia: Should One Kill a Child in Mercy or Is Life, However Hard, Too Dear to Lose?," *Life*, August 10, 1962.

35. British Pathé, "Liege: Mercy Gets the Verdict," aired November 15, 1962, http://www.britishpathe.com/video/mercy-gets-the-verdict/query/thalidomide. *Svenska Dagbladet* reported on the "Deafening Ovation" ('öronbedövande ovationer'), while *Dagens Nyheter* wrote that "the courtroom erupted with joy when the judgment was read out" ["Rättssalen jublade då domen lästes upp"], November 11, 1962. See also Parker, "From Immorality."

36. *Dagens Nyheter*, "Belgiskt rättsdrama om neurosedynmord."

37. Olof Lagercrantz, "Kvinnan i Liège," *Dagens Nyheter*, November 9, 1962.

38. Harald Ofstad, "Respekten för livets värde," *Dagens Nyheter*, November 11, 1962.

39. Juhlin, *Rikskuratorn*, 41.

40. Sonja Gaspard, "Ett barn har dödats men många lever . . . ," *Vecko-Journalen*, November 16, 1962.

41. E. N., "Applåder för mordet i Liège!," *Svensk vanföretidskrift* 12 (1962): 12.

42. Christina Palmgren, "Rätten att leva," *Vi* 47 (1962): 11.

43. See *Expressen*, August 17, 1962, 7, and Gaspard, "Ett barn har dödats," 40.

44. Kajsa Ohrlander, "Idéer och värderingar runt institutioner för barn med handikapp under 100 år," in *Barnhus: Om räddningsanstalter, barnhem, idiotanstalter, uppfostringsanstalter i Norden från 1700-talet till våra dagar*, ed. Kajsa Ohrlander (Stockholm: Allmänna barnhuset, 1991); Staffan Förhammar and Marie C. Nelson, eds., *Funktionshinder i ett historiskt perspektiv* (Lund: Studentlitteratur, 2004). See also Reagan, *Dangerous Pregnancies*, 66.

45. Palmgren, "Rätten att leva."

46. *Aftonbladet*, April 25, 1962.

47. *Aftonbladet*, April 25, 1962.

48. Jan Wiberg inquiry, "Utredning rörande det eventuella sambandet mellan fosterskador och läkemedel," published in four articles in *Svenska läkartidningen* 61 (1964). The terms of the inquiry were general, but the role of thalidomide was to be looked at in particular. The issue of abortion was raised with regard to two drugs other than thalidomide, but no connection could be established.

49. Editorial, "Neurosedynet," *Svenska Dagbladet*, September 4, 1962. The National Board of Health's representation is given in *Kungl.Maj:ts proposition*, no. 100, 1963: 5–6.

50. Between July 1, 1951, and June 30, 1952, it is estimated that 276 abortions were carried out as a result of rubella. The National Board of Health's representation is given in *Kungl.Maj:ts proposition* no. 100, 1963: 5–6.

51. *Kungl.Maj:ts proposition* no. 100, 1963: 6.

52. Brita Rudberg, "Förhastad lagstiftning?," *Svenska läkartidningen* 60, no. 11 (1963): 579.

53. *Kungl.Maj:ts proposition* no. 100, 1963: 11–12.

54. *Kungl.Maj:ts proposition* no. 100, 1963: 10, 12.

55. Roland Rosendahl, "Humanitet på avvägar," *Svensk vanföretidskrift* 11 (1962): 6.

56. Parliamentary motion from MP Elisabet Sjövall, Motioner i Andra kammaren, no. 836 (1963): 19, Riksdagstrycket.

57. *Kungl.Maj:ts proposition* no. 100, 1963: 15.

58. For eugenics and sterilization policy in Sweden, see Tydén, *Från politik till praktik.*

59. *Svenska Dagbladet* supported the bill in several leading articles and argued that any complaint that the proposal was based on a new principle was unreasonable and misleading since the law was intended to prevent suffering, not to rank people. See "Abortfrågan," May 9, 1963; and "Abortlagen ändras," May 23, 1963. *Dagens Nyheter* was on the same wavelength: see "Märklig abortstrid," May 8, 1963; and "Tvetydigt om abort," May 22, 1963.

60. Reagan, *Dangerous Pregnancies,* 49.

61. Lennerhed, "Sherri Finkbine's Choice," 15.

62. For more information on both Sherri Finkbine and the Poland Affair, see Annulla Linders and Danielle Besset, "Freeing Abortion in Sweden," in *A Fragmented Landscape: Abortion Governance and Protest Logics in Europe,* ed. Silvia De Zordo, Joanna Mishtal, and Lorena Anton (New York: Berghahn Books, 2017), 46–65.

[2]

From Heathrow Airport to Harley Street

The ALRA and the Travel of Nonresident Women for
Abortion Services in Britain

CHRISTABELLE SETHNA

FOUNDED IN 1936 by a few women who leaned toward socialism, feminism, and eugenics, the Abortion Law Reform Association (ALRA) was a key player in the British campaign for abortion law reform. After three decades of lobbying, the organization celebrated the passage of the 1967 British Abortion Act, applicable to England, Scotland, and Wales. The act, which Gayle Davis et al. explore in detail in this volume, had no residency requirements. It permitted women to have a legal therapeutic abortion up to 28 weeks of pregnancy once two physicians agreed in good faith that the pregnancy risked the life of the woman, her mental or physical health, any of her existing children, or the birth of a child with serious mental or physical disabilities. Physicians could take the woman's present or foreseeable environment into account. They also had to carry out abortions in an approved facility and provide the chief medical officer of the Department of Health and Social Security with a detailed notification form within seven days of the abortion. Coming into effect in late April 1968, the act was presented as at last resolving the issue of "backstreet," meaning illegal, abortions, especially for married working-class women. However, it was soon subjected to a furious attack about its purported abuses, compelling the ALRA to transition from campaigning for abortion law reform to defending the act itself.[1]

A mushrooming scandal featuring abortion travel was central to the early criticism of the act. Nonresident women, understood most often as nationals of other countries, began traveling to Britain and, in particular, to the city of London—where Britain's private sector was concentrated—to access abortion services. Ineligible for free-of-charge medical services under the public sector National Health Service (NHS) because they were not British citizens, nonresident women sought help from Britain's private sector. To meet the demand, commercial and volunteer "pregnancy referral agencies" and "pregnancy advisory bureaux" (hereafter "abortion referral agencies") sprang up in Britain and in other countries, raising concerns that nonresident women were being funneled to physicians for abortions in the private sector, likely for financial gain.[2] The travel of nonresident women posed a dilemma to the ALRA. The organization sympathized with nonresident women from countries in which abortion was illegal or otherwise unavailable. Yet it had to weigh their influx into Britain against growing opposition that threatened the act itself. This juggling act took place against the backdrop of larger questions about the British medical profession and changes to Britain's place in the world.

The geopolitical and biopolitical transnational dimensions of the ALRA's campaign for abortion law reform, defense of the Abortion Act, and response to the travel of nonresident women to Britain for abortion services are interrelated, substantial, and deserve closer examination. However, it must be noted that although the travel of women for abortion services is far from rare, it has been understudied in British abortion history, possibly because this vast literature deals most often with the long march toward the reform of birth control laws and terminates with the passage of the act.[3] Post-1967 scholarship is slanted toward the impact of legal abortion and the birth control pill on sexual behavior, the medical profession's responses to legal abortion, and the role of lobby groups in defending or rejecting legal abortion.[4] Also prominent is the role of feminist activism in regard to the act[5] as well as the influence of the act on abortion laws in Commonwealth countries and in Western European Roman Catholic countries.[6]

One early assessment of the Abortion Act holds briefly that the influx of nonresident women seeking abortion services was exaggerated, while another acknowledges the influx of nonresident women as a noteworthy outcome of the Abortion Act, but only in passing.[7] Because women seeking abortion services needed only to provide a British address to be counted as a resident, it is likely that the available quantitative data is problematic because it does not capture completely the extent of nonresident women's travels.[8] Additionally, because statistics show that considerably fewer abortions were performed on nonresident women than on residents, it is argued that the media coverage was misleading.[9] However, in a very useful article, Ashley Wivel shows that the 1971 Committee on the Working of the Abortion Act, colloquially known as the Lane Committee, deliberated on nonresident women's access to abortion services in Britain, while Anthony Horden acknowledges the travels of nonresident women in relation to those of resident women who also desired legal abortion services in Britain under the act.[10]

The Global Context of Abortion Law Reform

In their own history of abortion law reform in Britain, Keith Hindell and Madeleine Simms, the former a board member of a volunteer abortion referral service and the latter an editor of the ALRA newsletter, classified Britain as a laggard. They noted that as of 1948, Japan had a Eugenic Protection Law that provided abortions to a million women annually, while Russia and some Eastern European and Scandinavian countries had liberalized their abortion laws even earlier, as authors Lena Lennerhed, Anna Bogic, and Ewelina Ciaputa demonstrate in this volume. In the mid-1960s, Dr. Malcolm Potts, an ALRA member, visited Eastern Europe, where he learned for the first time about vacuum aspiration abortions, later commenting on the thrill of discovery in a way that also smacked of the stereotypical gender relations of the era: "I was absolutely astonished that you could do an abortion at eight weeks [gestation], and the woman could go home two hours later and make her husband's dinner."[11] Potts realized that statistics provided by Eastern European countries with liberal abortion laws, examples of which Anna Bogic and Ewelina Ciaputa discuss in this volume in relation to the former Yugoslavia and Poland, respectively, were sometimes dismissed by British physicians because of the presumed duplicity of communists. Nevertheless, the data showed that safe and legal abortions were not harmful to women; Hungary, which was said to have abortion on demand, had extremely low rates of maternal mortality. Higher rates of maternal mortality in Sweden were explained by the slow-moving bureaucracy in that country, leading to more abortions after the first trimester, when the procedure was more complicated and potentially more harmful to the woman.[12]

The ALRA had long promoted the argument that the woman most likely to benefit from abortion law reform in Britain would be the poverty-stricken "decent mother of a family who has as many children as she can cope with." Yet this argument, which was intended to propagandize abortion as a respectable choice rather than a sordid backstreet affair, was often subsumed by the popular notion that abortion was closely associated with the sexual immorality of single women.[13] The organization, and a network of physicians, politicians, and lawyers supporting it, had long-standing ties to the eugenics movement. The role of the rubella virus in causing damage to the fetus encouraged broader support for abortion. But in the decade before the passage of the act, it was thalidomide, a sedative of German origin pegged as the source of severe birth defects in utero, that fueled the general public's support for abortion law reform as never before. Pregnant women who swallowed the drug in more than 40 countries, among them Britain, Australia, Canada, and Germany, miscarried, had stillbirths, or gave birth in the thousands to children with damaged limbs. Two such mothers captured international headlines for their subsequent actions: accompanied by her husband, Robert Finkbine, Sherri Finkbine traveled to Sweden from the United States of America (USA) for an abortion, while Suzanne Vandeput, a Belgian woman, killed her afflicted infant but was acquitted of murder. In this volume, Lena Lennerhed deals with both of these examples in her reading of the impact of thalidomide on Swedish abortion provision and its relationship to disability. She likewise finds that respectable, white, married women's "dangerous pregnancies" spread global anxiety about disabled children and positioned abortion as a sensible public health solution. Thereafter, the putative association between abortion and the sexual immorality of single women was somewhat weakened.[14]

Hindell and Simms agree that the widespread eugenic revulsion spawned by the thalidomide tragedy drove up membership in and donations to the ALRA and paved the way toward the passage of the Abortion Act.[15] But once the act was passed, the ALRA recognized that its task was to make the new law work on the ground, using the same amount of "vigour and determination" that was required to bring it about.[16] In a pamphlet produced to inform the public about the new law before it went into effect, the ALRA urged women not to have an illegal abortion and cautioned them not to delay seeking an abortion past the first trimester. Any woman refused a legal abortion by the NHS was encouraged to contact another physician or pay for a legal abortion via the private sector route. Evidence of the difficulties British women continued to experience even after the passage of the Abortion Act is presented by Davis et al. in their contribution to this volume. They argue that access to NHS abortions varied enormously by region, a fact that led resident women to travel domestically to large cities such as London, Birmingham, and Liverpool, where private sector and charitable abortion provision was more plentiful. Anticipating that British women would continue to approach the ALRA as they had in the past for referrals to abortion services, the pamphlet stated "THIS ASSOCIATION CANNOT ARRANGE ABORTIONS NOR CAN IT GIVE NAMES OF DOCTORS WILLING TO DO THEM," in uppercase letters for added emphasis. The pamphlet did provide the names of other organizations for assistance purposes, the Family Planning Association, and Brook Advisory Centres.[17]

Money Makes the World Go 'Round

The ALRA and other supporters of the act praised it as "having brought about a revolution" in Britain because "it has changed medical practice. It has exposed the extent of unwanted pregnancy and made motherhood more of a voluntary occupation. It has reduced the number of illegitimate births and it will, in time, affect the birth rate. Whether or not one approves of the Act, one cannot deny its significance."[18] That significance was apparently not limited solely to Britain. The act was believed to have triggered the liberalization of abortion laws in several American states and in some Commonwealth countries, morphing into a global exemplar of abortion law reform.[19]

But by the ALRA's own admission, these plaudits had to be tempered by three main criticisms: the act was too permissive; put pressure on NHS hospitals, physicians, and staff to provide abortions; and attracted large numbers of nonresident women to Britain for abortion services.[20] In a discussion of these matters at a symposium held in London by the Council of the Medical Protection Society in February 1969, J. A. Stallworthy, professor of obstetrics and gynaecology at Oxford University, was scathing in his opinion of the act. Stallworthy, and some other physicians present, believed it had swung open the doors to abortion on demand, a provision that the ALRA, and many in the medical profession, rejected.[21] Worse, he declared that a minority of physicians had become involved in providing abortions to nonresident women for financial profit. Stallworthy pointed dramatically to "a procession of unhappy women who after a short visit [to Britain] leave these shores without the foetus which entered unnoticed through the immigration barrier and minus the requisite number of Deutschmarks, Swiss francs, and American dollars. Only time will be able to assess the gravity of this complication in terms of its effect on international regard for British medicine and British ethics."[22]

Stallworthy's praise for the high standards of British medicine and British ethics appears more performative than patriotic. Strict anti-abortion laws in place long before the Abortion Act came into effect meant that a trade in backstreet abortions by medical and nonmedical personnel flourished, and criminal trial records indicate that women from other parts of the country traveled to big cities such as London specifically to buy them. Backstreet abortions were often deployed strategically by those who opposed *and* supported abortion. They were heavily racialized, which contributed to their sordid reputation. Portrayed as dangerous and dirty, and allied with poverty and immorality, backstreet abortions were linked to shady Eastern European or West Indian immigrants who were unlicensed physicians, or who posed as physicians.[23] A shift occurred when Aleck Bourne, an eminent gynecologist who performed an abortion on a young rape victim for no fee, was acquitted in 1938. Thereafter, physicians determining whether an abortion was justified began taking into consideration a woman's physical and mental health, and, once the Abortion Act was passed, her present and foreseeable environment. These developments ensured that the medical profession, made up mainly of men, would maintain an even greater gatekeeping role over access to legal abortion services, thereby medicalizing and masculinizing the procedure.[24]

Although many women continued to turn to backstreet abortion after the Bourne decision, wealthy, white, middle-class married and single women had recourse to physicians who would sign off on a legal abortion. Even the Department of Health was said to have "turned a blind eye" to women referring themselves for abortions in London's prestigious West End.[25] Just one year before the act's passage, *Observer* journalist Paul Ferris published an exposé with all the characteristics of a potboiler. Ferris thanked his wife for doing much of the research and acknowledged the ALRA, the Family Planning Association, and the International Planned Parenthood Federation for providing him with information but kept his interviewees anonymous. In this volume, Cathrine Chambers, Colleen MacQuarrie, and Jo-Ann

MacDonald distinguish four intersecting pathways that women from Prince Edward Island, Canada, take in order to access abortion services. In a similar fashion, the crux of Ferris's exposé was the four abortion pathways that he determined British women with unwanted pregnancies might follow. Backstreet abortions were illegal. So too were those performed on the sly by licensed general practitioners. Legal "West End" or "Harley Street" abortions were performed by a variety of licensed physicians. Finally, NHS abortions were legal, but difficult to obtain.[26]

Ferris asserted that Harley Street abortions had "grown into a comfortable industry" that ran on money, dishonesty, hypocrisy, and which sometimes included the verbal and sexual abuse of patients. With licensed physicians cashing in on the celebrated London locale, he estimated that every year 10,000 women from wealthy families and the middle classes, as well as the more "humble" sort (e.g., typists, students, and secretaries), had an abortion for an average price of £100. Furthermore, he contended that a considerable number of physicians involved in the abortion industry were Eastern European or Jewish, conjecturing that because abortion was more readily available than reliable contraception in Eastern Europe, immigrant physicians "found a market for their special skill" in performing abortions. Ferris's claims are debatable; however, both Anna Bogic and Ewelina Ciaputa, in their respective contributions to this volume, illuminate the complicated relationship between contraception and abortion in the former Yugoslavia and Poland, respectively, as well as the predominance of abortion as a method of birth control. Ferris also threw into question just how far abortion law reform could proceed when abortion continued to be associated with the sexual immorality of single women. For this reason, the ALRA, he maintained, produced propaganda that focused deliberately on married women's unwanted pregnancies, ignoring mention of single women who had abortions.[27]

The claims Ferris made in his exposé may or may not have reflected his own xenophobia, anti-Semitism, class prejudice, or sexual conservatism; regardless, they contributed toward the casting of the Harley Street abortion industry as greedy, seedy, and foreign, and not unlike the disreputable illegal backstreet abortion trade. Above all, abortion law reform needed to appear respectable to the British public, not only in terms of the social status of the woman seeking an abortion but also of the physician performing the procedure.

Up in the Air

The influx of nonresident women to Britain for abortion services, and to London in particular, after the passage of the Abortion Act magnified the negative image of the legal Harley Street abortion industry that Ferris had conjured in his exposé. That image was further tarnished when, as David Paintin, ALRA consultant and member of the Royal College of Obstetricians and Gynaecologists, recalls, nonresident women who were not eligible for a legal abortion under the NHS "found their way to the private gynaecologists, particularly the entrepreneurs who had set up their own clinics. Many women came to London not knowing where to get help and sought advice from staff at the stations or airport, or from the taxi drivers waiting outside."[28] Abortion referral agencies facilitated the journeys of nonresident women, a matter that Hayley Brown and Agata Ignaciuk each pursue in this volume. In Britain, some of the homegrown agencies were volunteer organizations with ALRA connections founded to help British women access abortions under the new act. Others were commercially based and advertised their services and prices inside and outside Britain. The large size of London's private sector meant that it managed most of the abortions performed on nonresident women.[29]

The journeys of nonresident women did not go unnoticed. In contrast to the sympathetic reportage about white, respectable married women, like Sherri Finkbine, who underwent abortions in reputable surroundings, as Lena Lennerhed establishes in this volume, international media carried lurid stories of "foreign girls" traveling to London to terminate their pregnancies, sometimes under dodgy circumstances.[30] Adjective and noun performed double duty. This dynamic duo implied that nonresident women were young, single, and vulnerable to exploitation in the British private sector. But it also reinforced the swirl of unpleasant racialized connections between abortion, sexual immorality, money, and otherness. This was especially pertinent when it was alleged that commercial abortion referral agencies charged nonresident women referral fees, and private clinics paid these agencies for referrals. Both fees and advertisements for patients were illegal. In the early 1970s, the Pregnancy Advisory Service, an abortion referral service, set up a discrete office at Heathrow Airport to assist nonresident women coming to London in search of abortion services. Volunteers who spoke a number of European languages provided these women with abortion counseling in another London office,[31] driving home the value of providing information about abortion services in translation, as Anna Bogic, Ewelina Ciaputa, and Agata Ignaciuk each do in this volume.

The Abortion Act's lack of residency requirements led Tory politician Norman St. John-Stevas to propose an amendment to the act that would impose a six-month residential qualification for women seeking abortion services. An editorial in *New Society* countered, establishing that only a tiny number of nonresident women had abortions in Britain, and even suggested that some of the abortions were NHS provided, speculating that these women were "probably semi-resident, au pair girls, nurses, and the like." The editorial asked why abortion services for nonresident women had generated so much consternation when innumerable nonresidents of various nationalities traveled regularly to Britain to purchase a wide range of medical services in the private sector, in effect, participating in a version of medical tourism. The editorial posed additional valuable questions that pointed to the impracticalities of policing residential qualifications should the proposed amendment succeed: "Are doctors to turn detectives to make sure that if the girl says she has been in England for the statutory period, she really has? Or is the government to set up a new department for this purpose similar to the one in the Inland Revenue? The prospect of increasing the amount of bureaucracy and snooping, and multiplying forms, in order to harass a thousand desperate foreign girls each year, is not an attractive one."[32]

Such a sensible challenge to unstable concepts of nationality and residency was no match against accounts of young Danish women coming to London in droves for abortion services in the private sector, which were supposedly arranged as a package deal between a Danish underwear manufacturer and an unidentified London clinic.[33] The account led Jane Carter, a journalist for a tabloid newspaper, the *Daily Express*, to ask readers: "How easy is it for a foreign girl knowing no one in Britain, to get in touch with an abortion clinic?" Stationing herself outside Heathrow Airport with a suitcase, a phony American accent, and a fictitious tale starring a reluctant boyfriend and an unwanted pregnancy, Carter posed as a newly arrived foreign girl seeking an abortion. She said that she approached an airport taxi driver who did not take her to the (false) clinic address she requested. Rather, in just under an hour, he drove her to a clinic around the corner from Harley Street, where a nurse met her and made arrangements for an abortion. Carter recorded all the costs involved, from the taxi fare to the fees for consultation, nursing, and the operation itself, going on to specify that the journey from airport to clinic had been repeated many times over by other nonresident women and expedited by taxi drivers who received financial kickbacks from physicians.[34] Carter's investigation was followed by her coauthored report headlined "Abortion Hotel." Apparently familiar to clinics and taxi drivers, the hotel housed nonresident women who had come to London for abortion services. It would be a mistake to assume that all such women were financially privileged. A married Canadian woman staying at the hotel declared she was now "penniless" after paying for travel, accommodation, and the abortion procedure itself. The report's claim that the hotel was run by a woman of "Polish descent" intensified the hotel's unsavory aura of outsiderness.[35]

Despite energetic denials in Parliament that London was fast becoming the "abortion capital of the world," offering "weekend abortions" to nonresident women,[36] pressure to review the new law culminated in the striking of the Lane Committee.[37] Figures based on the compulsory notification forms for abortions performed under the Abortion Act that the committee later tabulated illustrate the rapid rise in abortions on nonresident women between 1968 and 1972. In 1968, abortions on nonresident women accounted for only 5.5 percent of total terminations. By early 1972, that number had jumped to 30.8 percent. Nonresident women from France and Germany constituted the two largest groups of nonresident women, with others arriving from Belgium, the Netherlands, and Switzerland.[38] Data confirmed that the private sector was absorbing most of the nonresident women, more of whom were single than married, and that their abortions were generally performed in large cities such as London, Birmingham, and Liverpool.[39]

The ALRA was not pleased with the prospect of an official review, insisting that the new law was working smoothly with the exception of "sensational publicity, mainly the alleged influx of foreign girls, and the so-called 'abortion racket' involving a mere handful of physicians whose misconduct should be dealt with by their professional bodies and by the General Medical Council, not by inserting restrictive clauses in the Act." The ALRA warned that some who had called for the inquiry were deeply opposed to the Abortion Act to begin with, while others had been swayed by adverse and unfounded publicity. It classified Britain once again as a laggard, this time in comparison to recent abortion law reforms in several American states, to tamp down concerns about Britain's global status as "the abortion capital of the world."[40]

Desperate Women

Before the passage of the 1967 British Abortion Act, the ALRA received hundreds of letters from British women and men asking for information about how to get a legal abortion. In analyzing such letters, Emma Jones reflects that the correspondents were keen to signal their "desperation" and express it in epistolary terms. Married women and couples raised the economic, health, and physical hardships they faced, while single women and men highlighted the many personal and professional challenges of having a child outside marriage. The ALRA made "significant rhetorical use" of that desperation in their pamphlets, one of which was titled "In Desperation," and distributed them to encourage support for abortion law reform. Perhaps because it suspected it was under surveillance by authorities, the organization was circumspect and took pains to dismiss any notion that it acted as an abortion referral agency rather than a lobby organization; still, in a few cases, individual ALRA members did give correspondents the names of licensed physicians they knew and trusted.[41] Some of the correspondents also inquired about the possibility of traveling to Sweden, Japan, or Denmark for abortion services, leading the ALRA to discourage them, cautioning that these countries had abortion laws that were not as liberal as they first appeared. Nor were they as welcoming to other nationals seeking pregnancy termination, especially when they arrived without reliable contacts.[42]

These kinds of inquiries spotlighted not only the personal agency of the correspondents but also the global attention abortion law reform attracted. After 1967, the ALRA encountered a similar situation, but in reverse. Over the decades, it had become the go-to organization where abortion law reform matters were concerned. Now, after the passage of the Abortion Act, individuals and organizations from far and wide contacted the ALRA about arranging abortion services for nonresident women in Britain. Keen to ensure that there was no confusion between the role of the ALRA and the services offered by commercial and volunteer abortion referral agencies, General Secretary Diane Munday, who handled the ALRA's incoming and outgoing correspondence, had to fire off several letters when it was discovered that some journalists, airline officials, and even embassy staff had given some nonresident women contact information for the ALRA. The tone of her letter to Sir Frank Roberts, British ambassador to the Federal Republic of Germany, reflected both sternness and sympathy:

> The British embassy in Bonn has given our name and address as an organisation that can help arrange for unwanted pregnancies to be terminated. Unfortunately, this is not true and although we recognise the compassionate motives of those giving this advice in Bonn, we feel that overall the women are being done a considerable disservice. . . . When women arrive clutching a piece of paper giving our telephone number our Association is put in a very difficult position as on the one hand we are quite unable to help, and on the other we feel under a strong emotional obligation not to dash the hopes which have driven women into making this journey.[43]

The same combination of sternness and sympathy characterized Munday's responses to individual correspondents asking for help. But they also betrayed the ALRA's unease that the Abortion Act was not functioning as it should, even for British women. When a married man from Belgium asked for assistance in arranging an abortion for his 42-year-old wife, Munday replied: "It is unfortunate that people overseas have been led to believe that it is easy to obtain a legal abortion in Britain. In fact, it is still very difficult in some parts of the country for British women to obtain abortions. Attacks have been made in Parliament on the new law because some foreign women have been obtaining abortions here, and therefore although I am sorry for you and your wife, I am afraid there is nothing I can do to help."[44] Similarly, after receiving questions from a single woman from France about fees for an abortion in the private sector in Britain, Munday stated: "Because the opponents of liberal abortion find easy and sensational headlines in those desperate women who come from overseas for the operation, we have had to establish the principle of giving no advice to any of these. I do hope you understand this and not think us unsympathetic."[45]

Munday rarely appeared to relent. Nevertheless, she admitted that she was moved when she received a letter from Spain; as Agata Ignaciuk specifies in this volume, London was well known to Spaniards as a destination hub for abortion services. The letter writer wrote poignantly to Munday about his wife in hesitant English: "My wife has had three babies in four years. To look after them and to do her work as housewife has, naturally, altered her nerves. Now, unfortunately, she is in the first month of a new period of gestation. We know that in England, liberal and comprehensive country this situation can be saved due to the Abortion Act Reform. For this reason we want to go to London, but before making the travel we would appreciate very much if you could advise us about hospitals or clinics and the correct way to do it."[46] In private, Munday allowed that the letter had touched her "soft streak" and put the Spanish letter writer in contact with the secretary of a London physician connected to the ALRA.[47] The secretary offered him and his wife an upcoming appointment, but not before warning him about unscrupulous taxi drivers at the airport, saying: "You must refuse to go with any of them and ignore any advice or suggestions they make" about any other clinic.[48]

Munday's soft streak may have been triggered in this particular instance because of the praise the Spanish letter writer heaped on the Abortion Act, or because he and his wife fit the respectable profile favored publicly by the ALRA. It is more likely that she felt a special camaraderie with this correspondent because his situation mirrored the one she and her husband faced in 1961. As a wife and mother to three young children, a diabetic Munday became pregnant for the fourth time. Having known a woman who died because of a backstreet abortion, she sought a legal abortion free of charge under the NHS but claimed she was treated "like dirt." Munday and her husband then managed to scrape together enough money for a Harley Street abortion with a well-qualified physician. Her postabortion insight—"it was because I had a cheque book to wave in Harley Street that I was alive"— motivated her to become even more involved in the ALRA.[49] Such experiences are not only reminiscent of the very public travails of Robert Finkbine and Sherri Finkbine, a couple that Lena Lennerhed studies in this volume; they signpost as well the involvement of husbands in matters of access to abortion services and, glaringly, the ability or inability of couples or individual women to fund that access.

A savvy Munday hoped that letters from overseas correspondents, such as the aforementioned missive, could be used beneficially as propaganda. The ALRA had splashed the desperation of British letter writers throughout its materials in support of abortion law reform in Britain. But Munday hoped to use the desperation of overseas correspondents in the service of better family planning in *their* own countries, while discouraging nonresident women's abortion travel to Britain. In response to several letters from West Germany from married women with families who described, as she put it, "really desperate situations," Munday wondered if these letters could be utilized as family planning propaganda in Germany and suggested contacting "family planners in these areas [where the correspondents lived]" to ask them "if they could insert something in their local newspapers stating that ALRA is not in a position to help women obtain abortions and then continue with propaganda for family planning."[50]

The ALRA did produce a fact sheet formatted as a call-and-response dialogue between a generic individual and the ALRA. When the individual questioned why the numbers of abortions had risen to such a great extent in Britain after the Abortion Act came into effect, the ALRA responded reassuringly to preempt any criticism that the act had introduced abortion on demand into Britain. Official details on legal abortions on British women were now being recorded; there were no reliable numbers on illegal backstreet abortions performed before the act came into effect; and "more foreign patients are coming from mainly Roman Catholic countries of Western Europe." These women were having abortions in the private sector . . . because they know that abortion in Britain is safe while backstreet abortion in their own countries, where the law has not yet been changed, is dangerous."[51] The ALRA would broadcast a similar message to the Lane Committee.

A Baggage Carousel

The travel of nonresident women figured extensively in the deliberations of the Lane Committee (which Davis et al. also address in this volume) into the way the Abortion Act functioned. These occurred just as Britain was negotiating once again to join the European Economic Community (EEC), its application having been twice turned down earlier by France. Closer integration with Europe was promoted as a way to boost the slack British economy, although this argument was disputed in Britain and Europe.[52] The EEC would be subsumed under the European Union in the early 1990s. One set of the Lane Committee's deliberations is especially pertinent to this chapter, for they showcase just how worrisome border control entanglements could be, anticipating on many levels Niklas Barke's contribution to this volume on the potential impact of Brexit on abortion travel in the current day.

Subcommittee 2 of the Lane Committee laid out five reasons for placing restrictions on nonresident women seeking abortions: public concern; the belief that the dignity of the medical profession was at stake; the possibility that fees for abortion services in the private sector were artificially elevated; the decline in the international reputation of British medicine, especially if nonresident women were breaking abortion laws in their own countries when having abortions in Britain; and the likelihood that abuses of the act where nonresident women were concerned could be addressed in other ways, such as extending the NHS "to undercut the private sector" rather than banning the travel of nonresident women outright.[53]

Members of Subcommittee 2 returned to the possibility of applying a residential qualification based on nationality to restrict the travel of nonresident women for abortion services in Britain, but documents illustrated that it would be virtually impossible to manage. The 1963 Ministry of Health "Memorandum of Guidance to Hospital Authorities Hospital Treatment for Visitors from Overseas" generally allowed that medical services under the NHS were available to an individual "normally living" in Britain or an individual from a country with which Britain had a reciprocal arrangement, while visitors seeking medical services had to "pay for it as private patients, though if they fall ill while here they may receive treatment for that illness under the National Health Service." The problem was that it was impractical to identify at ports of entry who was and was not eligible for medical services under the NHS. There were no immigration checks on Republic of Ireland (hereafter Ireland) nationals, and checks were less lenient for Commonwealth visitors.[54]

As it turned out, determining who was a British national or resident was a herculean task; in its repeated attempts to restrict the flow of nonwhite immigrants, the British government had created exclusionary entry categories that were, in effect, race based.[55] However, nonresident women traveling to Britain for abortion services were largely white and European. They were not necessarily seen as marked by race. Additionally, international flows of migrants from many parts of the globe complicated nationality and residency status. Subcommittee 2 prepared for witnesses a list of 16 questions that signposted the pitfalls ahead. It included queries such as: What period of residency would be sufficient? Would the lack of a residential qualification constitute an offence committed by the nonresident woman or by the physician treating her? Which authority would take responsibility for enforcing the residential qualification? Significantly, to whom should the residential qualification apply? The answer to this last question, according to Subcommittee 2, might include "a British subject resident overseas permanently" or "a British subject resident overseas on a tour of duty." It might also extend to a citizen of Ireland, au pairs, students, an immigrant, or a resident worker in some instances.[56]

More detailed answers to this question and others muddled matters even further, as representatives from the Home Office indicated to the members of the subcommittee. One representative versed in immigration issues stated: "Girls arriving here for an abortion are treated no differently . . . [than] . . . those arriving for other medical treatment" but laid out a host of complications that could ensue, were they to be interrogated directly about the purpose of their visit. Due to the sheer volume of arrivals, which would include leisure tourists, at ports of entry such as Heathrow Airport, "it would be impossible to ask every woman of child-bearing age whether or not she was pregnant." Neither was it "obvious when a woman was coming for an abortion" or if she was a student or working as an au pair. Nor was the address on a landing card a woman completed upon arrival necessarily synonymous with the address of an abortion clinic.[57] A second representative elaborated on the vagaries of citizenship in relation to Britain's far-flung colonies, the nationality of parents and grandparents, birth and marriage certificates, the role of adoption and illegitimacy, the status of the Irish, and the introduction of the 1971 Immigration Act, which distinguished between patrials, meaning individuals who had the right to live in the United Kingdom (England, Scotland, Wales, and Northern Ireland), and nonpatrials. The overall exercise "required skilled interpretation." Proof of length of residency, which might require passports, national insurance contributions, and employer certificates, was another frustrating affair, and the time required to collect and verify the documents could seriously delay an abortion.[58]

A third representative invited to speak about criminal law was no more helpful, offering: "If the large number of foreign girls seeking abortions here were really affecting international relations the Foreign and Commonwealth Office should be asked their views." He determined that the criminalization of abortions on nonresident women would be very difficult to enforce. Arrest warrants would need to be issued to prevent nonresident women who had abortions from leaving Britain, and the Department of Health and Social Security (DHSS) might have to carry out raids on physicians' offices to determine the residential qualifications of the patients.[59] In the end, a fourth representative, this time from the DHSS, supplied the subcommittee with a prescient vision of Britain's future within the embrace of Europe and the practice of medical tourism. Thinking ahead to the country's plans to join the EEC, he presumed that nationals of EEC member states might be able to come to Britain for medical care, possibly including abortions, via international healthcare insurance agreements. In any case, hospitals and medical professionals had received no guidance on what constituted proof of residence, and one's nationality had "never been a criterion for treatment" under the NHS, showcasing still another conundrum.[60]

The ALRA presented its own brief to the Lane Committee. In it, the organization acknowledged that like all new legislation, the act brought with it a number of unforeseen problems. The need for abortion had been underestimated, NHS abortions were available on an uneven basis, commercial abortion referral agencies had emerged, and the "lengths to which women of other countries would go to seek relief" were not anticipated. Still, the ALRA clung to the notion that the act's "defects" should not overshadow its "benefits" as "one of the most important measures of social legislation in Britain since the War."[61] The brief insisted that physicians, commercial abortion referral agencies, and abortion clinics that charged referral fees and advertised for patients inside or outside Britain should be investigated and disciplined. Notably, it rejected any residential qualification, but in contrast to the cautious tone of Munday's replies to overseas correspondents requesting the ALRA's assistance with abortion services, the brief boldly backed nonresident women's access to abortion services while nodding to British medical prowess. Nonresident women were no different from other patients who sought medical care in Britain's private sector, thereby enhancing Britain's coffers and reputation: "This is no less so in the case of abortion and we have no reason to be ashamed of it. It was to be expected that foreign women would prefer to come to Britain for a legal abortion than run the risk of an illegal abortion in their own countries." The brief also contained several letters in an appendix from British women who experienced difficulties accessing abortion services under the terms of the

Abortion Act. However, letters from nonresident women were excluded, no doubt deliberately.[62]

A remarkable sentence in the brief encapsulated the ALRA's position on nonresident women: "For Britain to fail to tackle this problem with humanity and compassion would be a much worse reflection than being labelled 'the Abortion Capital of the World'."[63] Glanville Williams, ALRA president, Vera Houghton, ALRA chair of the Executive Committee, and Munday repeated the same moral in a face-to-face meeting with the Lane Committee. They even proposed that "charitable organisations" could establish "reasonably priced special clinics" for nonresident women because the private sector was now unable to cope with the demand. Moreover, Munday drew a parallel between nonresident women and British women, saying that the ALRA's primary concern was the exploitation of nonresident women: "In the same way as our concern in the early 'sixties [sic] was that the British women should not be exploited . . . I think once a woman arrives in this country desperate you cannot say 'Go back to your own country.' But I think we should not be positively encouraging them to come, as has happened."[64]

The three-volume *Report of the Committee on the Working of the Abortion Act* was published in 1974. One critic noted that the quality of the report was "uneven" and that on occasion "the level of argument and the assumptions upon which it is based, descend to reflect the underlying ideology and homely wisdom found in women's magazines." Still, he pronounced it "a lucid and impartial exposition."[65]

The report found that abortions on nonresident women from European countries had increased between 1968 and 1972, with France and Germany leading the way. In 1968, 56 nonresidents from France had abortions in Britain, while in 1972 it was 25,189. During the same time period, the numbers for German nonresidents stood at 620 and 17,531, respectively. In 1972, abortions on women from Belgium were recorded at 2,536; Ireland at 972; Spain at 730; and Switzerland at 675. Considerably smaller numbers of nonresident women arrived from Canada and the USA. Abortions on Canadian nonresidents were the highest at 376 in 1969 but fell to 52 in 1972, whereas abortions on American nonresidents reached a maximum of 1,601 in 1970 and then dropped to 131 in 1972. The decline in these numbers was attributed to the liberalization of abortion laws in both these countries.[66]

Broadly speaking, the report asserted that nonresident women from other countries who had abortions in Britain under the terms of the

Abortion Act committed no crime under British law. Moreover, the issue as to whether nonresident women who had abortions in another country, or physicians who helped women seek abortions in another country, were breaking their own countries' laws was pertinent, but prosecutions were said to be rare. The report also clarified that the British public's consternation over nonresident women was not directed at the women themselves but at their exploitation in the private sector. Finally, it confirmed that abortion, like sterilization and contraception, was now a part of British medical practice. Thus, a physician's "first duty" was to the patient, irrespective of nationality or residence. Were abortion services in Britain to be restricted on the basis of nationality or residence, it would be the *only* medical service to be dealt with in this fashion.[67]

A year before the report was published, Britain's membership in the EEC became official, a development that the Lane Committee had to factor into its conclusions and recommendations. The report reiterated the practical difficulties of restricting nonresident women's access to abortion services in Britain on the basis of nationality, speculating that it could now be illegal to exclude a national of an EEC member country. Furthermore, a restriction of abortion services on the basis of nationality risked excluding non-British nationals who were already living in Britain "more or less permanently."[68] A legally prescribed period of residency also had to be ruled out because it could negatively affect British women living overseas who returned home for a short time to access abortion services. Similarly, requiring nationals from EEC member countries to abide by a residency requirement could constitute "an infraction" of EEC law, a point that the Lane Committee did not have the expertise to decide on. The report also posited that a legal residency period would mean that a nonresident woman who broke the law would likely have already left the country after the abortion was completed, or additional legislation would have to be enacted to ensure that she stayed in the country for a specific postabortion length of time in order for prosecution to take place. In turn, these constraints would place great pressure on physicians and clinics, who would have to defend themselves in a court of law. A period of residency could also result in more late-term and illegal backstreet abortions for nonresident women in Britain or elsewhere, placing their health at undue risk.[69]

Based on the evidence it gathered, the Lane Committee acknowledged that profiteering had occurred in the private sector involving the usual suspects: a minority of physicians, commercial abortion referral agencies, and taxi drivers. However, the report stated categorically that any attempt to introduce statutes restricting access to abortion services based on nationality or residency could lead individuals to evade the law because "so great are the profits to be made from the abortion of foreign women coming here." The report speculated that even greater abuses of the Abortion Act could result because there would be more competition for smaller numbers of nonresident women. Like the ALRA, the report put its faith in already-existing disciplinary bodies to root out and punish profiteering, arguing that nonresident women should not be restricted from accessing abortion services in Britain unless the overall situation worsened.[70]

Conclusion

The distance between Heathrow Airport and Harley Street was both literal and symbolic. The geopolitical and biopolitical transnational dimensions of the ALRA's campaign for abortion law reform, defense of the Abortion Act, and response to the travel of nonresident women to Britain for abortion services highlight the futility of dealing with abortion strictly in a local context. Although the ALRA was reinvigorated by the international thalidomide crisis and inspired by the examples of more liberal abortion laws in Eastern European and Scandinavian countries at the time, juggling requests from overseas correspondents seeking abortion services in Britain conflicted with the organization's post-1967 determination to defend the act against its critics. The lurid stories about nonresident women traveling to Britain for abortion services skimmed the surface of more deeply anchored, racialized tales about avarice and outsiders in the private sector that conflicted sharply with cherished notions about the international standing of the British medical profession. They spoke profoundly to the desperation and agency of women seeking to terminate unwanted pregnancies. And, in the case of a changing Britain that created race-based categories of immigrants, while seeking at the same time to enter the EEC, they exposed the complexity and impracticality of policing access to abortion services on the grounds of nationality and residency. These grounds not only threatened to implicate nonresident *and* British women. They also begged yet one more tantalizing question: Just who could be considered British in a profoundly entwined world?

The lack of concerted attention paid to the travel of nonresident women for abortion services represents a lost opportunity to investigate several matters that are as pertinent today as they were then, including the multifaceted value of mobility for many women. The cross-border travel of nonresident women in the late 1960s and early 1970s can be seen as an early example of abortion tourism and part and parcel of a long-standing flow of medical tourists to Britain. It also heralded what was to come. Governments around the world continue to engage in a cost-benefit calculus, supposing that in the face of domestic opposition to abortion, the political cost of providing safe and legal abortion services for their own resident nationals is too great a cost to assume at all. Numerous federal governments have, therefore, exported the provision of safe and legal abortion services to other nations internationally or have downloaded them onto a number of domestic jurisdictions. Consequently, politicians can choose not to court controversy in dealing with abortion issues; hospitals can choose not to allot space for abortion services; medical schools can choose not to include abortion training in the curriculum; and physicians can choose not to provide abortion referrals, perform abortions, or face anti-abortion harassment violence. Meanwhile, women have little choice but to travel, pregnant, with the risky burdens of life and death.

Acknowledgments
Many thanks to Lesley Hall, Anthony Day, Emma Jones, Agata Ignaciuk, and Jesse Olszynko-Gryn. I am grateful to the Social Sciences and Humanities Research Council of Canada for funding this research.

Notes

1. Keith Hindell and Madeleine Simms, *Abortion Law Reformed* (London: Peter Owen, 1971). See also Barbara Brookes, *Abortion in England, 1900–1967* (London: Croom Helm, 1988); Stephen Brooke, *Sexual Politics: Sexuality, Family Planning, and the British Left from the 1880s to the Present Day* (Oxford: Oxford University Press, 2011); and Gayle Davis and Roger Davidson, "'The Fifth Freedom' or 'Hideous Atheistic Expediency'? The Medical Community and Abortion Law Reform in Scotland, c. 1960–1975," *Medical History* 50, no. 1 (2006): 29–48.

2. Hindell and Simms, *Abortion Law Reformed*, 216. For definitions of "pregnancy referral agencies" and "pregnancy advisory bureaux," see *Report of the Committee on the Working of the Abortion Act, Vol. I: Report* (London: Her Majesty's Stationary Office, 1974), 136.

3. See Angus McLaren, *Birth Control in Nineteenth-Century England* (London: Croom Helm, 1978); Brookes, *Abortion in England*; Kate Fisher, *Birth*

Control, Sex, and Marriage in Britain 1918–1960 (Oxford: Oxford University Press, 2006); Emma Jones, "Abortion in England, 1861–1967" (unpublished PhD diss., University of London, 2007); and Lesley Hall, *The Life and Times of Stella Browne: Feminist and Free Spirit* (London: I. B. Tauris, 2012).

4. Hera Cook, *The Long Sexual Revolution: English Women, Sex, and Contraception 1800–1975* (Oxford: Oxford University Press, 2004); Gayle Davis and Roger Davidson, "'Big White Chief', 'Pontius Pilate' and the 'Plumber': The Impact of the 1967 Abortion Act on the Scottish Medical Community, c.1967–80," *Social History of Medicine* 18, no. 2 (2005): 283–306; John Keown, *Abortion, Doctors and the Law: Some Aspects of the Legal Regulation of Abortion in England from 1803 to 1982* (New York: Cambridge University Press, 1988); Sally Sheldon, *Beyond Control: Medical Power and Abortion Law* (London: Pluto Press, 1997); and Martin Durham, *Sex and Politics: The Family and Morality in the Thatcher Years* (Basingstoke: Macmillan Education, 1991).

5. Dorothy McBride Stetson, "Women's Movements' Defence of Legal Abortion in Great Britain," in *Abortion Politics, Women's Movements, and the Democratic State: A Comparative Study of State Feminism*, ed. Dorothy McBride Stetson (Oxford: Oxford University Press, 2003 [2001]), 135–56; Lesley Hoggart, *Feminist Campaigns for Birth Control and Abortion Rights in Britain* (Lewiston, NY: Edward Mellen Press, 2003); and Jesse Olszynko-Gryn, "The Feminist Appropriation of Pregnancy Testing in 1970s Britain," *Women's History Review* (2017): 1–26, https://www.tandfonline.com/doi/full/10.1080 /09612025.2017.1346869.

6. Colin Francome, *Abortion Freedom: A Worldwide Movement* (London: Allen and Unwin, 1984); and Colin Francome, *Abortion Practice in Britain and the United States* (London: Allen and Unwin, 1986).

7. See Hindell and Simms, *Abortion Law Reformed*, and Malcolm Potts, Peter Diggory, and, John Peel, *Abortion* (Cambridge: Cambridge University Press, 1977).

8. *Report of the Committee on the Working of the Abortion Act, Vol. I: Report*, 138.

9. Brooke, *Sexual Politics*.

10. Ashley Wivel, "Abortion Policy and Politics on the Lane Committee of Enquiry, 1971–1974," *Social History of Medicine* 11, no. 1 (April 1998): 109–35; and Anthony Hordern, *Legal Abortion: The English Experience* (Oxford: Pergamon Press, 1971).

11. Malcolm Potts, interviewed in *Abortion Law Reformers: Pioneers of Change*, ed. Ann Furedi and Mick Hume (BPAS, 2007 [1997]), 40.

12. Hindell and Simms, *Abortion Law Reformed*, 49–50.

13. Rachel Conrad, review of *A Law for the Rich: A Plea for the Reform of the Abortion Law* by Alice Jenkins (London: Gollancz, 1960), *Eugenics Review* 52, no. 4 (January 1961): 242.

14. Hindell and Simms, *Abortion Law Reformed*, 108–12; Brookes, *Abortion in England*, 150–53. For more information about the impact of the rubella virus in the USA, see Leslie J. Reagan, *Dangerous Pregnancies: Mothers, Disabilities and Abortion in Modern America* (Berkeley: University of California Press, 2010). For her own story about joining the ALRA in relation to thalidomide, see

Madeleine Simms, interviewed in *Abortion Law Reformers*, 15. The impact of thalidomide in South Africa is explored by Susanne M. Klausen and Julie Parle in "'Are We Going to Stand By and Let These Children Come Into the World?' The Impact of the 'Thalidomide Disaster' in South Africa, 1960–1977," *Journal of Southern African Studies* 41, no. 4 (2015): 735–52.

15. Hindell and Simms, *Abortion Law Reformed*, 108–12. Kate Gleeson, "Persuading Parliament: Abortion Law Reform in the UK," *Australasian Parliamentary Review* 22, no. 2 (Spring 2007): 34, makes the same point. Ann Farmer, *By Their Fruits: Eugenics, Population Control and the Abortion Campaign* (Washington, DC: Catholic University of America Press, 2008), sees the campaign for abortion law reform as one driven by negative eugenics throughout its history, resulting ultimately in the weakening of family ties and the spread of more crime, disorder, and abortion.

16. *ALRA Annual Report 1967–1968*, 10, Library and Archives Canada (LAC), MG 28 I350 Vol. 4, File 5, Resource Material, Great Britain, 1966–1970.

17. ALRA pamphlet, "The Abortion Law: How It Affects You before and after 26 April 1968," n.d., LAC, MG 28 I350 Vol. 4, File 5, Resource Material, Great Britain, 1966–1970.

18. Jean Morton Williams and Keith Hindell, "Abortion and Contraception: A Study of Patients' Attitudes," *PEP* 38, no. 536 (March 1972): 1.

19. Hindell and Simms, *Abortion Law Reformed*, 225–28.

20. Williams and Hindell, "Abortion and Contraception," 1.

21. Drew Halfmann, "Historical Priorities and the Responses of Doctors' Associations to Abortion Reform Proposals in Britain and the United States, 1960–1973," *Social Problems* 50, no. 4 (2003): 570–71; and John Keown, *Abortion, Doctors and the Law: Some Aspects of the Legal Regulation of Abortion in England from 1803 to 1982* (Cambridge: Cambridge University Press, 1988), 111.

22. J. A. Stallworthy, "Complications of Therapeutic Abortion: Immediate and Remote," in *The Abortion Act 1967: Proceedings of a Symposium Held by the Medical Protection Society, in Collaboration with the Royal College of Obstetricians and Gynaecologists, London, 7 February 1969*, ed. Royal College of Obstetricians and Gynaecologists (Great Britain), Royal College of General Practitioners (Great Britain), and Medical Protection Society (England) (London: Pitman Medical Publishing Company, 1969), 48.

23. Amy Helen Bell, "Abortion Crime Scene Photography in Metropolitan London 1950–1968," *Social History of Medicine* 30, no. 3 (2017): 661–84.

24. Sally Sheldon, "The Decriminalisation of Abortion: An Argument for Modernisation," *Oxford Journal of Legal Studies* 36, no. 2 (June 2016): 334–65; and Emma Jones and Neil Pemberton, "Ten Rillington Place and the Changing Politics of Abortion in Modern Britain," *Historical Journal* 57, no. 4 (2014): 1100–1.

25. David Paintin, *Abortion Law Reform in Britain 1964–2003: A Personal Account* (Stratford-upon-Avon, Warwickshire: BPAS, 2015), 55.

26. Paul Ferris, *The Nameless: Abortion in Britain Today* (London: Hutchinson and Co., 1967 [1966]), dedication, 19–33.

27. Ferris, *The Nameless*, 9, 14–15, 101–2, 123–24, 154–56. See also Fisher, *Birth Control, Sex, and Marriage in Britain 1918–1960*. For information on the immigration of medical professionals to Britain, see Karola Decker, "Divisions and Diversity: The Complexities of Medical Refuge in Britain," *Bulletin of the History of Medicine* 77, no. 4 (Winter 2003): 850–73.

28. Paintin, *Abortion Law Reform in Britain*, 65.

29. Hindell and Simms, *Abortion Law Reformed*, 216–18.

30. For just three examples of media coverage, see Alvin Schuster, "Abortions in Britain Increase after Reforms," *Globe and Mail*, September 3, 1968, 12; Garry Lloyd, "Foreign Girls Come to London," *Times* (London), December 30, 1968; and Michael Steemson, "Abortion 'Touting' Quiz," *Daily Express*, July 7, 1969, 5.

31. Potts, Diggory, and Peel, *Abortion*, 299–303; and Paintin, *Abortion Law Reform in Britain*, 67–70.

32. "Abortion Backlash," *New Society*, July 10, 1969, 43.

33. "$221 Plus Travelling," *Globe and Mail*, July 2, 1969, 18.

34. Jane Carter, "It's All So Easy," *Daily Express*, July 3, 1969, 1.

35. Jane Carter and George Hunter, "Abortion Hotel," *Daily Express*, July 4, 1969, 1.

36. See Abortion (Amendment) House of Commons Debates, July 15, 1969, vol. 787, cc411–24; Lloyd, "Foreign Girls Come to London," 4; and "Time to Act on US Abortion Rush MP says," *Times* (London), May 31, 1969, 3.

37. Wivel, "Abortion Policy."

38. Nonresident women of other nationalities continued to flow into London from as far away as South Africa well into the 1980s. See Rebecca Hodes, "The Medical History of Abortion in South Africa, c. 1970–2000," *Journal of Southern African Studies* 39, no. 3 (2013): 534. See also Susanne M. Klausen, *Abortion Under Apartheid: Nationalism, Sexuality, and Women's Reproductive Rights in South Africa* (London: Oxford University Press, 2015), 52–53.

39. *Report of the Committee on the Working of the Abortion Act, Vol. II: Statistical Volume* (London: Her Majesty's Stationary Office, 1974), 202–8; *Report of the Committee on the Working of the Abortion Act, Vol. I: Report*, 137; Potts, Diggory, and Peel, *Abortion*, 299.

40. ALRA, "The First Two Years: A Review of the Working of the Abortion Act, 1967," October 1970, 9, LAC, MG 28 I350 Vol. 4, File 5, resource material, Great Britain, 1966–1970.

41. See also Ferris, *The Nameless*, 121–22.

42. Emma Jones, "Attitudes to Abortion in the Era of Reform: Evidence from the Abortion Law Reform Association Correspondence," *Women's History Review* 20, no. 2 (2011): 286, 291–92.

43. Diane Munday to H. E. Sir Frank Roberts, ambassador to the Federal Republic of Germany, June 2, 1969, Wellcome Library (WL), SA/ALR/U.30, supplementary papers, "Abortion: Other Countries c. 1965–1977 E-H."

44. Diane Munday to Anonymous #1, September 4, 1969, WL, SA/ALR/U.30, supplementary papers, "Abortion: Other Countries c. 1965–1977."

45. Diane Munday to Anonymous #2, May 17, 1971, WL, SA/ALR/U.30, supplementary papers, "Abortion: Other Countries c. 1965–1977."

46. Anonymous #3 to Diane Munday, May 27, 1971, WL, SA/ALR/H.32, supplementary papers, "Abortion: Other Countries c. 1965–1977."

47. Handwritten note, D. Munday to B. Fish [?], n.d., WL, SA/ALR/H.32, supplementary papers, "Abortion: Other Countries c. 1965–1977."

48. B. Fish to Anonymous #3, June 11, 1971, WL, SA/ALR/H.32, supplementary papers, "Abortion: Other Countries c. 1965–1977."

49. Diane Munday, interviewed in *Abortion Law Reformers*, 8–9.

50. Diane Munday to Joan Rettie, June 25, 1969, WL, SA/ALR/U.30, supplementary papers, "Abortion: Other Countries c. 1965–1977."

51. "Abortion—Some Facts," LAC MG 28 I350 Vol. 4, File 4, Resource Material, Great Britain, n.d.

52. John W. Young, *Britain and European Unity, 1945–1999*, 2nd ed. (New York: St. Martin's Press, 2000 [1993]).

53. "Note of Meeting No. 3 of Subcommittee 2," March 14, 1972, 1–4, WL, SA/ALR/C.12, ALRA Lane Committee, Subcommittee 2-Meetings: agendas, notes, papers nos. 1–6, Jan.–June 1972.

54. Ministry of Health, "Memorandum of Guidance to Hospital Authorities Hospital Treatment for Visitors from Overseas," 1963, WL, SA/ALR/C.12, ALRA Lane Committee, Subcommittee 2-Meetings: agendas, notes, papers nos. 1–6, Jan.–June 1972.

55. Ian R. G. Spencer, *British Immigration Policy since 1939: The Making of Multi-racial Britain* (London: Routledge, 1997).

56. "Some Questions on Residential Qualifications for the Subcommittee and Witnesses," March 14, 1972, WL, SA/ALR/C.12, ALRA Lane Committee, Subcommittee 2-Meetings: agendas, notes, papers nos. 1–6, Jan.–June 1972.

57. "Note of Meeting No. 3 of Subcommittee 2," 2.

58. "Note of Meeting No. 3 of Subcommittee 2," 2–3.

59. "Note of Meeting No. 3 of Subcommittee 2," 3.

60. "Note of Meeting No. 3 of Subcommittee 2," 3.

61. "Evidence to the Committee of Inquiry into the Working of the 1967 Abortion Act," 1972, 7, 26, LAC MG28 I350 Vol. 6, File 7, Evidence to the Committee of Inquiry into the Working of the 1967 Abortion Act from Abortion Law Reform Association 1972, Abortion Law Reform Association.

62. "Evidence to the Committee of Inquiry into the Working of the 1967 Abortion Act," 9.

63. "Evidence to the Committee of Inquiry into the Working of the 1967 Abortion Act," 9.

64. "Committee on the Working of the Abortion Act, Note of a Meeting," May 24, 1972, 19, WL, SA/ALR/C.12, ALRA Lane Committee, Subcommittee 2-Meetings: agendas, notes, papers nos. 1–6, Jan.–June 1972.

65. J. Temkin, "The Lane Committee Report on the Abortion Act," *Modern Law Review* 37, no. 6 (November 1974): 657.

66. *Report of the Committee on the Working of the Abortion Act, Vol. I: Report*, 139.

67. *Report of the Committee on the Working of the Abortion Act, Vol. I: Report,* 139.

68. *Report of the Committee on the Working of the Abortion Act, Vol. I: Report,* 141.

69. *Report of the Committee on the Working of the Abortion Act, Vol. I: Report,* 138–40.

70. *Report of the Committee on the Working of the Abortion Act, Vol. I: Report,* 142, 143–46.

[3]

The Trans-Tasman Abortion Travel Service

Abortion Services for New Zealand Women in the 1970s

HAYLEY BROWN

D URING THE 1970s, New Zealand women had to travel to Australia for abortions. This travel was necessary because either abortion was illegal or appropriate services were not available. Given New Zealand's geographical location, Australia provided the only practical travel destination for the provision of abortion services when these were not available in New Zealand, and the similarities between the two countries and their cultures meant that the travel was less difficult than it might otherwise have been. While there is a growing international literature on abortion travel, very little has been written within the New Zealand–Australian context, with the obvious exception of Barbara Baird's contribution to this volume, which surveys women's access to abortion services across Australia since the 1970s.[1] However, in recent years, there has been a growing body of historical work on the Tasman world and the shared history of Australia and New Zealand, a relationship to which the history of abortion travel arguably adds an important new dimension.[2]

The travel that took place during the 1970s illuminates several aspects of the comparative histories of these countries that have been previously ignored by historians. These include the limitations of the New Zealand and Australian healthcare systems during the 1970s as well as the severe crisis in the New Zealand system caused by restrictive legislation enacted in 1977 that forced women to seek the approval of two doctors registered as certifying consultants before obtaining an abortion. While the two countries, with their shared histories as white British settler societies, were similar in demographic and legal terms, they had different healthcare systems. New Zealand operated a publicly funded national healthcare system, whereas in Australia only Queensland operated a free public healthcare system before the introduction of Medibank, a universal health insurance system, in mid-1975. As abortions were rarely performed in public hospitals in New Zealand before 1978, women had to pay the full cost of treatment, whereas in Australia, once Medibank was introduced, a patient only paid 15 percent of the doctor's fee, unless the doctor believed that the patient could not pay at all, in which case the government covered the entire cost. A variety of funding arrangements for abortion services, including out-of-pocket payments, can be seen in several chapters in this volume.

An examination of abortion travel also adds a feminist dimension to the Australian–New Zealand relationship, which tends to be characterized by the masculine concept of "mateship," as exemplified in the mythology surrounding the Anzac spirit, by highlighting the interactions between feminist groups in Australia and New Zealand.[3] Abortion rights were a central issue for feminists in 1970s New Zealand and Australia, and many groups that advocated for changes to the legislation pertaining to abortion had an explicitly feminist perspective.[4] In New Zealand, the main feminist group advocating for abortion access was the Women's National Abortion Action Campaign (WONAAC), and in New South Wales (NSW), Australia, it was the Women's Abortion Action Campaign (WAAC). Both organizations allowed only women members. Additionally, prominent in advocating for abortion law reform was the Abortion Law Reform Association of New Zealand (ALRANZ) and the Abortion Law Reform Association (ALRA) in NSW, which—despite having feminist members—supported abortion law reform from a civil liberties, rather than an explicitly feminist, perspective.[5] These latter two organizations were influenced by their British namesake, the Abortion Law Reform Association, which was founded in the 1930s, and which Christabelle Sethna discusses in this volume. But in contrast to the British version of this organization, which was reluctant to assist nonresident women coming to Britain, several abortion law reform organizations in New Zealand and Australia did become involved in assisting New Zealand women's travels to Australia.

Feminist organizations in both countries had effective communication links and discussed many issues pertinent to the women's liberation movement, and groups in New Zealand could draw on these networks to help women travel to Australia with the support of feminist groups in Australia, particularly those in Sydney, who were able to offer advice and support to New Zealand women. New Zealand women had a variety of experiences seeking and obtaining abortions in Sydney, and the diversity of experience was due in large part to the range of abortion services provided in that city. The circumstances of this travel may be particular to the New Zealand–Australian context. However, it also demonstrates that this aspect of New Zealand–Australian history forms part of a wider international history of abortion travel that likewise includes transnational abortion referral networks such as those described by Agata Ignaciuk in her contribution on Spain to this volume.

The abortion travel that took place between New Zealand and Australia in the 1970s demonstrates the failure of New Zealand lawmakers to enact a clear and workable law, the determination of women to access abortions, and the willingness of feminist groups on both sides of the Tasman to work together to help women. Traveling to access abortion services, however, was far from a perfect situation, as it excluded those who could not afford the costs involved and often meant that women received less than ideal medical care. While the 1977 act gradually became more workable, the need for women to travel to access abortions has not been removed, and there remains a considerable number of New Zealand women traveling domestically to access abortion services. This chapter examines how Australia, and particularly Sydney, became a destination for New Zealand women seeking abortions, the difficulties they faced in traveling internationally for an abortion, and why the number of women making this journey fluctuated during the 1970s. In many cases, these women were assisted by feminist groups in either New Zealand, Sydney, or both to access abortions.

New Zealand Women's Access to Abortion in Early 1970s Australia

Barbara Baird, in this volume, remarks on the difficulties that Australian women experienced, and continue to experience, in accessing abortion services within Australia. Still, New Zealand women have been traveling to Australia to have abortions ever since South Australia legalized abortion in 1969. This was the case despite the fact that there was a residency clause, which required that a woman be a resident in South Australia for at least two months prior to having an abortion.[6] Before this development, a very small number of women had traveled to Japan for abortions, where abortion had been legal since 1948, but most had accessed abortions in New Zealand either through individual doctors or "backstreet abortionists" who worked in clandestine and illegal conditions.[7] In an article in the *New Zealand Herald* in November 1971, it was claimed that of the 2,354 women who obtained legal abortions in South Australia since the law change, New Zealand women would have been among the 5 percent in the "unclassified" category, as well as among the 14 percent of British-born women.[8]

Soon afterward, the law was clarified in Victoria in *R v. Davidson* in 1969, and New Zealand women began to travel to Melbourne.[9] Other than in South Australia, the law in the Australian states and in New Zealand was presumed to be based on the English Bourne ruling of 1938, in which it was decided that if the likely result of continuing with a pregnancy would make the woman a physical or mental wreck, then the doctor may be considered as performing the termination to preserve the life of the mother, which was the only ground for abortion under English law at the time.[10] This was tested in Victoria in *R v. Davidson*, and in a decision that became known as the Menhennitt ruling, the principles outlined in the earlier Bourne case were upheld.[11] Once it became possible to go to Melbourne, this option was preferred because of New Zealand's proximity to that Australian city. Geographical proximity to abortion services in a neighboring jurisdiction has been a boon to many women, including Irish women who have traveled to Britain to terminate their pregnancies, as Mary Gilmartin and Sinéad Kennedy observe in this volume. A similar decision to the Menhennitt ruling, known as the Levine ruling, was made in NSW in 1971.[12] Following the 1971 Levine ruling, women began to go to Sydney, although some continued to travel to Melbourne.[13] With the founding of the Auckland Medical Aid Centre (AMAC) in May 1974 by the Auckland Medical Aid Trust, the trans-Tasman abortion travel slowed down, but then increased rapidly after the passing of the 1977 New Zealand Contraception, Sterilisation, and Abortion Act.

Once abortions became available in Sydney, New Zealand women were more likely to go there for abortion services rather than Melbourne. One reason for this preference was suggested by Julia Freebury of ALRA, who noted that abortions in Sydney cost A$80, whereas the operation was more expensive in Melbourne.[14] The trans-Tasman abortion traffic was also becoming much more public in New Zealand, increasing women's awareness of the possibility of traveling to Australia to access abortion services, and in 1974 *New Zealand Truth*, a tabloid newspaper, published a list of the names, addresses, and phone numbers for eight doctors who could perform abortions in Australia. Four of the doctors were based in Sydney and four in Melbourne.[15] The use of print media to publicize abortion services is duly noted elsewhere in this volume, as in Agata Ignaciuk's chapter on Spain.

It is difficult to be certain about the number of women who traveled to Australia for an abortion prior to the law change in December 1977, as estimates vary. In 1974, it was estimated by Julia Freebury that 4,000 New Zealand women flew to Australia for abortions each year, mostly to Sydney and Melbourne.[16] In 1975, a study of the numbers of women going to Melbourne and Sydney for abortions was completed for submission to the New Zealand Royal Commission on Contraception, Sterilisation and Abortion. The author of the study contacted all the clinics, hospitals, and individual doctors in Sydney that were known to her organization, ALRANZ Christchurch. They were asked to give the number of New Zealand women seen in the period July 1974 to June 1975.[17] Some organizations claimed that they kept no records and thus were unable to provide the necessary information. The details provided by the remaining clinics are shown in table 3.1. It was estimated that approximately 770 New Zealand women had an abortion in Sydney during this twelve-month period, while a further 195 abortions were carried out in Melbourne, giving a total of 965.[18]

While AMAC greatly reduced the need for New Zealand women to travel to Australia, it did not stop the trans-Tasman traffic completely. The decision of the Auckland Medical Aid Trust to found AMAC rested on the assumption that the 1938 Bourne ruling in England was applicable to New Zealand and that the clinic would operate on this basis. The courts in New Zealand, with its English-inherited common law system, placed great weight on the doctrine of precedent, particularly decisions from English courts, which is why it was assumed that the Bourne ruling would be used to interpret New Zealand's abortion legislation. The effect AMAC had on women's choices about where to go for an abortion, particularly for those living in the Auckland area, is clear from the data in table 3.2. Not only did the numbers of women contacting the Family Planning Association about abortions increase significantly in the two years from June 1973, but once AMAC was operational, more than half were referred to the clinic, and the proportion of women going to Australia for abortions dropped dramatically.

Table 3.1. Abortions performed in Sydney on New Zealand women, July 1974–June 1975

Abortion Provider	Number of Abortions
Population Services International, Potts Point	147
Populations Services International, Arncliffe	52 (from Sept. 3, 1974)
The Women's Hospital, Crown Street	1
Dr. Leslie Smoling	130–140
Dr. N. Marinko	234
Dr. George Smart	83
Preterm Clinic	30

Table 3.2. Referrals from a city clinic of the Auckland Medical Branch of the Family Planning Association in New Zealand

Months	Patients requesting an abortion	Referred to Australia	Referred privately	Referred to National Women's Hospital	Referred to Auckland Medical Aid Centre	Not referred
June-July-Aug 1973	18	8 (45%)	4 (22%)	4 (22%)	—	2 (11%)
Feb-Mar-Apr 1974	69	39 (57%)	21 (30%)	2 (3%)	—	7 (10%)
June-July-Aug 1974	76	10 (13%)	19 (25%)	1 (1%)	39 (52%)	7 (9%)
Feb-Mar-Apr 1975	95	8 (8%)	9 (5%)	4 (5%)	61 (63%)	13 (14%)

There were several problems with New Zealand women traveling to Australia to have abortions rather than being able to access safe, legal abortions in their home country. These problems were often publicized by feminists or medical professionals who supported abortion law reform. The submission made by the Auckland Medical Aid Trust to the Royal Commission on Contraception, Sterilisation and Abortion, which sat between 1975 and 1977, highlighted the problems New Zealand women often experienced when they traveled to Australia for an abortion. Variations of the following problems appear in many chapters in this volume.

The single biggest problem for such women was the financial cost. Rex Hunton, the director of AMAC, announced at the ALRANZ annual meeting on April 8, 1975, that New Zealand women spent about NZ$2,000,000 per year on abortions in Australia.[19] Most of this was spent on airline tickets, although a considerable portion was also spent on Australian medical fees. From July 1, 1975, however, New Zealand women were able to have free or heavily subsidized abortions in Australia under the Medibank scheme. This change was beneficial to New Zealand women, particularly those who lived in the South Island and had to fly to Auckland to have an abortion. Once this change occurred, there was little difference in trans-Tasman prices because the medical fees in New Zealand were not covered by the government-funded healthcare system.[20]

Some doctors, particularly in Sydney, were prepared to offer discounts to New Zealand women because they were aware of the expense the women had already incurred. Other clinics, however, felt that this was unprofessional and that medical fees should not be offered at a discounted rate. In 1975, a Sydney doctor, George Smart, announced that he charged New Zealand women only A$60 for abortions because they had to pay for their airfares and also were not covered by medical insurance, unlike most Australians.[21] He publicized that he was going to ask the Australian government to organize cheap airfares for New Zealand women going to Australia for abortions, as normally women could not get discounted airfares because they did not purchase their tickets far enough in advance.[22] However, this commitment does not seem to have been followed up.[23]

The second concern, as outlined in the Auckland Medical Aid Trust's submission about women traveling to Australia, was that the service was not available to all; in particular, Pacific Island women were excluded.[24] Until 1981, New Zealand citizens did not need a passport to enter Australia, although those Pacific Islanders who were not New Zealand citizens needed a passport and a visa. This requirement, combined with the fact that Pacific Island women were also less likely to have the money to pay for a trip to Australia due to socioeconomic factors, and the fact that most Pacific Island communities at this time were strongly Christian, made very slim the likelihood of a Pacific Island woman wanting an abortion and being able to have one in Australia.

While, according to the submission, very few women had difficulty obtaining abortions in Australia, some were too advanced in their pregnancies, which meant normally they were over 18 weeks.[25] Many women going to Sydney or Melbourne were in their second trimester because of the delay in organizing such a trip. This limited the number of doctors who could perform an abortion, it made the operation more complicated, and it meant women needed more time to recover before they could fly safely again. In 1972, ALRA in Melbourne wrote to ALRANZ about its unease with New Zealand women going to Melbourne for an abortion when they were in their second trimester. At that time, there was only one doctor in the city who would perform second-trimester abortions.[26] It was also claimed that the standard of care provided in Australian clinics varied considerably, and while attempts were made to contact women when they returned, it was difficult to be sure of the standard of care provided by Australian doctors.

The third concern with women traveling to Australia was about the feelings of the women involved.[27] The submission allowed: "There is no doubt that women who bear the weight of the unwanted pregnancy often feel suppressed anger, guilt and fear as they travel to another country to terminate their pregnancies."[28] Many women had to make the trip alone because of financial constraints, contributing to their feelings of isolation, particularly in a country with which they were unfamiliar. There were two major medical issues that the submission highlighted to the New Zealand commission. The first was the lack of follow-up provided for New Zealand women, especially those who went to Australia without a referral.[29] The other issue was the medical dangers involved in having an operation followed by a flight of several hours. This was particularly a problem for women who had a termination in the second trimester, as later terminations were potentially more complicated and more likely to be performed under general anesthetic.[30]

There were further problems with women going to Australia, in addition to those highlighted in the submission. Sometimes the clinics in Melbourne and Sydney were overloaded with Australian patients, and were thus unable to help those from New Zealand. This was particularly a problem in the early 1970s, when abortion clinics were only beginning to open. Similar concerns emerged in Britain in respect to resident and nonresident women accessing abortion services in both the public and private sectors, as Gayle Davis et al. scrutinize in this volume. On September 13, 1972, the ALRA in Melbourne wrote to ALRANZ and asked that they stop referring patients to them, as they were "inundated" with their own problems.[31] Others, including Dr. Margaret Sparrow, felt that the fact that women had to travel to have an abortion indicated a public health problem, and that those women should be receiving treatment in New Zealand.[32] No one would have tolerated New Zealanders traveling to Australia for other basic medical procedures, she argued.

The Contraception, Sterilisation, and Abortion Act (1977)

The Contraception, Sterilisation, and Abortion Act severely restricted access to abortion by making the procedure for obtaining an abortion far more complicated than it had been previously. First, a woman had to acquire a referral from her general practitioner. Then, two certifying consultants had to approve her termination. If this were achieved, a certificate would be issued. Doctors had to apply to become certifying consultants, and doctors with extreme views, either conservative or radical, were not permitted to be consultants. One of the consultants had to be an obstetrician or a gynecologist. The woman then had to find someone who was willing to perform the operation in either a public or a private hospital. Abortions performed in public hospitals were free, whereas abortions performed in private hospitals had to be paid for out of pocket. The Abortion Supervisory Committee (ASC) was established under the act to review continuously all the provisions of the abortion law, as well as the operation and effect of the provisions in practice. There were several grounds under which abortions were permitted: to save the life of the woman, to preserve the physical health of the woman, to preserve the mental health of the woman, and in cases of fetal impairment or incest. Not surprisingly, most abortions were granted on the grounds of preserving the mental health of the woman, though the interpretation of this term varied considerably, and at first it was interpreted conservatively.

After the act's passing, feminists throughout New Zealand almost immediately set up an organization called the Sisters Overseas Service (SOS). Its purpose was to help women who needed an abortion. It informed women of the law in New Zealand and then gave them the option of either trying to get an abortion in New Zealand or traveling to Sydney. Feminist organizations like these continue to assist women transnationally, as is evident, for example, in Ewelina Ciaputa's chapter on Poland and Agata Ignaciuk's chapter on Spain in this volume. "The Knitting Needle Bill" (figure 3.1), a satirical song commissioned in 1976 by Dr. Erich Geiringer, a prominent supporter of abortion law reform in New Zealand and opponent of the Society for the Protection of the Unborn Child (SPUC), critiques the need for women to travel to Australia to access abortion services, particularly as the cost of the travel excluded poorer women.[33] A number of anti-abortion politicians are named in the song, including then prime minister Robert Muldoon, and

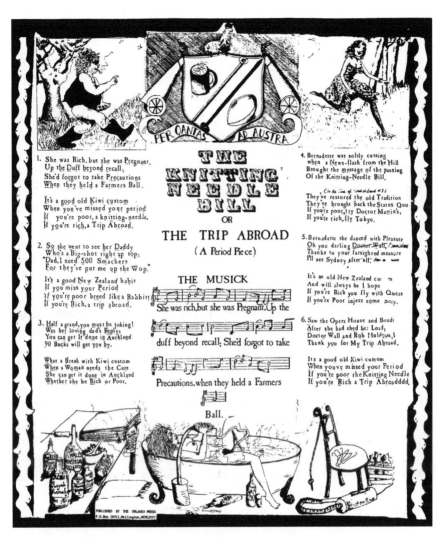

Figure 3.1. "The Knitting Needle Bill or The Trip Abroad (A Period Piece),"
song written by Dr. Erich Geiringer. Alexander Turnbull Library, EPH-C-ROTH-
ABORTION-1976-01. Wellington: Orlando Press, 1976.

an amendment by hand has been made to include Commodore Frank
Gill, a cabinet minister. Geiringer sent a copy of this song sheet along
with a cover letter in October 1977 to every MP who had critiqued the
proposed legislation, which was ultimately passed into law in December of that year. He reproduced his correspondence with National
Party MP Jim McLay in the *New Zealand Observer*.[34] He also sang this

song publicly many times, including on a talk radio program on Radio Windy.[35]

Doctors referred many patients who had become ineligible for an abortion in New Zealand to SOS.[36] The organization was active in New Zealand in the late 1970s and early 1980s, until its services were no longer needed. The anti-abortion movement opposed the actions of SOS, with the Otago University right-to-life group asking the minister of justice to outlaw SOS, as it believed that its activities were illegal.[37] Nothing, however, eventuated from this complaint. It is impossible to know exactly how many women went to Sydney and Melbourne for abortions after the passing of the Contraception, Sterilisation, and Abortion Act. Estimates vary widely depending on what organizations were consulted. In August 1978, eight months after the act had been passed, SOS in Auckland claimed that it had sent 1,078 women to Australia for an abortion, at a cost of at least NZ$500,000. Clinic fees totaled NZ$100,000, New Zealand travel tax NZ$32,000, airport tax NZ$2,000, and airline tickets NZ$352,000.[38] Many more women flew to Australia without contacting SOS, though it is difficult to know how many. The lack of accurate data on abortion travel is likewise pertinent to Christabelle Sethna's and Niklas Barke's respective contributions to this volume. In *Abortion Is a Woman's Right to Choose*, a Sydney periodical publication, it was estimated that in 1978, 125 New Zealand women traveled to Sydney each week for an abortion, with an annual figure of 6,500 women, a particularly high number considering that some women would also have gone to Melbourne.[39] The Auckland Medical Aid Trust estimated that between January 3 and January 27, 1978, 247 New Zealand women went to the four main abortion clinics in Sydney, with another 55 women going to Melbourne.[40]

Over the course of a year, assuming such numbers were maintained, 5,200 traveled to Australia for an abortion. In February 1979, it was reported in the *Journal of the Nurses Society* that for every woman having an abortion in New Zealand, two were traveling to Australia.[41] It was suggested that 3,337 women traveled to Australia for abortions in 1978. In a report on abortion prepared for the ASC, author Janet Sceats stated that at the beginning of 1978 the number of abortions being performed in New Zealand reduced dramatically, while at the same time the number of women traveling to Australia increased.[42] After the Trust-run clinic was reopened in Auckland in September 1979, the number of women traveling from Auckland and Wellington to Australia fell.

However, very few Christchurch women attended the Auckland clinic because of the two-week waiting list and instead paid the extra NZ$200 to go to Australia.

Another problem for women going to Australia was the decision of the Australian government that all New Zealanders entering Australia after July 1, 1981, had to have a passport. The requirement that non-residents provide entry documents is yet another potential obstacle to international abortion travel, a point that Niklas Barke factors into his chapter in this volume. By this time, only women seeking a second-trimester abortion were having to travel to Australia, but because it took about four weeks to obtain a passport, it would have delayed some women's travel, or prevented them from going altogether because their pregnancy would have been too far advanced by the time they acquired this vital travel document.[43]

Not everyone was convinced that it was necessary to travel to Australia to access abortion services. Some groups believed that women were being encouraged to go to Australia to have an abortion, rather than attempt to have one in New Zealand, so that the new law would appear unworkable. Bill Birch, National Party MP, one of the prominent supporters of the Contraception, Sterilisation, and Abortion Act, stated: "Women are suffering the cost and anguish of going to Australia for abortions because of Auckland doctors' emotional reaction to the new law. I am quite concerned about the climate in Auckland. Women are possibly being persuaded to go to Australia when it is not in their best interests to do so."[44] The ASC made similar allegations. It suggested that women were being encouraged to go to Australia so that the situation appeared worse than it was. In response, the Wellington branch of SOS claimed that between April 1978 and March 1979, they referred 110 cases to local practitioners as well as dealing with many women on the phone who also visited local doctors. More than half of the women it assisted in going to Australia were said to be over ten weeks pregnant when they first contacted the organization. A decision had been made in the Wellington region not to consider cases in which the woman had reached 12 weeks, despite the fact that the legislation did not include such a limit, and because the procedure to obtain an abortion involved visiting several doctors, none of those women would have been able to have an abortion in New Zealand.[45]

Just as the cost of going to Australia for an abortion had been a problem prior to the passing of the Contraception, Sterilisation, and Abortion

Act, it remained a major dilemma for women traveling in 1978 and 1979. In late 1977, the return fares were as follows: Christchurch to Melbourne NZ$354, Christchurch to Sydney NZ$320, Auckland to Melbourne NZ$372, and Auckland to Sydney NZ$320.[46] In addition, women had to pay for the operation, accommodation, and transport costs. It was estimated that a woman would need at least NZ$500 to cover her expenses. While many women were able to obtain this money from friends or family or use savings, some could not. Chapters by Barbara Baird and Lori A. Brown in this volume suggest that marginalized, racialized women are especially vulnerable to the geographical and economic obstacles to abortion travel. Similarly, Donna Awatere and Rebecca Evans, two Maori women activists, highlight the particular difficulties many Maori women had while reinforcing racialized stereotypes of Maori men as violent toward women:

> Abortions are inaccessible to any woman in NZ now, inaccessible of course to those who haven't [NZ]$500. Despite the existence of SOS and any similar service, it is still no answer to a Maori or Polynesian woman living in a rented house in Ponsonby [suburb of Auckland], with six kids and a sexist husband who amonst [sic] other things works in a factory and helps the state control what his wife does with her womb—if she doesn't listen to what he says when he is asserting his ego and mana [power and prestige] by telling her to have more babies—she gets a hiding.[47]

Most women had to borrow the money from family members, their partner, or his family, while some obtained bank loans or used their savings. Most of this money went toward paying for the airfares. There were two main reasons for the unhappiness of SOS over the use of Air New Zealand. The first was that a prominent anti-abortionist and president of SPUC, Des Dalgety, was on the board of the airline, a presence many women found insulting. The second reason was it was felt that the government should not profit from its own bad legislation—the government being the major shareholder in the airline at the time.[48] However, because Qantas and Air New Zealand had an arrangement that they shared trans-Tasman air travel, only women in Auckland were able to use another airline, Pan American World Airways, which flew through Auckland.[49] Evidently, transportation systems, many of which cater to tourist traffic, are another major factor shaping the choices women can and cannot make in terms of abortion travel. They materialize in various contributions to this volume, including the work of Agata Ignaciuk and that of Cathrine Chambers, Colleen MacQuarrie, and Jo-Ann MacDonald.

In August 1979, the Aotea Clinic, formerly AMAC, was granted a license to perform abortions by the ASC.[50] It was estimated by a clinic trustee, Rex Hunton, that about 5,000 women per year were flying to Australia for abortions, and that the clinic would be able to cover those women, although the clinic would not perform as many abortions as it had done before its closure in December 1977.[51] In January 1980, the Aotea Clinic was forced to stop making appointments for a month because of such high demand. In Auckland, SOS anticipated that this would increase the number of women needing to travel for their abortions in the short term.[52] Another day clinic had opened in Auckland in 1978, known as the Epsom Day Hospital. As it was a public institution, there were no fees to use its services. It performed a large number of abortions, although not enough to prevent women from flying to Australia. Feminists believed that this was because the terms of the act were such that many women were not legally entitled to an abortion in New Zealand.[53]

Some women who were entitled to an abortion in New Zealand under the 1977 legislation still had to travel to Sydney and Melbourne due to the way that the act was interpreted by some doctors and the delays that were often involved in the process. The primary reason for this was that there were not enough certifying consultants in New Zealand to approve abortions in the first place. Even by 1985, women still had to travel overseas because of this shortage. However, by this time the ASC had agreed to cover the cost of travel, as other patients who had to go overseas for medical treatment were also entitled to be reimbursed, although other patients who traveled overseas were doing so to access specialist treatment not available in New Zealand, rather than for services that were underprovided.[54] Moreover, some general practitioners refused to refer women to a certifying consultant. When asked by SOS whether women had a legal right to be referred to a certifying consultant, the ASC responded that it was only an administrative body and could not interpret the legislation.[55]

In July 1979, Marilyn Waring, National Party MP, told the ASC that three-quarters of women from Hawke's Bay and Auckland who wanted an abortion had gone to Australia for the procedure in the previous 12 months because they could not obtain the procedure in their region. In comparison, 56 percent of women from Christchurch who sought an abortion had been compelled to go to Australia. This suggests that the law was not being interpreted consistently throughout the country.[56] On average, 61 percent of New Zealand women who had abortions went to Australia, according to Waring. She estimated that for the year ending March 31, 1979, 3,857 women had traveled to Australia for an abortion.[57] Waring had obtained these statistics from SOS, and she assumed that the proportion of women going to Australia rather than having abortions in New Zealand was the same for women who had contacted the SOS as it was for those who had not.

In Christchurch, as well as other parts of the country, SOS organizers were prepared to accommodate women living far outside major cities before they could fly to Australia for an abortion. One supporter explained, "During 1978 I billeted about twenty women for SOS on their way to Sydney and safely home again to Wyndham [a rural town], or deepest darkest Southland [New Zealand's southernmost region]."[58] In October 1980, SOS changed its name to Health Alternatives for Women and expanded its role to include contraceptive advice and assistance with nutrition, self-defense, and drug abuse.[59]

As well as managing the bookings for women going to Australia and providing funding where necessary, SOS also attempted to make the experience as tolerable as possible. Elizabeth Sewell, who ran the Christchurch branch of SOS, asked women if they wanted to travel with others who were also going to Australia for a termination. Companionship during the voyage was particularly important because the high cost meant that most women could not take a family member or friend with them. Sewell explained, "We try to arrange compatible groups, mixing older, married women who are more composed about it all with any nervous teenagers. Comforting them takes the older women's minds off their problems, and it helps the young ones a lot."[60]

There were also disputes between SOS and hospitals as to whether school-age girls were automatically entitled to have an abortion. The superintendent of Christchurch Women's Hospital stated that only under the "most unusual circumstances" would a school-age female be refused an abortion. However, SOS had helped five school girls go to Australia for abortions, all of whom had been assessed by doctors in Christchurch. It was believed that those who could afford to go to Australia did so because the environment there was more supportive, their privacy would be preserved, and they would be guaranteed an abortion.[61]

In 1981, one woman from the Nelson branch of SOS told the Women's Electoral Lobby conference that New Zealand women could claim a "staggering political victory" in the abortion issue because they had managed to obtain terminations despite the passage of the Contraception, Sterilisation, and Abortion Act.[62] In 1984, WONAAC contacted some abortion clinics in Sydney to see if New Zealand women were still making the trans-Tasman journey for an abortion. The Bessie Smyth Feminist Abortion Clinic reported that nobody could remember any New Zealand patients after 1979.[63] Geoffrey Davis from Population Services International (PSI) stated that the monthly average from early 1980 to mid-1982 was 24, and from that date until the time of his letter (September 1984) the monthly average was about eight. He stated that most referrals to the clinic for New Zealand women were late second-trimester operations because the service was not provided adequately in New Zealand.[64]

Support from Sydney Feminist Groups and Sydney Abortion Services

Australian women's liberation groups declared themselves happy to offer their support for New Zealand women after the passing of the Contraception, Sterilisation, and Abortion Act, despite the additional pressure that New Zealand women traveling to Australia would place on abortion services there. It was feared that if a repressive law could be passed in New Zealand, then it was possible that such a law could also be passed in any of the Australian states.[65] Although most of the support came from groups in Sydney, others across Australia also offered encouragement. For example, the Adelaide branch of WAAC suggested that an Australian and New Zealand Abortion Action Campaign with the acronym ANZAAC, a play on ANZAC, be launched on International Woman's Day.[66] However, groups in New Zealand felt that the public was already too confused with so many groups being involved in the abortion campaign: ALRANZ, WONAAC, Repeal, SOS, Coaction, and Cohab, among others.[67] The New Zealand groups were happy for Australian groups to use the name ANZAAC, and they did. Groups in Australia believed that an anti-abortion backlash had been launched in Australia following the passing of the laws in New Zealand, and this backlash had to be countered.[68]

Sydney women's groups were also involved in protesting against New Zealand's abortion laws. On February 6, 1978, more than 100 Sydney women protested outside both the New Zealand Government offices and the New Zealand Tourist Bureau, both located in Sydney, strengthening the connections between abortion travel, abortion legislation, and the tourism industry. Both were closed because of Waitangi Day (New Zealand's national holiday).[69] The following week, National Party prime minister and known anti-abortionist Robert Muldoon was in Sydney for the Commonwealth Heads of Government regional meeting. About 50 demonstrators waited for him outside the Hilton Hotel. One of the protestors held a sign asking Muldoon whether he, too, was in Sydney for an abortion.[70] Not all the protests were limited to Sydney. Just as the New Zealand Tourist Bureau had been a target for protestors in Sydney, so it again became a target in Brisbane. In September 1978, the offices were targeted by protestors, and this resulted in one woman being arrested.[71] These combined acts demonstrated that Australian women shared the anger of many New Zealand women over the Contraception, Sterilisation, and Abortion Act, and that some of those women were prepared to act on their feelings and show their support for New Zealand women.

Not all New Zealand women were able to access adequate abortion services in Australia. One woman who went to Sydney for an abortion in the 1970s explained:

> My friends and I used to borrow each other's [oral contraceptive] pills. I got pregnant when I was 23. You could not get an abortion in New Zealand so I went off to Sydney. I arrived with a list of doctors and I can remember standing in a phone booth ringing them up. The abortion itself was the most frightening experience I have ever had. The doctor said, "If you don't stop shrieking I'll throw you into the street." I remember later standing in a post office sending postcards to my friends in New Zealand with blood dripping on to the floor.[72]

Communication between SOS and the women it referred to Australia continued even after they returned to New Zealand. If the women reported receiving inadequate treatment from a doctor, SOS would no longer refer other women to that abortion provider. Control, a Sydney feminist referral organization, also worked closely with SOS. Control did not run its own abortion clinic; rather, it monitored clinics in Sydney and provided a counseling service for women using clinics that did not have their own service. The counselor would also accompany the women on their visits to the doctor.[73] Its members helped make bookings for New Zealand women in Sydney clinics, arranged accommodation for them while they were in Sydney, and provided them with transport to and from the airport.[74] Accommodation was normally at a cheap hotel, although Control had a list of people willing to house women who did not want to stay in a hotel, or could not afford to do so.[75]

Control was an organization designed primarily to help women in NSW, although it was also willing to help women from New Zealand and Queensland. However, this willingness could have resulted in problems for the organization because there was often a shortage of spaces available at abortion clinics, particularly those that Control preferred to use. Control never complained about the impact that out-of-state women had on the services that were provided to NSW women. They made it clear that more clinics were needed but were always supportive of all women requiring their assistance.[76]

Control saw itself as a safeguard against doctors who had set up small clinics to perform abortions because it was profitable, but whose service was often inadequate, thereby hoping to halt the exploitation of pregnant women for financial gain, as is described further within the British context by Gayle Davis et al. and by Christabelle Sethna in this volume. Control also challenged the types of medication that were prescribed to women. For example, in 1978 some New Zealand women traveled to Australia with Depo-Provera, a contraceptive to be injected after their operation.[77] At the time, Depo-Provera was commonly available in New Zealand and recommended to young women. However, Depo-Provera had been very controversial, particularly so in NSW among feminist organizations, and Control refused to allow the women to be injected with it. The Family Planning Association in New Zealand refused to refer women through Control and also put pressure on SOS to do the same. Despite this, SOS continued its contact with Control, and in many ways the controversy brought them closer together.[78]

As president of ALRA, Julia Freebury indicated to New Zealand women that she was prepared to help:

WE CAN HELP NZ women to have an abortion in Sydney. You can ring 32 2244 (anytime) and I will be able to immediately book you into a <u>first-class</u> clinic for a termination of pregnancy. You can stay at the clinic overnight and there is no charge.

We can offer reduced fees for NZ women:
- one stage operation (up to 12–14 weeks)   A$80
- later one stage operation (up to 16 weeks)   A$100
- two stage operation 1–2 nights (20 weeks)   A$180

One stage operation requires a stay of approximately 3 hours in the clinic.[79]

Some women were able to return to New Zealand on the same day as their operation, while others stayed the night in cheap accommodation organized for them by Control.

There was some debate over the quality of medical care provided at a number of Sydney's abortion clinics. *Broadsheet*, a New Zealand feminist publication, reported that several SOS branches were referring women to the Arncliffe Clinic, which was run by PSI, and that the clinic only operated under general anesthetic, whereas many other clinics gave women the choice of a local anesthetic when the operation was being performed in the first trimester.[80] Sydney feminists later launched a campaign against the PSI clinics.[81] In December 1976, six women health workers, including counselors, a doctor, and a telephone receptionist, resigned from PSI.[82] Feminist groups accused PSI of failing to take into account women's needs when supplying them with oral contraceptives. The company received sample packs from a variety of drug companies, which they then sold to the women instead of supplying them for free. Women were given no choice as to which contraceptive pill they were prescribed.[83] The clinic also prescribed antibiotics to patients at a cost greater than a pharmacy, because there were concerns that complications might arise from the treatment.[84] Sydney feminists believed that PSI offered New Zealand women discounted rates to get their business. The clinic justified their actions by stating that New Zealand women organized their own blood tests and drugs, whereas Australian women received these from the clinic.[85] Children by Choice, the Brisbane referral agency, also sent women to PSI.[86] However, because all the women from Queensland arrived together, the clinic was often overbooked. Women were block-booked, rather than having individual appointments, and this meant that many had to wait hours before seeing a doctor.[87]

The other two main clinics in Sydney were Preterm and the Bessie Smyth Feminist Abortion Clinic.[88] Preterm did not have many New Zealand patients and only performed abortions up to ten weeks, with a local anesthetic. This may explain why so few New Zealand women used the clinic, especially if they were unsure how advanced their pregnancy was.[89] Bessie Smyth was the only clinic that Sydney feminists would endorse. However, it was run on a small scale and only saw 12 women per day. Because of the traffic caused by the Christchurch flight, each Tuesday in the late 1970s was known as "New Zealand Day."[90] Preterm had originally received considerable support from the feminist movement, but during the 1970s the organization of the clinic changed and it became more conservative. *Mabel*, a Sydney feminist newspaper, believed that Preterm had developed "into a cash-flow business venture with little regard for the needs of individual women."[91] This change was particularly noticeable in 1977 when the three research and education assistants at the clinic were fired. The three women had been working for Preterm since the clinic had opened in 1974. *Mabel* wrote, "The sackings [firings] seem to represent an attempt to remove almost the last survivors of the early feminist orientation from the organisation."[92] As abortion services were unregulated in NSW, the quality of these services varied considerably, and New Zealand women were often more vulnerable than their Australian counterparts, given the distance they had to travel and the fact that they were more likely to require late-term abortions.

Conclusion

The trans-Tasman abortion traffic that existed during the 1970s was evidence both that adequate abortion services were not being provided in New Zealand and that inadequate services did not stop women from having abortions; instead, women had to go elsewhere to access the services. Prior to the 1970s, this had been with recourse to backstreet abortionists, but after the change in laws in some of the Australian states, particularly NSW and Victoria, women who could afford to travel went to Australia. The dramatic increase in abortion travel in 1978 after the change to New Zealand law was able to be absorbed by the Australian clinics, although the quality of care was not always of the highest standard. The number of women traveling to Sydney during this period meant that feminist organizations in New Zealand and Sydney had to work together to ensure that women were able to access the services they needed. Despite not being able to prevent a restrictive law change in New Zealand in 1977, many feminist groups saw it as a victory that they had been able to help so many women go to Australia for a termination of pregnancy.

Nevertheless, by the early 1980s the trans-Tasman traffic had slowed, and most women were able to access abortion services in New Zealand. This was not without opposition. Anti-abortion groups who had seen the 1977 act as an initial success were upset that the number of abortions in New Zealand was increasing, and they made their objections public, predominantly by protesting outside abortion clinics. This meant that even though women could access abortion services in New Zealand, they still had to fight to retain these services. Unlike abortion travel that occurred in other locations, the travel from New Zealand to Australia has largely been ignored until now, despite the close relationship between the two countries being examined by historians in many other contexts. Focusing on this travel adds a feminist dimension to the Australia–New Zealand relationship, which has often been defined in the masculine terms of mateship.

The end of trans-Tasman abortion travel in the early 1980s does not, however, indicate that adequate abortion services were secured in New Zealand but rather that doctors became more comfortable interpreting the 1978 law, and consequently the number of certifying consultants increased and services became more widely available. The 1977 law, however, remains in place, along with the certifying consultant system and the ASC, and abortion remains unavailable in some regions of New Zealand (particularly second-trimester abortions), resulting in domestic abortion travel, a feature explored in detail in the next section of this volume. Currently, the New Zealand Law Commission is preparing a ministerial briefing paper, reviewing the abortion law of New Zealand at the request of the minister of justice, who along with the prime minister, Jacinda Ardern, has signaled the central government's intention to treat abortion as a health issue.[93]

Notes
1. For the international literature on abortion travel, see Christabelle Sethna, "All Aboard? Canadian Women's Abortion Tourism, 1960–1980," in *Gender, Health, and Popular Culture: Historical Perspectives*, ed. Cheryl Krasnick Warsh

(Waterloo: Wilfrid Laurier University Press, 2010), 89–108; Beth Palmer, "'Lonely, Tragic, but Legally Necessary Pilgrimages': Transnational Abortion Travel in the 1970s," *Canadian Historical Review* 92, no. 4 (2011): 637–64; Christabelle Sethna and Marion Doull, "Accidental Tourists: Canadian Women, Abortion Tourism, and Travel," *Women's Studies* 41, no. 4 (June 2012): 457–75; I. Glenn Cohen, "Medical Tourism and Ending Life: Travel for Assisted Suicide and Abortion," chap. 8 in *Patients with Passports: Medical Tourism, Law, and Ethics* (New York: Oxford University Press, 2015). A recent history of the abortion rights struggle in New Zealand does acknowledge the existence of Sisters Overseas Service and the need for New Zealand women to travel to Australia for abortion in the 1970s but does not examine this travel in any detail or consider it from a transnational perspective. See Alison McCulloch. *Fighting to Choose: The Abortion Rights Struggle in New Zealand* (Wellington: Victoria University Press, 2013): 186–90.

2. For examples of transnational histories of Australia and New Zealand as well as discussions relating to the advantage of such an approach, see Katie Pickles and Catharine Coleborne, eds., *New Zealand's Empire* (Manchester: Manchester University Press, 2015); Philippa Mein Smith, Peter Hempenstall, and Shaun Goldfinch, *Remaking the Tasman World* (Christchurch: Canterbury University Press, 2008); Philippa Mein Smith and Peter Hempenstall, "Australia and New Zealand: Turning Shared Pasts into a Shared History," *History Compass* 1, no. 1 (January 2003): 1–8; Donald Denoon and Philippa Mein Smith with Marivic Wyndham, *A History of Australia, New Zealand and the Pacific* (Oxford: Blackwell, 2000). For a discussion of the limitation of a trans-Tasman approach, see Steven Loveridge, "The 'Other' on the Other Side of the Ditch? The Conception of New Zealand's Disassociation from Australia," *Journal of Imperial and Commonwealth History* 44, no. 1 (2016): 70–94.

3. The term "mateship" has been used extensively in both Australia and New Zealand to describe the nature of masculine relationships, particularly those forged by soldiers both within the context of national histories, that is, homosocial relationships between New Zealand men and between Australian men as well as across national borders. It is often bound up with the mythology of the Australian and New Zealand Army Corps (ANZAC) and the common popular belief that the Gallipoli campaign of World War I (which Anzac Day commemorates) marks the birth of both the Australian and New Zealand nations. For a history of how this relationship was depicted in cartoons, see Philippa Mein Smith, "The Cartoon History of Tasman Relations," in Smith, Hempenstall, and Goldfinch, *Remaking the Tasman World*, 31–55. For a critique of the emphasis on the Anzac myth in the Australian context, see Marilyn Lake and Henry Reynolds, *What's Wrong with Anzac? The Militarisation of Australian History* (Sydney: University of New South Wales Press, 2010).

4. For a brief overview of the pronatalist histories of New Zealand and Australia, see Philippa Mein Smith, "Blood, Birth, Babies, Bodies," *Australian Feminist Studies* 17, no. 39 (2002): 305–23. Countering this history of women as mothers of the nation was one of the challenges faced by feminists in New Zealand and Australia.

5. For more details of these groups, see Hayley M. Brown, "'A Woman's Right to Choose': Second Wave Feminist Advocacy of Abortion Law Reform in

New Zealand and New South Wales from the 1970s" (master's thesis, University of Canterbury, 2004).

6. "Doctors Turning Away NZ Women Seeking Abortions," *Dominion*, October 18, 1971, 79-016-1/05, Alexander Turnbull Library (ATL), Wellington.

7. For further details of women accessing abortions in New Zealand prior to having the option of traveling to Australia, see Margaret Sparrow, *Abortion Then and Now: New Zealand Abortion Stories from 1940 to 1980* (Wellington: Victoria University of Wellington Press, 2010). For a critique of the term "backstreet abortionist" and a reevaluation of abortions provided outside of the medical profession, see Barbara Baird, "'The Incompetent, Barbarous Old Lady Round the Corner': The Image of the Backyard Abortionist in Pro-Abortion Politics," *Hecate* 22, no. 1 (1996): 7–26.

8. "New Zealanders May Be Getting Abortions," *New Zealand Herald*, November 1, 1971, 79-016-1/05, ATL.

9. R v. Davidson [1969], *Victorian Law Reports*, 667.

10. R v. Bourne [1939] 1 KB 687 [1938] 3 All ER 615, CCA.

11. R v. Davidson [1969] VR 667.

12. R v. Wald [1971] 3 DCR (NSW) 25.

13. For further details on the abortion law in the various Australian states, see Karen Coleman, "The Politics of Abortion in Australia: Freedom, Church and State," *Feminist Review*, no. 29 (Summer 1988): 75–97.

14. "NZ Women Fly for Abortions," *Auckland Star*, June 7, 1974, Scrapbook XVII, MLMSS 7012/6, ATL.

15. "The Docs Who Are 'Suitable,'" *NZ Truth*, May 28, 1974, 79-016-2/11, ATL.

16. "NZ Women Fly for Abortions."

17. Submission 28: Mrs. J. Steincamp, p. 1, Box 27, Com 26, Archives New Zealand (ANZ), Wellington.

18. Submission 28: Mrs. J. Steincamp, pp. 4–5, Box 27, Com 26, ANZ. The approximation was before Preterm altered their number from 100 to 30.

19. "$(NZ)2m for Abortions in Australia," *Evening Post*, April 9, 1975, 80-386-1, ATL.

20. "Aust. Abortion Free for NZ Women," *Press*, July 3, 1975, 80-386-1, ATL.

21. "Sydney Medic Admits Abortion Traffic," *Dominion*, April 3, 1975, 80-386-1, ATL.

22. "Girls Fly for Weekend Abortions," *Sunday Telegraph*, August 25, 1974, Scrapbook XVII, MLMSS 7012/6, Mitchell Library, Sydney.

23. George Smart was later suspended from practicing medicine by the Australian Medical Association because he advertised to most New Zealand doctors, and some Australian doctors, that he performed abortions.

24. Submission 440: AMAC, p. 29, Box 32, Com 26, ANZ.

25. Submission 440: AMAC, p. 30, Box 32, Com 26, ANZ.

26. Beatrice Faust to the Secretary, ALRANZ, September 5, 1972, 79-016-1/02, ATL.

27. Submission 440: AMAC, p. 30, Box 32, Com 26, ANZ, 32.

28. Submission 440: AMAC, p. 30, Box 32, Com 26, ANZ, 9.

29. Submission 440: AMAC, p. 31, Box 32, Com 26, ANZ.

30. Submission 440: AMAC, p. 32, Box 32, Com 26, ANZ.

31. Patricia Martin (ALRA Victoria) to the Secretary, ALRANZ, September 13, 1972, 79-016-1/02, ATL.

32. "Abortions Done in Australia Point to a Big Public Health Problem Here," 80-386-1, ATL. Dame Margaret Sparrow is a doctor who was and still is involved with the Family Planning Association, and is a former president of ALRANZ.

33. For a more detailed example of Geiringer's views, see Erich Geiringer, *Spuc 'em All! Abortion Politics 1978* (Martinborough: Alister Taylor, 1978).

34. Erich Geiringer, "Prescriptions: Abortion Offensive," *New Zealand Observer*, November 1977, 37.

35. Carol Shand, correspondence, February 7, 2018.

36. "Seekers of Aust. Abortions Almost Doubled," item 39, folder 47, box 12, ARC 1993.4, Canterbury Museum (CM), Christchurch.

37. "Plea to Outlaw SOS," item 39, folder 47, box 12, ARC 1993.4, CM.

38. "Abortions Cost $.5m," *Dominion*, August 21, 1978, 91-123-2/2, ATL.

39. Emmi Snyder, "Control Expands Service," *Abortion Is a Woman's Right to Choose*, no. 15 (1978): 2.

40. "'Staggering' Number of Women Get Abortions," *Evening Post*, February 8, 1978, 91-123-2/1, ATL.

41. "Abortions Pattern Changed," February 20, 1979, 91-123-2/3, ATL.

42. Janet Sceats, *Induced Abortion in New Zealand, 1976–1983* (Wellington: Government Printer, 1985), 19.

43. Sandra Coney, untitled, *Broadsheet*, no. 90 (1981): 8.

44. "Abortion Law Felt in Sydney," *Dominion*, January 12, 1978, 91-123-2/1, ATL.

45. "Principal Abortion Agencies Clash," *Dominion*, May 24, 1979, 91-123-2/3, ATL.

46. "Australia Awaits an Abortion Upsurge," *Christchurch Star*, December 17, 1977, 89-326-1/20, ATL.

47. Donna Awatere and Rebecca Evans, "Maori Women," 89-326-2/03, ATL.

48. Sandra Coney, "The Tasman Traffic," *Broadsheet*, no. 58 (1978): 10.

49. "No Boycott in Chch," *Press*, March 4, 1978, 80-326-2, ATL.

50. After the passing of the Hospitals Amendment Act in 1975, all abortions had to be performed in a licenced hospital, and so AMAC had to move to the Aotea Hospital. It has since reverted to its original name, AMAC, and continues to operate in Auckland.

51. "Aotea Set for Influx," *Dominion*, August 9, 1979, 91-123-2/3, ATL.

52. "Pressure on Abortion Clinic Grows," *New Zealand Herald*, January 15, 1980, 91-123-2/3, ATL.

53. "'Wait and See' on Abortions," *New Zealand Herald*, October 26, 1978, 80-386-2, ATL.

54. "Abortion 'Lacks' Concerns," *Dominion*, March 18, 1985, 91-123-4/1, ATL.

55. "Abortion Plaint," *Dominion*, April 28, 1975, 80-386-1, ATL.

56. "Abortion Talks 'Waste of Time,'" *Hawke's Bay Herald Tribune*, July 12, 1979, MSX-2794, ATL.

57. "Most Abortions Still Done in Australia?," *Evening Post*, July 12, 1979, 91-123-2/3, ATL.

58. "Tribute to Elizabeth Sewell," 88–159, ATL.

59. "New Name, New Role for SOS," *Evening Post*, October 8, 1980, 91-123-3/2, ATL.

60. "28 a Week for Abortion," *Press*, undated, 89-326-1/20, ATL.

61. "Girls' Abortions 'Could Have Been Done Here,'" 89-326-1/20, ATL.

62. "Staggering 'Win' over Abortion Law Claimed," *Evening Post*, June 22, 1981, 91-123-3/2, ATL.

63. Bessie Smyth Foundation to WONAAC, September 3, 1984, 91-123-4/1, ATL.

64. Dr. Geoffrey Davis (Project Director PSI) to Sue Clement (WONAAC), September 25, 1984, 91-123-4/1, ATL.

65. WAAC Adelaide to Sisters in New Zealand, undated, 91-123-2/2, ATL.

66. WAAC Adelaide to Sisters in New Zealand, undated, 91-123-2/2, ATL. ANZAC is an acronym for the Australia and New Zealand Army Corps, and Anzac Day (April 25) is a public holiday in both Australia and New Zealand that commemorates those who have served and died in war. For a critique of the importance ascribed to this day and the masculine culture often associated with the Anzac spirit, see Marilyn Lake, "Mission Impossible: How Men Gave Birth to the Australian Nation—Nationalism, Gender and Other Seminal Acts," *Gender and History* 4, no. 3 (1992): 305–22.

67. Fern Hickson (WONAAC Coordinator) to WAAC Adelaide, April 6, 1978, 91-123-2/2, ATL. The passing of the Contraception, Sterilisation, and Abortion Act had increased the number of different groups and organizations formed to support women's access to abortion and oppose the legislation. Many of these groups were short-lived.

68. National Coordinator of WONAAC to Auckland University Students' Association, July 15, 1978, 91-123-2/2, ATL.

69. "Sydney Protest at NZ Law," *New Zealand Herald*, February 7, 1978, 80-386-2, ATL. See also "Abortion Rally in Sydney," 91-123-2/1, ATL.

70. "Mr. Muldoon Makes Backdoor Entry to Talks," *Evening Post*, February 13, 1978, 91-123-2/1, ATL.

71. "Abortion Rally Arrest in Brisbane," *New Zealand Herald*, September 18, 1978, 80-386-2, ATL.

72. Quoted in Mary Varnham, "Who'll Marry Her Now?," in *Heading Nowhere in a Navy Blue Suit: And Other Tales from the Feminist Revolution*, ed. Sue Kedgley and Mary Varnham (Wellington: Daphne Brasell Associates Press, 1993), 105. For other examples of women's experiences, see Sparrow, *Abortion Then and Now*, 97–98, 162–65.

73. Snyder, "Control Expands Service," 2.

74. "28 a Week for Abortion."

75. Snyder, "Control Expands Service," 2.

76. "Reactionary Laws Attack New Zealand Women," *Abortion Is a Woman's Right to Choose*, no. 15 (1978): 5.

77. It was not uncommon for New Zealand women to take their own medication with them, as it was cheaper than buying it in Australia.

78. Rebecca Albury, "Women's Health—Man-Made Medicine," *Scarlet Woman*, no. 13 (1981): 10.

79. Open letter to the women of New Zealand from ALRA (NSW), item 7, folder 7, box 2, ARC 1993.4, CM.

80. Untitled, *Broadsheet*, no. 57 (1978): 19.

81. Rosemary McLeod, "The Sydney Procedure," *New Zealand Listener* 88, no. 1997 (1978): 22.

82. Control, *Abortion: Our Bodies Their Power* (Chippendale, NSW: Control, 1977): 1.

83. Control, *Abortion*, 2.

84. Control, *Abortion*, 4.

85. McLeod, "The Sydney Procedure," 22.

86. "Children by Choice" was formed in Queensland after the Levine Ruling to help women go to Sydney for abortions. It operated in a similar way to SOS. Children by Choice was able to negotiate a deal with Ansett to fly women to Sydney on discounted fares, which helped make the process more affordable to women.

87. Control, *Abortion*, 3.

88. Bessie Smyth had been a campaigner for birth control in Melbourne during the nineteenth century.

89. McLeod, "The Sydney Procedure," 23.

90. McLeod, "The Sydney Procedure," 23.

91. "Preterm Sacks Workers," *Mabel: Australian Feminist Newspaper* 8 (1977): 7.

92. "Preterm Sacks Workers," 7.

93. See http://lawcom.govt.nz/abortion, accessed May 29, 2018. For a recent discussion of the limitations of New Zealand's current law, see Alison McCulloch and Ann Weatherall, "The Fragility of De Facto Abortion on Demand in New Zealand Aotearoa," *Feminism and Psychology* 27, no. 1 (2017): 92–100.

PART II DOMESTIC TRANSGRESSIONS

[4]

All Aboard the "Abortion Express"

Geographic Variability, Domestic Travel, and
the 1967 British Abortion Act

GAYLE DAVIS, JANE O'NEILL, CLARE PARKER, AND SALLY SHELDON

THE 1967 Abortion Act was a landmark piece of legislation that liberalized access to abortion in Britain and sparked a wider wave of global reform. Crucially, the act placed abortion firmly under medical control, since two registered medical practitioners were required to certify that appropriate indications existed.[1] It can be contrasted with the "abortion on request" system that many European countries have since chosen to adopt for at least the first trimester of pregnancy. It has been argued that the "medicalization," or enforced medical monopoly, of British abortion policy has been a decidedly mixed blessing, for it has "depoliticised the extension of women's access to abortion services" and "defused political conflict," but it has also left women "dependent on the vagaries of medical discretion and goodwill."[2]

The legislation succeeded where six previous bills had failed, yet this did not secure goodwill on its passing. In fact, criticism of the British Abortion Act and its operation began to build from the moment it came into effect on April 27, 1968, stimulating the government's 1970 announcement that it would establish an official inquiry to review the act's operation, though not its wording or principles.[3] A 15-member Committee on the Working of the Abortion Act was assembled, better known as the Lane Committee since it sat under the chairmanship of Justice Elizabeth Lane (1905–88), the first female High Court judge in England. It began to take evidence in August 1971—in both written and oral form—from a wide variety of private individuals and organizations from the fields of medicine, law, education, welfare, and religion. This was to be the first and most thorough review of the workings of the Abortion Act,[4] and the comprehensive witness testimony collected provides a unique opportunity to examine the perceived deficiencies of the act when it was initially implemented.

This chapter focuses on one of the most prominent strands of criticism presented to the Lane Committee: a profound geographic variability in British abortion provision, as well as the associated need for women to travel to another part of the country in order to access services.[5] By the early 1970s, it had already become apparent that there were pronounced geographical variations in how the act was being interpreted, and ironically so as the 1967 Abortion Act was the first piece of abortion-related legislation to cover Britain—Scotland, England, and Wales—collectively. The act did not extend to Northern Ireland, resulting—within the geographical context of the United Kingdom (UK)—in the much better-known, and ongoing, phenomenon of travel to Britain that is touched upon in this volume by Mary Gilmartin and Sinéad Kennedy. Using the witness testimony and final reports of the Lane Committee in conjunction with a wider range of medical, governmental, and newspaper archives, this chapter maps the "postcode lottery" of British abortion provision in the early years of the act's operation and—particularly through the work of psychiatrist I. M. Ingram—explores the tensions that constrained access to abortion in certain parts of the country and propelled women elsewhere.

Scotland

Even before the 1967 Abortion Act came into effect, Scotland was noted for the geographic variability of its abortion provision. In Scotland, abortion constituted a common law offense without strictly defined limits. In the decades before 1967, the Scottish legal establishment considered abortion a matter of medical discretion and advised that it was possible for a medical practitioner to terminate a pregnancy when acting in "good faith" in the interests of the health or welfare of his patient.[6] In short, abortion was only a crime if "criminal intent" could be proved, doctors otherwise having freedom to practice in accordance with their clinical judgment. Yet, the oral testimony of retired Scottish medical practitioners suggests that most Scottish doctors failed to exploit the flexibility of Scottish law in this sphere because they were unaware of their legal rights.[7] Neither the nuances of abortion law nor the differences between English and Scottish law were made clear to medical students,[8] so graduates generally believed that performing an abortion was a crime unless the woman's life was in imminent danger.

In only one area of Scotland do doctors appear to have taken full advantage of the potential flexibility of Scottish abortion law in the decades before the 1967 act, and that was in Aberdeenshire in northeast Scotland, under the guidance of the chief gynecologist Dugald Baird. Employed initially as a gynecology registrar at Glasgow Royal Infirmary, it was in that city, the largest and also the most Catholic in Scotland,[9] that Baird witnessed the excessive childbearing, high maternal mortality, and highly restrictive access to fertility limitation (contraceptives and abortion) that was to shape his future career. These factors, and most notably his frustration with the city's Catholic administration—which in one case caused him to remove a priest from the hospital by "tak[ing] him by the back of the neck and march[ing] him down the stairs and chuck[ing] him out onto the street"[10]—propelled him out of Glasgow. In 1936, he accepted an appointment to the Regius Chair of Midwifery at the University of Aberdeen, located in a city with a supportive medical and political infrastructure, and a "liberal" population in political and religious terms.[11]

Conscious of the tenuous legal standing of abortion in Scotland, Baird sought the advice of Thomas Smith, professor of law at the university, for clarification on the issue. Smith reportedly explained that there was little likelihood of prosecution against doctors who terminated a pregnancy unless the authorities were convinced of "criminal intent."[12] Armed with this assurance, Baird and his colleagues adopted an active "therapeutic abortion" policy under which they chose to recognize an increasing number of social as well as medical indications that might adversely affect a woman's health. When the young politician David Steel put forward the bill that would become the 1967 Abortion Act, some questioned the involvement of a Scottish politician in the matter given the greater flexibility of Scottish abortion law. However, according to Steel, Baird made him aware that he was "the only person" who—thanks to his "considerable [professorial] status and the security which that brings"—felt able to take advantage of Scottish common law to "follow his professional conscience."[13] As such, Baird was invited to become a medical adviser to the Abortion Law Reform Association (ALRA), the most notable of the activist groups working to liberalize access to abortion, some of whose activities are explored in detail in this volume by Christabelle Sethna.[14] Baird enthusiastically accepted the appointment.

Working for the "other side" was Baird's Glasgow-based equivalent. Ian Donald, an English obstetrician who in 1954 had accepted the Regius Chair of Midwifery at the University of Glasgow, was a founding member of the Society for the Protection of Unborn Children (SPUC), the most organized anti-abortion activist group working in opposition to Steel's bill. An active member of the Scottish Episcopal Church, Donald characterized most abortions as "legalised murder" performed for "flimsy reasons" and lamented: "I joined this profession to save life not to kill babies."[15] Donald's campaigning was highly effective in combination with the medical technology that he had developed: obstetric ultrasound. At a time when ultrasound was not used routinely in the management of pregnancy, he employed these images and recordings of the fetal beating heart as a powerful anti-abortion device, both at public rallies and in his own institution, the Queen Mother's Hospital, in a deliberate attempt to deter women seeking an abortion.[16]

The divergence in opinion between Baird and Donald is reflected in their cities' abortion statistics. In the decade before 1966, Aberdeen had the highest abortion rate of any Scottish city, and Glasgow the lowest; according to the press, one pregnancy in 50 was terminated in Aberdeen compared to one in 3,750 in Glasgow.[17] In 1968, the year the act was implemented, the rate ranged from 4.6 per 1,000 women in the Northern Hospital Board Region (where Aberdeen was situated) to 1.6 per 1,000 women in the Western Hospital Board Region (where Glasgow was situated).[18] This pronounced variation was to continue throughout and beyond the life of the Lane Committee: the abortion rate per 1,000 women aged 15 to 44 for the last quarter of 1974 was 12.6 in the Northern region, compared with 7.4 for Scotland as a whole.[19] It should be noted that the vast majority of these abortions were performed under the public sector's National Health Service (NHS): almost 99 percent in 1973.[20] Indeed, there was very little private medicine in general in Scotland.

So striking were the variations in these figures that a popular tabloid, the *Scottish Daily Record*, devoted a special "shock issue" to the subject. It reviewed abortion provision in the major Scottish cities and deplored the fact that obtaining an NHS abortion was highly dependent on where one happened to live, despite its founding principle as a free and universal healthcare provider.[21] Glasgow was said to have "diehard pro and anti-abortion forces . . . battling it out in the various theatres of war," while the capital city of Edinburgh seemed to leave abortion "pretty much to the consciences of individual doctors." In Dundee, it was estimated that more than 700 abortions were being carried out yearly, the highest rate per head of population in Scotland. As one of the city's senior gynecologists observed: "It has reached the stage where we carry out abortions almost on request. Though we don't shout it from the rooftops." Finally, Aberdeen was said to be a "leading" abortion provider, although only women living in the hospitals' catchment areas were considered. As the *Daily Record* concluded, the working of the act was "a giant lottery and if your number [came] up you [could] thank lady luck for the privilege."[22]

Concerns over geographical variation in abortion provision were expressed similarly in witness testimony to the Lane Committee. The Scottish General Medical Services Committee claimed that facilities were "sporadic and unevenly distributed throughout the country" due to doctors' individual attitudes.[23] As the Scottish Association of Executive Councils noted: "Variation in the application of the Act . . . sometimes result[ed] in 'shopping around' to find a gynaecologist whose interpretation of the criteria [was] liberal and who [was] prepared to agree to termination of a pregnancy."[24] Indeed, the Board of Management for the Glasgow Royal Infirmary, along with several other medical organizations, lamented the fact that it was this very shopping around that was responsible for their gynecological waiting list having doubled in just one year[25] Donald's grip on Scotland's largest city was obviously weakening, as various witnesses described "the anomalous situation of being able to refer a patient in one area [of Glasgow] to a hospital serving that area with the reasonable prospect that she will be judged suitable for termination of her pregnancy and at the same time having to advise a woman living in another area, whose grounds for termination are at least as strong, that it is pointless to refer her to the hospital serving her area."[26]

Due in large part—though not exclusively—to this geographical inequality, significant numbers of women normally resident in Scotland were reported to be obtaining abortions in England, and the vast majority in non-NHS premises. From 1972 onward, about 7,500 abortions were carried out each year in Scotland, while as many as 1,000 women traveled south to England for an abortion.[27] As the medical secretary of the Glasgow Local Medical Committee lamented: "Much against his inclination," a doctor in certain parts of Glasgow might feel obliged to advise a woman with an unwanted pregnancy to use "the private services operated in England."[28] He deplored the fact "that one patient [could] have certain services provided free under the NHS" while another living nearby, and whose grounds for termination were at least as strong, would have "to be put to the expense of travelling to England and paying privately for the same service." Doctors had reportedly complained to the Glasgow Local Medical Committee that they "felt it their duty to assist" such women "by making the necessary arrangements for her to be seen at such a [private] clinic."[29] Furthermore, as the Medical and Dental Defence Union of Scotland warned, the family doctor of any women who traveled for an abortion was unlikely to be notified, and it was "utterly wrong that her doctor should be kept in ignorance as he may very well be called in to deal with post-abortion complications."[30]

Birmingham, Liverpool, and London appear to have been the most popular destinations for Scottish women seeking a private abortion, for reasons discussed later in this chapter. Indeed, the Glasgow-Liverpool train was reportedly nicknamed "the Abortion Express" in recognition of this traffic south by women forced to pay for the operation because a free NHS abortion had been denied them. One particular "cut price" clinic in Liverpool dealt with 720 Scottish girls in 1972 alone.[31] One doctor working in the West of Scotland deplored the fact that "the Act might as well not have been passed as far as my patients are concerned. . . . In all but a few specialised cases I have to send them south and they have to pay. . . . However you feel about abortions, this is not justice, not law, and not what the National Health Service is supposed to be about."[32] To a much lesser extent, Edinburgh also witnessed attempts by Glaswegian women to access abortion services. As a growing number of women took the "abortion shuttle that stops at Edinburgh," local doctors complained increasingly of the associated "crisis" of stretched hospital resources.[33] As one consultant gynecologist protested: "I don't think Edinburgh should be solving their problems." Anecdotal evidence suggests that Scottish women might also try their luck in Aberdeen, with the euphemistic claim that they were "going to see Uncle Dugald."[34]

It should be noted that the post-1970 statistics indicate that Scottish women who obtained an abortion in England were on average younger than the women who remained in Scotland, with a particular overrepresentation of women in their early 20s in the traveling group. It is, therefore, possible that some women who left Scotland did so as a matter of personal preference, perhaps to safeguard their confidentiality rather than through problems of local access per se. As the Lane Committee reported, the private sector enabled patients who could afford it "to have treatment in the privacy and with the amenities they desire."[35] However, evidence also suggests that doctors in Scotland were more willing to terminate the pregnancies of respectable married women who already had a family than the younger generation with very different standards of sexual behavior than their parents and, more specifically, their doctors.[36] One Scottish study found that those recommended for an abortion had a mean age of 31 years, and those refused an abortion had a mean age of 24, young single women "provok[ing] the most moralistic response" from their doctors.[37] Indeed, in their evidence to the Lane Committee, the Royal College of Physicians of Edinburgh noted that some doctors opposed abortion for this group as it would remove "a natural barrier to promiscuity."[38] Similarly, Christabelle Sethna's chapter in this volume notes that the ALRA's campaign for abortion law reform was willing to publicize the plight of the respectable married woman seeking an abortion, rather than the unwed.

A final relevant factor when analyzing the significance of age is the fact that young women were more likely to be constrained by fear, parental disapproval, denial of pregnancy, or—for those living in the Scottish Highlands and Islands—practical difficulties in accessing a family doctor, and were thus more likely to request an abortion at a later stage of their pregnancy. As the fetus was approaching viability, and with a higher risk of complications, doctors may have felt greater reluctance to approve an abortion request.[39] For all of these reasons, it is important to note that while the vast majority of abortions in Scotland were performed under the NHS, the private sector in England clearly served Scottish women and continues to do so. This appears to have become the case in recent decades for women of all ages who seek an abortion for nonmedical reasons in Scotland after 18–20 weeks' gestation. Despite the fact that the official time limit for an abortion in Britain is currently 24 weeks, these women tend to be denied an NHS abortion in Scotland and forced to travel to England, where they must pay their own costs up front, often without knowledge that their local NHS Board should reimburse them retrospectively.[40]

England and Wales

Prior to 1967, any attempt to procure an abortion in England and Wales by a pregnant woman or by anyone else, "whether she be or be not with Child," was outlawed by the 1861 Offences Against the Person Act.[41] The crime was not the abortion itself but the committing of an act with intent to procure a miscarriage "unlawfully," hence the woman did not actually have to be pregnant if the abortion were performed by a third party. A 1938 judicial ruling, *Rex v. Bourne*, provided that in prohibiting "unlawful" procurement of miscarriage, the framers of the 1861 act must logically have envisaged circumstances in which the procurement of miscarriage was lawful. The judge in the case thus found that there was an exception for those cases in which abortion was deemed necessary to save the life of the mother,[42] with this condition met where "the probable consequences of the continuance of the pregnancy [were] to make the woman a physical or mental wreck."[43] Given the exceptional nature of the Bourne case—in which a London obstetrician terminated the pregnancy of a 14-year-old girl who had been raped by a group of soldiers, then invited the law to prosecute him—most doctors remained deeply uncertain over the legalities of abortion and were thus highly wary of involvement in that sphere. Nonetheless, as the ALRA campaigner Alice Jenkins's provocatively titled *Law for the Rich* suggested, women from well-to-do families seemed able to find a doctor who would provide a safe abortion in a private facility,[44] while working-class women played "Russian roulette" with more affordable backstreet abortionists or attempted to self-induce an abortion. Thus, as in Scotland, abortion provision was highly variable, though perhaps more for reasons of wealth than location.

When the Abortion Act came into force in April 1968, English critics quickly focused on a set of concerns that was rather distinct from those articulated in Scotland, since the relative dominance of the private sector in England tended to be portrayed across Britain as "the cause of all the subsequent troubles in the south."[45] Certainly, witness testimony to the Lane Committee supports this contention. In addition to the troublingly prominent and profiteering role of the private sector were the related concerns of British abortion services being advertised abroad and access by nonresident women to British abortion services, a topic examined in this volume by both Christabelle Sethna and Agata Ignaciuk.[46] It was also noted in the committee's final reports that comparisons between England and Scotland tended to be "affected by the non-resident component" in the former.[47] Nonetheless, geographical variation and the consequent need for women to travel, "forced to pay for abortions when they had legitimate medical grounds for termination of pregnancy under the Act," was a leitmotif in those testifying across Britain.[48]

A review of NHS abortion rates in the first year of the act illustrates an already-significant variation in provision. Per 1,000 females aged 15 to 44 years, the abortion rate ranged from 2.36 in North West London and 2.04 in Newcastle to 0.85 in Birmingham and 0.71 in Liverpool. Wales sat sixth highest in the rankings at 1.65 per 1,000 women. By 1971, on the eve of the Lane Committee's establishment, positions had changed slightly, from South East London (8.34), Newcastle (7.96), and North West London (7.70) to Liverpool (4.16), Leeds (3.94), and— bottom of the league table for NHS provision—Birmingham (2.34). This was a striking rise in the number of women who successfully sought an abortion across all regions of England and Wales in a mere four years, though this differed fairly dramatically from an increase of 175 percent (Birmingham) through to 511 percent (Sheffield).[49]

It is worth noting that, outside London, very few NHS abortions were performed outside the patient's area of residence. That is, many hospitals were choosing to implement a local residency requirement. Their motivation might have been the fact that no additional facilities had been made available for the significantly increased demand on NHS resources, with a consequent growth in the waiting list for other routine gynecological procedures. Also worth noting is the percentage of these women who were sterilized after their abortion—from 15.7 percent in North West London to 40.2 percent in both Birmingham and Liverpool[50]—and the potentially dire health consequences: in 1969, it was reported that the mortality rate for abortion was 11.4 percent per 100,000 operations, but for combined abortion/sterilization it was 107.9 percent.[51] Finally, in the NHS sector, it was found in a 1971 survey of general practitioners that one-fifth or more of family doctors working in Birmingham, Liverpool, and Sheffield declared a conscientious objection to abortion—as many as 32 percent in Liverpool—compared to 5 percent in South East London and 4 percent in East Anglia.[52]

Non-NHS (i.e., private- *and* charitable-sector) abortions were noted by the Lane Committee "to have taken place in large numbers in relatively few regions," those being North West London, South West London, and Birmingham.[53] In 1968, 11 out of the 15 regional hospital boards for England and Wales notified that more than 90 percent of their abortions were performed in NHS hospitals. Yet by 1971, this had fallen to six boards (Newcastle, Leeds, Sheffield, Oxford, Wales, and Manchester), while in North West London only 11 percent of abortions were performed in an NHS facility.[54] Birmingham saw quite a change in this regard: in 1968, 95.2 percent of its abortions were performed in NHS facilities, but by 1971 this figure had dropped dramatically, to 16.2 percent.[55] Those regions that experienced a drop in the rate of NHS abortions tended to note "a substantial and rising" proportion of private operations in other parts of England,[56] as well as the establishment of other "approved" (i.e., private) clinics in their regions, most notably those opened by the Birmingham (renamed British) Pregnancy Advisory Service (BPAS) in Birmingham (1968) and Liverpool (1970). By 1971, the media was reporting that of the 126,000 abortions performed in England and Wales, almost 60 percent were carried out in the private sector: 40 percent by profit-making enterprises, and 20 percent by nonprofit charities, most notably BPAS.[57]

As with the cities of Aberdeen and Glasgow, the senior gynecologist was exerting considerable influence on NHS abortion provision in Birmingham. Professor Hugh McLaren was a leading medical opponent of abortion who joined Donald as a founding member of SPUC. McLaren reportedly prevented the doctors working under him from performing an abortion in all but a fraction of cases.[58] He disparaged "those who believe that abortion like the [birth control] pill is their right," and lamented the sizable incomes of those performing abortions in the private sector, urging the president of the Royal College of Obstetricians and Gynaecologists, John Peel, to deny them a college fellowship.[59]

Many English women living in cities such as Birmingham were thus forced to travel outside their area of residence in search of an abortion. In 1968, 29.1 percent of women resident in England and Wales obtained an abortion outside their home region,[60] though, again, figures differed significantly across the country. Thus, 96.9 percent of Newcastle residents—the highest proportion in England—obtained an abortion locally; at the other end of the table, the equivalent figures for Birmingham and South West London were 57.9 and 31 percent, respectively.

By 1971, while Newcastle remained at the top of the table (92.6 percent), Birmingham had risen to second place (jointly with East Anglia); in both cities, 83.8 percent of residents obtained their abortion locally. The BPAS provision had clearly made a significant impact in a short space of time. At the other end of the scale, 49.9 percent of Leeds residents obtained their abortion in another region, and 69.5 percent for South West London. In their oral evidence to the Lane Committee, BPAS staff suggested that while McLaren—"the head of all this side of the work in our teaching hospital"—had declared "he would not sit in the same bus as the people who support" BPAS because of his personal opposition to abortion, "a good many of the local doctors who might otherwise be under pressure" were "quite pleased to see that [BPAS was] relieving them of this particular responsibility."[61] When asked whether they saw BPAS as "a permanent structure" or "something which in all conscience the health service should aim ultimately to replace," François Lafitte, professor of social policy and administration at the University of Birmingham and chair of BPAS (1968–88), noted their initial wish to exist purely as a "temporary voluntary group working in Birmingham alone," but that while they would "rather not be in business," staff had begun to accept "that we shall have to continue at any rate for some years, and that the scale of our work is growing and reaching the point where we have to think about pension schemes for our employees."[62]

BPAS benefited many British women living in such "restrictive" areas as Birmingham because, unlike the NHS, it did not limit its services to those living nearby. In her oral evidence to the Lane Committee, one gynecologist complained that catchment areas were set by NHS hospitals for only a few select services, including abortion, whereas those who sought a chest operation or even plastic surgery could "go anywhere else for a preferred surgeon."[63] Similarly, a doctor based in London condemned his NHS colleagues who had introduced catchment areas only for their abortion services, which constituted "a selective discrimination in medical matters against human dignity" since these patients fulfilled the act's clinical requirements "as strictly interpreted."[64] As he concluded, "the Abortion Act works fully and successfully for the socially privileged but help for the working woman without means is very scarce and many unnecessary obstacles are put in her way." Indeed, class was not the only variable to take into consideration. As the lengthy written submission from the Royal College of Obstetricians and Gynaecologists explained, the private sector recorded a much higher proportion of single women than the NHS; 69 percent of the single women who received an abortion in 1968 had to, or chose to, pay for a private abortion.[65]

Media exposés lambasted the "opportunity given to private entrepreneurs" in the "abortion market" during these early years and speculated about their level of profiteering.[66] BPAS charged between £51 and £65 per abortion and still managed to cover the cost of a free abortion for women who could not afford to pay. With British women charged between £100 and £120 on average for an abortion, private entrepreneurs might make a profit of £50 per resident woman (and up to £120 per nonresident woman) from those able to afford these services.[67] While some private providers of abortion were acknowledged to be providing a "high standard of medical care," some were accused of "operating on a scale and at a rate which suggest that high profit may form a stronger motivation than medical care," leaving commentators "gravely concerned that women [were] receiving less than optimal treatment."[68] Poor treatment, as the Department of Health reported, might include "absence of any pre-operative examination" and premature discharge or otherwise "unsatisfactory post-operative treatment," forcing the NHS to deal with any complications.[69]

"Abortion Games"

The complex dynamics of doctors engaged in the abortion decision-making process in the early years of the 1967 act, and resulting need for women to travel across Britain, were neatly summed up by I. M. Ingram, a psychiatrist based at the Southern General Hospital, Glasgow. His controversial 1971 article "Abortion Games: An Inquiry into the Working of the Act," published in the *Lancet* medical journal, arguably constituted one of the most damning medical indictments of the legislation.[70] Ingram was here inspired by Californian psychiatrist Eric Berne's "transactional game analysis," which defined "game" not as a "frivolous" activity but as "an ongoing series of superficially plausible transactions with a concealed or dishonest motivation."[71] Ingram argued that the Abortion Act had "created an arena for the development and multiplication of a variety of games," the concealed function of which was to "abolish or minimise personal responsibility for decisions made for or against termination."[72] The psychiatrist was quick to point to the source of the conflict: the "compromise wording" of "a meaningless Act" that left "the scrupulous and cynical doctor alike . . . obliged to give opinions on matters which he considers to be non-medical," since the pregnant woman was "not ill in a strict medical or psychiatric sense," and that asked the doctor "to take life when his natural feelings and training predispose him to conserve it."

Doctors could stymie a woman's chances of accessing a timely abortion, a point that Agata Ignaciuk likewise raises in her chapter on Spain in this volume. In Ingram's assessment, the family doctor acted as the gatekeeper to abortion services and had a variety of options open to him in order to devolve responsibility. The obvious strategies entailed trying to discourage the pregnant woman from seeking an abortion or refusing to refer her anywhere. Alternatively, he could obligingly refer her to a local hospital but rather than make his own recommendation for or against the procedure, simply write a neutral letter committing himself to no decision and thus evading responsibility for whatever would follow. Ingram referred to this game as "Pontius Pilate." Alternatively, the family doctor could covertly disapprove of an abortion but evade a confrontation with the pregnant woman by apparently agreeing to her request and referring her to a specialist known to be antagonistic, the game of "Bounced Cheque."

Donald, the anti-abortion, Glasgow-based obstetrician, illustrated the "streaming phenomenon" that lay behind this last strategy, whereby family doctors "quickly came to know which [hospital] units would readily carry out abortions and which were 'likely to prove sticky.'"[73] As Donald noted, due to the "strict line" that he took in his own unit, most abortion requests came to him from doctors "seeking support in their view that the request for termination of pregnancy should be refused." Thus, the family doctor could effectively harness his knowledge of local gynecologists' attitudes toward abortion, enabling him to refer the woman to that consultant whose decision coincided most neatly with his own views, whether sympathetic or hostile. Since, under the NHS, the patient first had to consult a family doctor for referral to the specialist, this procedure afforded that practitioner a great deal of discretion in how the Abortion Act was interpreted.

The gynecologist had, according to Ingram, a greater and more complex range of "games" open to him. Using terminology based on unfortunate colonial stereotypes, Ingram argued that for those in positions of authority, "Big White Chief" was a particularly popular and effective game, played by a professor or head of department who imposed on his staff an extreme policy for or against termination. Ostensibly, his justification was "logical and medical," although "covert ethical, religious, and personal motives" could often be inferred.[74] This extreme view would prejudge all individual cases, thus simplifying decision-making in this area, and would be enforced in an authoritarian way with all the prestige that Big White Chief commanded, in some cases spreading to whole cities and regions. A dominating senior gynecologist, such as Baird in Aberdeen, Donald in Glasgow, or McLaren in Birmingham, could exert significant influence on his "Little Indian" junior staff, be it to encourage very restrictive or liberal access to abortion.

This game had far-reaching effects. Since the general practitioner would know the consultant's views and refer or divert patients accordingly, within a short time Big White Chief would see only those patients he wanted to see. His neighboring colleagues, who were likely to see many more patients as a result, might play a corresponding defensive game of "Catchment Area." Thus in 1973, Baird's successor, Professor Ian MacGillivray, had to state publicly that only women living in a hospital's catchment area would be considered for a termination, and that "a woman who [could not] get an abortion elsewhere in Scotland [would not] get one in Aberdeen."[75] Similarly, as a result of Donald's restrictive influence on abortion provision in certain areas of Glasgow, those liberal gynecologists now operating in the city—most notably Professor Malcolm Macnaughton at the Glasgow Royal Infirmary—came under increasing pressure to refuse patients who lived outside the hospital catchment area. And such a system would be particularly problematic in smaller or more remote areas, as Baird complained, where there might be great difficulty in obtaining an alternative opinion.[76]

Another game said to be popular among gynecologists was "Plumber." Here, the doctor would claim to be merely "a technician, an honest, simple craftsman whose abilities [were] bounded by the female pelvis," and who would maintain that psychiatric and social factors did not fall within his competence, thus devolving responsibility to the family doctor, social worker, or psychiatrist.[77] The obverse of this game was "Amateur Psychiatrist," where the gynecologist "turn[ed] his hand enthusiastically to psycho-social diagnosis and treatment," a task for which he was "ill-suited by training and temperament." Other, more obvious, gynecologist strategies were noted to include "Waiting-list," where the patient had to wait months for an appointment, perhaps until it was too late, and "Sterilization," where the pregnant woman was provided with the desired abortion only on the condition that she simultaneously allow herself to be sterilized.[78] Ingram mentioned an additional game, "Cash before Delivery," but considered this more of "a business game . . . than a medical one," and one "largely confined to the Home Counties" (the English countries that surround the city of London).[79]

Finally, Ingram did not absolve his own specialty from blame and, in fact, claimed that psychiatrists, with their "specialist training in game theory and practice," had demonstrated "more sophistication—or sophistry—in their choice of gambits."[80] The best documented was named "Sim's Position," where the doctor adopted the stance that there were no psychiatric indications for abortion, based on evidence that the major psychoses were not worsened by pregnancy and that suicide was rare during pregnancy. The main assumption here—and it was "a big one" according to Ingram—was that the reference to mental health in the act meant the absence of psychotic illness and no more. The psychiatrist playing this game would thus maintain that the vast majority of women requesting an abortion did not fall within his province, and, like Big White Chief, he would be unlikely to be troubled much on this subject once his views became widely known. While "Sim's Position" is a type of gynecological examination position, the game itself was named after the Birmingham psychiatrist Myre Sim's refusal to bow to pressure brought to bear on the psychiatrist to recommend a termination. He reportedly felt it more appropriate to "nurse the patient through her unstable phase."[81]

A second psychiatric game involved an opposite reading of the act's wording. The doctor chose to interpret mental health in the widest possible sense and maintained that if a woman was "forced to bear an unwanted child," then her mental health "must automatically suffer."[82] The wording of the legislation could effectively be interpreted as justifying abortion on request. The act permitted an abortion where "the continuance of the pregnancy would involve risk . . . greater than if the pregnancy were terminated."[83] As the Royal College of Psychiatrists noted in the year following Ingram's article, this justified a doctor to recommend an abortion in every case presented to him, since the danger of death as a consequence of legal abortion (21 per 100,000 cases in the first year of the act) was lower than that of dying during childbirth (24 per 100,000 cases).[84] Ironically, this clause had been added in the final stages of debate in the House of Lords by opponents of abortion, who labored under the false assumption that early termination was more dangerous than a full-term pregnancy.[85] Ingram named this game

"Woman's Lib.," since the object was "to place the ball of decision firmly in the woman's court, in part removing the decision from the doctor."[86]

The final "player" was the pregnant woman herself, who might "play games spontaneously or in response to medical games."[87] She was often obliged to play "Obstacle Race," where each of the aforementioned games constituted a potential hindrance to be overcome in her search for a legal abortion. This race is pertinent to every chapter in this volume. The pregnant woman required "luck and determination . . . to succeed," and, as Ingram warned, "honesty may not be rewarded." The woman prepared to play "Psychiatric Case," producing "the symptoms that the doctor seeks" to feel he can justify an abortion, was likely to be more successful than the "intelligent woman" who made her decision "rationally and calmly." Another popular game, "Class Warfare," referred to the evidence that those from a higher social class were more likely to be successful in their request for an abortion. Middle-class patients were "usually more knowledgeable about the law" and "better able to put their case convincingly," while doctors tended to sympathize more readily with girls "who might easily be their own daughters." Thus, as Baird and his Aberdeen colleagues argued, doctors tended to see abortion as "a second chance" for the better-educated girl who was "anxious that [her] future should not be imperilled by one mistake."[88] Thus the poorer patient suffered on two counts: she was both less likely to elicit sympathy in her family doctor and less likely to be able to afford the travel, accommodation, and private abortion if local NHS provision was denied her.

Conclusion

Ingram's *Lancet* article brought into sharp relief the inherent, and deeply damaging, ambiguities of the 1967 British Abortion Act as well as the resulting inconsistencies in decision-making across Britain. Women with an unwanted pregnancy who sought a termination after 1967 were not "ill" in any medical or psychiatric sense yet were compelled to obtain permission from two registered medical practitioners, in part since doctors were the only people considered technically qualified to carry out the operation at a time when abortion was largely a surgical procedure. Doctors were arguably not qualified to lead—or even participate in— the decision-making process, though some were more enthusiastic or transparent than others in taking on this duty and in influencing those around them to adopt a similar approach. Their ability to interpret the legislation so variably goes a long way in explaining the pronounced geographical disparities in British abortion provision and the consequent need for many women to seek—and often finance—an abortion away from home. It also shines a slightly ironic light on the many nonresident women who sought an abortion in Britain (the focus of Christabelle Sethna's contribution to this volume), hardly a permissive haven for resident women. British women who had to travel in search of, and find the money to pay, a private abortion provider appeared to experience little or no advantage in being a "resident" whose taxes funded the NHS.

And this was all to remain the case. The Lane Committee completed its investigations in 1974 with the publication of a three-volume report that suggested a variety of administrative measures to tighten the regulations and thereby improve the act's effectiveness. However, unexpectedly—given the scathing criticisms expressed by witnesses of the "considerable" problems identified—the report concluded by noting that the committee members were "unanimous in supporting the Act and its provisions."[89] It recommended that "the wording of the Act laying down the criteria for abortion be left unamended"; that "doctors should continue to make the decision as to abortion"; and that "abortion work should not be restricted to the N.H.S." but "should continue to be performed in the private sector without statutory restriction upon the qualifications of registered medical practitioners undertaking the operations, and without statutory control of fees."[90] Thus the underlying conditions that created a market for abortion travel would remain in place.

As the 1967 Abortion Act approached its 50th anniversary, momentum began to build palpably for both the decriminalization and, to a more limited extent, demedicalization of abortion in Britain. The political architect of the act, David Steel, advocated decriminalization on the basis that British women are "miles behind our European neighbours who allow all women to access abortions on request."[91] The three most relevant medical bodies—the Royal College of Midwives, British Medical Association, and Royal College of Obstetricians and Gynaecologists—voted one by one in support for abortion to be regulated "in line with other medical procedures, rather than criminal sanctions."[92] Such statements have been welcomed by those who recognize the remaining impediments to local abortion access, and the emotional and financial cost of travel to obtain abortion provision away from home. They further recognize the increasing accessibility of abortifacients without the legal approval of medical gatekeepers—in particular, abortion pills sold online[93]—which has arguably made the prosecution of women with an unwanted pregnancy more likely.

The same audience has welcomed the Scottish government's October 2017 decision to allow women residing in Scotland to take the abortion pill misoprostol at home, albeit only when deemed "clinically appropriate," thus allowing women "to be in control of their treatment and as comfortable as possible during this procedure."[94] This effectively implemented a 2006–07 recommendation from the House of Commons Science and Technology Committee, though it fell short of their package of recommendations that would have significantly demedicalized abortion provision.[95] Women will still need to attend a medical facility to take the first pill (mifepristone), but by obtaining the second pill (misoprostol) at the same time, to be taken by the woman in her own home, this new judgment now removes the requirement for a return trip to the doctor's office. As Jillian Merchant, the vice chair of campaign group Abortion Rights UK, argues, this decision allows women to escape the "horrendous experience of abortions commencing on public transport due to outdated legislation, which takes no account of medical advances or the reality of women's lives."[96]

Acknowledgments
We wish to thank the Arts and Humanities Research Council for their support of our research project "The Abortion Act (1967): A Biography," AH/N00213X/1.

Notes

1. Full details of the act can be found at Public General Statutes, Elizabeth II, CH. 87.

2. Sally Sheldon, *Beyond Control: Medical Power and Abortion Law* (London: Pluto Press, 1997), 168.

3. National Records of Scotland (NRS), HH61/1315, Draft Memorandum by the Secretary of State for Social Services, 1970.

4. A later review of the act, also worthy of mention, is the House of Commons Science and Technology Committee, *Scientific Developments Relating to the Abortion Act, 1967: Twelfth Report of Session 2006–07*, https://publications.parliament.uk/pa/cm200607/cmselect/cmsctech/1045/1045i.pdf.

5. For a more complete overview of the Lane Committee's proceedings, see Ashley Wivel, "Abortion Policy and Politics on the Lane Committee of Enquiry,

1971–1974," *Social History of Medicine* 11, no. 1 (April 1998): 109–35; Roger Davidson and Gayle Davis, *The Sexual State: Sexuality and Scottish Governance, 1950–80* (Edinburgh: Edinburgh University Press, 2012), 110–16.

6. NRS, HH41/1146, Briefing Notes on Abortion Bill, February 2, 1954.

7. Interviews by Gayle Davis with retired general practitioners, gynecologists, and psychiatrists, April 2003–April 2004.

8. Indeed, textbooks such as John Glaister's *Medical Jurisprudence and Toxicology*, 12th ed. (Edinburgh: Churchill Livingstone, 1966), the "medico-legal bible" for generations of doctors in Scotland, failed to differentiate between abortion law in Scotland and England.

9. N. A. Todd, "Psychiatric Experience of the Abortion Act (1967)," *British Journal of Psychiatry* 119, no. 552 (1971): 491. Todd estimated that 30 percent of Glasgow's population was Roman Catholic, compared with 17 percent for Scotland as a whole and 8 percent for England and Wales.

10. University of Aberdeen Special Collections, MS3620/21/1-2, Interview by Elizabeth Olson with Sir Dugald Baird, April 3, 1985.

11. Davidson and Davis, *The Sexual State*, 100–101.

12. Gopika Bhatia, "Social Obstetrics, Maternal Health Care Policies and Reproductive Rights: The Role of Dugald Baird in Great Britain, 1937–65" (master's thesis, University of Oxford, 1996), 59.

13. *Observer*, February 6, 1966; *Observer*, January 30, 1966; Michael Kandiah and Gillian Staerck, eds., *The Abortion Act, 1967: Institute of Contemporary British History Witness Seminar* (London: Institute of Historical Research, 2002), 47.

14. Barbara Brookes, *Abortion in England, 1900–1967* (London: Croom Helm, 1988), 94–98; Stephen Brooke, "The Sphere of Sexual Politics: The Abortion Law Reform Association, 1930s to 1960s," in *NGOs in Contemporary Britain: Non-State Actors in Society and Politics since 1945*, ed. Nick Crowson, Matthew Hilton, and James McKay (Basingstoke: Palgrave Macmillan, 2009): 77–94.

15. *Scottish Daily Record*, May 16, 1973.

16. Wellcome Library (WL), SA/ALR/H.58, Note on a Public Abortion Meeting, Manchester, December 6, 1966; Malcolm Nicolson and John Fleming, *Imaging and Imagining the Fetus: The Development of Obstetric Ultrasound* (Baltimore: Johns Hopkins University Press, 2013).

17. *The Scotsman*, December 23, 1966.

18. *Report of the Committee on the Working of the Abortion Act, Volume 2: Statistical Volume, Cmnd. 5579* (London: Her Majesty's Stationery Office, 1974), 144.

19. Barbara Thompson, "Problems of Abortion in Britain—Aberdeen, a Case Study," *Population Studies* 31, no. 1 (1977): 153.

20. NRS, HH101/2877, Note by SHHD, February 4, 1975.

21. *Scottish Daily Record*, May 16, 1973; Charles Webster, *The National Health Service: A Political History* (Oxford: Oxford University Press, 2002).

22. *Scottish Daily Record*, May 16, 1973.

23. NRS, HH102/1232, Notes of Meeting between SHHD and Representatives of the Scottish General Medical Services Committee, September 24, 1974.

24. WL, SA/ALR/C.27, Proceedings of the Lane Committee (PLC), Submission of A. W. Smith, Scottish Association of Executive Councils, December 20, 1971.

25. WL, SA/ALR/C.35, PLC, Submission of Board of Management for Glasgow Royal Infirmary and Associated Hospitals, December 1971; SA/ALR/C.41, PLC, Submission of Lothian and Peebles Executive Council, Edinburgh, November 2, 1971.

26. WL, SA/ALR/C.68, PLC, Submission of William Fulton, Medical Secretary, Glasgow Local Medical Committee, March 9, 1973.

27. Hilary Homans, ed., *The Sexual Politics of Reproduction* (Aldershot: Gower, 1985), 84–85.

28. WL, SA/ALR/C.68, PLC, Submission of William Fulton, Medical Secretary, Glasgow Local Medical Committee, March 9, 1973.

29. WL, SA/ALR/C.68, PLC, Submission of William Fulton, Medical Secretary, Glasgow Local Medical Committee, March 9, 1973.

30. WL, SA/ALR/C.35, PLC, Submission of the Medical and Dental Defence Union of Scotland, December 28, 1971.

31. *Scottish Daily Record*, May 16, 1973.

32. *Scottish Daily Record*, May 16, 1973.

33. *Sunday Standard*, May 24, 1981.

34. Interview by Gayle Davis with practicing general practitioner, February 24, 2004.

35. *Report of the Committee on the Working of the Abortion Act, Volume 1: Report, Cmnd. 5579* (London: Her Majesty's Stationery Office, 1974), 183.

36. E. M. Briggs and A. E. Mack, "Termination of Pregnancy in the Unmarried," *Scottish Medical Journal* 17, no. 12 (December 1972): 398–400.

37. E. Hamill and I. M. Ingram, "Psychiatric and Social Factors in the Abortion Decision," *British Medical Journal* 1, no. 5901 (1974): 231.

38. WL, SA/ALR/C.25, PLC, Submission of Royal College of Physicians, Edinburgh, 1972.

39. Todd, "Psychiatric Experience of the Abortion Act," 492.

40. "Women Travelling to England for Abortions," *BBC News*, June 13, 2017, http://www.bbc.com/news/uk-scotland-scotland-politics-40257828; Carrie Purcell et al., "Access to and Experience of Later Abortion: Accounts from Women in Scotland," *Perspectives on Sexual and Reproductive Health* 46, no. 2 (2014): 101–8.

41. Public General Statutes, 24 and 25 Vict., CH. 100.

42. Public General Statutes, 19 and 20 Geo. V., CH. 34.

43. For further details of this case and its wider context, see John Keown, *Abortion, Doctors and the Law: Some Aspects of the Legal Regulation of Abortion in England from 1803 to 1982* (Cambridge: Cambridge University Press, 1988), 49–59.

44. Alice Jenkins, *Law for the Rich: A Plea for the Reform of the Abortion Law* (London: Victor Gollancz, 1960). For a fuller discussion of the perceived relationship between class and abortion in Britain, see Brooke, "The Sphere of Sexual Politics."

45. NRS, HH61/1315, R. M. Bell to J. Walker, March 31, 1970.

46. Wivel, "Abortion Policy."

47. *Report of the Committee on the Working of the Abortion Act, Volume 2*, 45.

48. *Report of the Committee on the Working of the Abortion Act, Volume 1*, 183.

49. *Report of the Committee on the Working of the Abortion Act, Volume 2*, 109.

50. *Report of the Committee on the Working of the Abortion Act, Volume 2*, 147–49.

51. Malcolm Potts, Peter Diggory, and John Peel, *Abortion* (Cambridge: Cambridge University Press, 1977), 212–14.

52. *Report of the Committee on the Working of the Abortion Act, Volume 2*, 111.

53. *Report of the Committee on the Working of the Abortion Act, Volume 2*, 135.

54. *Report of the Committee on the Working of the Abortion Act, Volume 2*, 138.

55. *Report of the Committee on the Working of the Abortion Act, Volume 2*, 139.

56. *Report of the Committee on the Working of the Abortion Act, Volume 2*, 140.

57. "Economics of the Abortion Market," *Daily Telegraph*, March 22, 1972.

58. Alex Mold, *Making the Patient-Consumer: Patient Organisations and Health Consumerism in Britain* (Manchester: Manchester University Press, 2015), 56–59.

59. Royal College of Obstetricians and Gynaecologists Archives (RCOGA), RCOG A16/10, Hugh McLaren to John Peel, President of the Royal College of Obstetricians and Gynaecologists, March 17, 1968.

60. *Report of the Committee on the Working of the Abortion Act, Volume 2*, 138.

61. WL, SA/ALR/C.81, PLC, Submission of Birmingham Pregnancy Advisory Service, June 28, 1972.

62. WL, SA/ALR/C.81, PLC, Submission of Birmingham Pregnancy Advisory Service, June 28, 1972.

63. WL, SA/ALR/C.75, PLC, Submission of Miss Dorothea Kerslake, Fellow of the RCOG, January 26, 1972.

64. WL, SA/ALR/C.113, PLC, Submission of W. Weinberg, M.D., London, November 10, 1971.

65. RCOGA, RCOG A16/6, Submission of Royal College of Obstetricians and Gynaecologists to the Lane Committee, n.d. (c.1971–2).

66. "Economics of the Abortion Market," *Daily Telegraph*, March 22, 1972.

67. "Economics of the Abortion Market."

68. WL, SA/ALR/C.13, House of Commons Report from a Working Party Reviewing the Operation of the Abortion Act 1967 in "Approved Places," March 19, 1970.

69. WL, SA/ALR/C.13, G. M. Bebb, Department of Health and Social Security, London, April 1970.

70. I. M. Ingram, "Abortion Games: An Inquiry into the Working of the Act," *Lancet* 2, no. 7731 (1971): 969–70.

71. See Eric Berne, *Games People Play: The Psychology of Human Relationships* (London: Grove Press, 1964), 44–45.

72. Ingram, "Abortion Games," 969.

73. Ian Donald, "Naught for Your Comfort," *Journal of the Irish Medical Association* 65, no. 1 (1972): 286.

74. Ingram, "Abortion Games," 969.

75. *Scottish Daily Record*, May 16, 1973.

76. Dugald Baird, "The Abortion Act 1967: The Advantages and Disadvantages," *Royal Society of Health Journal* 90, no. 6 (1970): 294.

77. Ingram, "Abortion Games," 969.

78. Ingram, "Abortion Games," 970.

79. Ingram, "Abortion Games," 970.

80. Ingram, "Abortion Games," 970.

81. Myre Sim, "Abortion and the Psychiatrist," *British Medical Journal* 2, no. 5350 (1963): 148.

82. Ingram, "Abortion Games," 970.

83. Public General Statutes, Elizabeth II, CH. 87.

84. "The Royal College of Psychiatrists' Memorandum on the Abortion Act in Practice," *British Journal of Psychiatry* 120, no. 557 (April 1972): 449.

85. Kandiah and Staerck, *The Abortion Act, 1967*, 50.

86. Ingram, "Abortion Games," 970.

87. Ingram, "Abortion Games," 970.

88. Baird, "The Abortion Act 1967," 293; Jean Aitken-Swan, *Fertility Control and the Medical Profession* (London: Croom Helm, 1977), 11.

89. *Report of the Committee on the Working of the Abortion Act, Volume 1*, 184.

90. *Report of the Committee on the Working of the Abortion Act, Volume 1*, 186–88.

91. David Steel, "I Introduced the Abortion Act 50 Years Ago This Week: This Is Why It Now Needs Extending," *Independent*, October 26, 2017.

92. See, for example, Denis Campbell, "Abortion Should Not Be a Crime, Say Britain's Childbirth Doctors," *Guardian*, September 22, 2017.

93. See, for example, "British Women are Ordering Abortion Pills Online Due to Difficulty Accessing Clinics," *Debrief*, September 21, 2017, https://thedebrief.co.uk/news/real-life/british-women-using-abortion-pills-due-difficulty-accessing-clinics/.

94. Libby Brooks, "Women in Scotland Will Be Allowed to Take Abortion Pill at Home," *Guardian*, October 26, 2017.

95. Most significantly, it was recommended that the requirement for two doctors' signatures be removed. See House of Commons Science and Technology Committee, "Scientific Developments Relating to the Abortion Act, 1967," 55.

96. Brooks, "Women in Scotland."

[5]

A Double Movement

The Politics of Reproductive Mobility in Ireland

MARY GILMARTIN AND SINÉAD KENNEDY

IN NOVEMBER 2013, the British Pregnancy Advisory Service took out an advertisement in the *Irish Times*, a daily newspaper in the Republic of Ireland (hereafter Ireland). The full text reads as follows: "As if deciding to have an abortion wasn't enough of a journey almost 4,000 Irish women have to travel to Britain for help every year. We'll care for your women until your government does."[1] The advertisement, predictably, was controversial in Ireland because it highlighted the ongoing reality of crisis pregnancies. It also explicitly addressed the ongoing movement of women from Ireland in order to access abortion services, because those services are unavailable in Ireland.

Abortion is one of a number of reproduction-related services that women, in many parts of the world, have to travel to access. Like others, we have difficulties with the use of the term "abortion tourism" to describe such travel.[2] We argue that the word "tourism," when used to describe women's travel for the purposes of accessing abortion services, or any other reproduction-related services, both trivializes the experience and ignores the broader structures that make such travel necessary. From our perspective, our term "reproductive mobility" is more appropriate. The "mobility turn" in the social sciences has directed our attention to the complexity of contemporary human and technological movement.[3] It has also highlighted the importance of immobility. The term "mobility" thus captures both movement and "stuckness," meaning the ways in which movement occurs and the attempts to regulate or prevent it.[4] In this chapter, our focus is on what we describe as "reproductive mobility," including travel for the purposes of accessing reproductive services, as well as the conditions that both enable and restrict this travel. The concept of reproductive mobility thus includes not only individual actions but also the broader context for those actions. We insist on the use of "reproductive mobility" as a term rather than focusing solely on travel for abortion services. As we show in this chapter, the specific context of Ireland clearly illustrates that the issue of accessing abortion services needs to be understood in conjunction with, rather than separate from, other reproduction-related services. This is because in Ireland, reproductive mobility, including both movement and stuckness, is used to regulate and discipline the act of reproduction, particularly as embodied in women's fertility. Reproductive mobility becomes a means of fixing fertility: dealing with, sorting out, and putting it right.

In this chapter, we discuss the politics of reproductive mobility in Ireland. We begin with an overview of the different forms of reproductive mobility that exist. This includes travel for the purposes of accessing abortion services, most often to Britain, but also includes a range of other types of reproductive mobility such as internal and international mobility during pregnancy or for childbirth. These different forms of reproductive mobility must be understood as attempts to discipline women's bodies and women's fertility in Ireland. We then discuss the act of disciplining in more detail, showing how women's reproductive mobility has been restricted through bans on travel, information, and immigration. However, reproductive mobility has also been a site of political protest, and this is our focus in the next section, where we reclaim reproductive mobility. The chapter concludes with a broader discussion of the politics of reproductive mobility in Ireland and beyond.

Reproductive Mobility in Ireland

Mobility has long been a way of dealing with problematic fertility in Ireland. From the early years following the foundation of the Irish Free State (1922), the state, in alliance with the Catholic Church, sought to restrict or prevent women's reproductive mobility as a means of regulating and disciplining female fertility. The 1937 Irish Constitution, authored by Ireland's founding patriarchs Éamon de Valera and Archbishop John Charles McQuaid, created a privileged position for heterosexual marriage and the family: "The State pledges itself to guard with special care the institution of Marriage, on which the Family is founded and to protect it against attack." The family imagined in this document is thus highly gendered, with the "special" role of "mothers" within the private home also elevated as an ideal: "The State shall, therefore, endeavour to ensure that mothers shall not be obliged by economic necessity to engage in labour to the neglect of their duties in the home."[5] The maintenance of this conservative ideal of motherhood required the regulation and control of women's reproductive capacity, a matter raised repeatedly in this volume by several authors, regardless of the era, region, or government involved.

For women who became pregnant outside marriage, regulation and control took a variety of forms. The first form of reproductive mobility was, in effect, a form of enforced immobility, as women were removed from their family homes and incarcerated in institutions for the duration of their pregnancy or, in some instances, for significantly longer. Following the report of the Commission on Relief of the Sick and Destitute Poor in 1927, a network of institutions—which included mother and baby homes, county homes, industrial and reformatory schools, and Magdelene asylums—were used to deal with women who were perceived to have transgressed sexual norms.[6] There was a hierarchy of institutions, with mother and baby homes used for women from well-off families who were pregnant for the first time and Magdalene asylums used to incarcerate poor women and women with more than one pregnancy, who were then forced to work in associated laundries. Many women never left the Magdalene asylums.[7] Those women were forced internal migrants, exiled from their homes and coerced to give up their children. In turn, many of those children were exported, with thousands sent to the United States of America (USA) from the early 1940s to the mid-1960s through an informal (and possibly illegal) overseas adoption scheme.[8] The Adoption Board, as the Adoption Authority of Ireland used to be known, signed off on more than 40,000 adoptions in Ireland since 1952.[9] More precise figures are difficult to attain. Mike Milotte, an investigative journalist who has researched the Irish "baby black market," found that in many cases birth certificates were altered, and the names of the adopted parents were recorded, rather than those of the birth mothers. The Irish State refers to adoptions based on this practice of falsified birth records as "informal adoption," a term that angers victims of these practices because it contributes to the idea that no crime was committed. The vast majority of these adoptions were arranged by religious-run adoption societies—in most cases closely aligned with mother and baby homes, such as the Bon Secours Mother and Baby Home in Tuam, County Galway, which are the subject of an ongoing official Commission of Investigation.[10]

Not all women who became pregnant were institutionalized. The second form of reproductive mobility was the migration, either on a temporary or permanent basis, of Irish pregnant women to Britain. As Lindsey Earner-Byrne writes, "Irish expectant single mothers emigrated to Britain in significant numbers during the twentieth century."[11] While the numbers are difficult to estimate, there are snapshots of the scale of this reproductive mobility. For example, Mary Daly reports that 1,693 pregnant Irish women applied for assistance from the Westminster Crusade of Rescue, in London, between 1950 and 1953, and Paul Michael Garrett comments that the acronym PFI (pregnant from Ireland) was "part of the everyday vocabulary of the social workers who dealt with unmarried mothers arriving from Ireland."[12] There were some attempts to repatriate Irish women prior to or immediately after giving birth, but these attempts were often resisted by women who wanted to avoid institutionalization in Ireland.[13]

The introduction of the 1967 British Abortion Act made a third form of reproductive mobility possible, although Irish women did travel to Britain for abortions before 1967.[14] Irish women, along with nonresident women of other nationalities, as examined by Christabelle Sethna in this volume, traveled to Britain after 1967 for abortion services, long before the medical migrants of the 1990s undertook their journeys. After 1967, the migration of Irish women for the purposes of giving birth was largely replaced by the shorter-term mobility of women in order to access legal abortion services in Britain, traveling mainly to the English cities of Liverpool and London. While statistics are incomplete, Diane Munday et al. estimated that, in the period from 1968 to 1989, 50,000 women from Ireland traveled to Britain for abortions.[15] From 1990 to 2014, the total figure was around 125,000.[16] Of course, these figures are incomplete, because they include only those women who gave an Irish address to the clinic where they were treated. The actual figure is likely to be higher. The future of these Irish journeys may or may not be immediately affected by the results of the May 2018 referendum on abortion that was introduced by Taoiseach Leo Varadkar, or even by the ongoing Brexit negotiations, about which Niklas Barke speculates in this volume.

The availability of legalized abortion coincided with a drop in the number of PFIs in Britain, suggesting that many women—when given the option—chose termination over giving birth. However, they had to engage in mobility practices to do so: leaving Ireland, traveling to Britain for a short stay, and then returning to Ireland. In many instances, Irish women remained silent about their choices, though this is now beginning to change.[17] Until recently, the experiences of women who traveled abroad for abortions were largely hidden and ignored. However, one of the many contradictions in Ireland's abortion laws is that reproductive mobility is assumed, and indeed expected. Similarly, Cathrine Chambers, Colleen MacQuarrie, and Jo-Ann MacDonald in their contribution to this volume observe that although travel for abortion services was an open secret for decades in Prince Edward Island (PEI), Canada, women maintained their silence about their off-island abortions.

Restricting Reproductive Mobility

Voluntary and involuntary mobility has long been a way of dealing with and disciplining problematic fertility in Ireland, but so too is the restriction of women's reproductive mobility. First, Ireland had a constitutional prohibition on abortion—Article 40.3.3 of the Irish constitution—that presupposed and simultaneously limited reproductive mobility. Abortion has been illegal in Ireland since the introduction of the Offences against the Persons Act in 1861. This prohibition was incorporated into Irish law and extended to a constitutional ban in 1983, when, following a referendum, the Irish constitution was altered to include a guarantee of life for the "unborn." This ban, known as the Eighth Amendment, has placed serious restrictions on women's reproductive mobility. Despite these laws, as we discussed earlier, significant numbers of women living in Ireland travel abroad to obtain abortions, that is, of course, when mobility is possible. In 1992, the Irish State attempted to prevent a 14-year-old girl who had been raped from having an abortion in Britain by obtaining a legal injunction from the High Court against the young girl and her parents, which prevented them from leaving the state. The judge, Justice Costello, in granting the injunction, held that Ms. X's right to travel had to give way to the right to life of the unborn.[18] The injunction was eventually overturned by the Supreme Court in Ireland, where three of its five judges ruled that a woman had a right to an abortion to save her life, either in Ireland or abroad. However, in a nonbinding aspect of the judgment, three out of five of the judges maintained that the state is entitled to prevent a pregnant woman from traveling abroad for an abortion, illustrating, as James Kingston argues, that Article 40.3.3 "did require the State to provide protection of the right to life of the unborn by ensuring that pregnant women did not travel out of the jurisdiction."[19]

Since the judgment could represent a "potential restriction on a woman's freedom of movement," a referendum was held on the issue in November 1992.[20] The result was that the electorate voted to guarantee a woman's freedom to travel, which includes the freedom—though not the right—to travel abroad for an abortion. If women had the right to travel, it would place a positive obligation on the state to ensure that women had the ability to travel; freedom to travel only ensures that the state cannot act to prevent travel. While that freedom is mostly upheld, there are occasional attempts to restrict it, such as the 1997 case of Ms. D., who was 17 years of age and in state care. Ms. D was four months pregnant with a diagnosis of fatal fetal abnormality. The Health Service Executive prevented her from leaving the country for an abortion, and she had to appeal this decision to the High Court in order to be able to travel.[21] More recently, in 2014, Ms. Y, an asylum seeker, was prevented from leaving Ireland in order to access an abortion and was forced to carry the pregnancy to term and give birth to the child, which was then placed in the care of the state.[22] The case of Ms. Y is also important because it highlights the ways in which many migrant women currently living in Ireland, in particular asylum seekers who can be forced to wait more than a decade to have their migrant status regularized, do not have freedom to travel because of their visa status and so are unable to access abortion services in Britain or elsewhere.[23] Their reproductive mobility continues to be restricted, and largely unacknowledged.

Both the Ms. D and Ms. Y cases also show how attempts to restrict mobility are most acutely experienced by the most vulnerable members of society. As addressed by Lori A. Brown in this volume, the reproductive mobility of undocumented migrants, poor women, rural women, and Latina and Hispanic women in Texas, many of whom occupy each of these categories at once, is also precarious when it comes to accessing abortion services. And in their contribution to this volume, Cathrine Chambers, Colleen MacQuarrie, and Jo-Ann MacDonald show that while those women unable to afford the costs of a journey from PEI to neighboring provinces might attempt to self-induce an abortion, or end up carrying an unwanted pregnancy to term, the authors label all women who travel considerable distances to secure abortion services "abortion refugees."

The second explicit attempt to restrict women's reproductive mobility relates to immigration. Growing levels of immigration to Ireland, from the 1990s on, led to a moral panic about so-called citizenship tourists, meaning migrant women giving birth in Ireland in order to secure Irish citizenship for their child and, by association, for the wider family. Media and other reports highlighted this racialized so-called crisis, with dramatic stories of pregnant migrant women of color arriving directly from the airport, ready to give birth.[24] These resemble the lurid newspaper accounts denigrating the travel of nonresident women to Britain for abortions in the 1960s and 1970s, as Christabelle Sethna points out in this volume. Stories of what is sometimes called "birth tourism" claimed that the number of pregnant migrant women placed an undue burden on Ireland's maternity services, put the women themselves at risk, and, in turn, posed a threat to Irish society. In response to this moral panic, the 2004 Citizenship Referendum changed the basis of Irish citizenship. Prior to the referendum, anyone born in Ireland was an Irish citizen; afterward, birthright citizenship was no longer guaranteed, and citizenship is now granted on the basis of descent.[25] The symbolic importance of this referendum, in a discussion of reproductive mobility, is to show how mobile pregnant women—whether leaving or coming to Ireland—continue to be constructed as a problem that needs to be fixed.

A third explicit attempt to restrict and control women's reproductive mobility involves the regulation of abortion information. Following the introduction of the constitutional prohibition on abortion in 1983, anti-abortion activists began targeting groups and organizations that provided women with information about abortion clinics in Britain. One of the explicit aims of the Society for the Protection of Unborn Children (SPUC) in Ireland in the aftermath of the 1983 amendment was to prevent women from accessing information about traveling to Britain for abortion services. SPUC set about closing Irish counseling agencies that referred women, securing injunctions in October 1986 against Open Door Counselling as well as the Well Woman Centre. In December 1986, High Court justice Hamilton ruled that it was now illegal in Ireland to provide information that would facilitate abortions in Britain. The agencies appealed the High Court judgment to the Supreme Court, but their appeal was rejected on the grounds that "there could not be an implied and unenumerated constitutional right to information about the availability of a service of abortion outside the state, which, if availed of, would have the direct consequence of destroying the expressly guaranteed constitutional right to life of the unborn." It is notable that before widespread internet access, restriction of information was a serious obstacle to women accessing abortion. Women's magazines such as *Cosmopolitan* and *Company* had to publish special Irish editions of their magazines without the pages of addresses of abortion clinics.[26] An edition of the *Guardian* newspaper that contained information on abortion was seized from the Belfast-Dublin train and taken to a nearby police station because it contained an advertisement for a clinic that performed abortions. Books on women's health were also removed from libraries and bookshops under the 1967 Censorship of Publications Act.[27] In 1988, on the strength of the Hamilton judgment, SPUC obtained an injunction against three student unions for publishing the addresses and phone numbers of British abortion clinics in their student handbooks. This potential restriction on a woman's freedom of movement gave rise to what Siobhán Mullally described as "the spectre of anti-abortion groups seeking injunctions to restrain pregnant women from traveling abroad," provoking "widespread protest."[28]

In Ireland, therefore, reproductive mobility has long been used as a way of dealing with unwanted fertility, for individuals, for families, and for society in general. Despite the clear usefulness of reproductive mobility for fixing problematic fertility, there is also a visible double movement that attempts to regulate access to reproductive mobility. This is most obvious in the various efforts to restrict access to abortion and information on abortion. It is important, however, not just to frame reproductive mobility as an action that is managed and controlled by the Irish State. Instead, as we argue in the next section, reproductive mobility is also a site of political protest and action.

Reclaiming Reproductive Mobility

Abortion rights activists have sought to exploit reproductive mobility for positive political change, highlighting the hypocrisy inherent in enforced and restricted mobility. One of the challenges in exploring activism around reproductive rights is that the history of this struggle is, albeit with some notable exceptions, largely unexplored.[29] In this volume, activism around reproductive rights is a salient aspect of Christabelle Sethna's chapter on Britain and Hayley Brown's chapter on New Zealand. The efforts of the PEI Reproductive Rights Organization, Abortion Access Now PEI, and the Women's Legal Education and Action Fund play a prominent role in the chapter by Cathrine Chambers, Colleen MacQuarrie, and Jo-Ann MacDonald on bringing abortion services to PEI. Additionally, authors Agata Ignaciuk, Anna Bogic, and Ewelina Ciaputa each showcase in their contributions to this volume the ways in which reproductive rights organizations, feminist groups, nonprofit abortion referral agencies, and the assistance of doctors and lawyers have been major actors facilitating access to information about abortion, as well as access to abortion services inside and outside Spain, the former Yugoslavia (and later, Serbia), and Poland, respectively.

In Ireland, the 2014 *Women to Blame* exhibition was an explicit attempt by activists to construct and preserve their own history. The exhibition visually represented the events before, during, and after the Eighth Amendment referendum, when Article 40.3.3. was inserted into the Irish Constitution.[30] The filmmaker, Cathal Black, who produced and directed a short film on the Irish Women's Liberation Movement (IWLM), tried unsuccessfully to produce a documentary on second-wave feminism in Ireland. He met Máirín De Búrca, a founding member of the IWLM, who asked him: "Why has no one done this before? We'll all be dead by the time they get around to talking to us about one of the most successful political movements in modern Irish history—its legacy is still being felt today."[31] Therese Caherty, one of the exhibition's curators, writes that *Women to Blame* was an attempt to bring together the scattered and fragmented story of the struggle for reproductive rights in Ireland. The exhibition demonstrates how "different generations of women [took] opportunities to express themselves on their right to bodily autonomy and to have reproductive justice. Their actions have ranged from actions of defiance, protesting censorship, innumerable court cases across Europe, to campaigns on five referendums."[32] Here, we highlight the relationship between reproductive rights activism and the Irish experience of migration, where activists draw on experiences of diaspora and exile to show the connections between forced migration and enforced reproductive mobility. We also show the explicit acts of defiance that make specific use of mobility in order to reclaim reproductive rights, while drawing attention to restrictions on and limits to reproductive mobility for women in Ireland.

Ireland has a long and sustained history of migration, and these experiences of exodus are woven deep, in often painful ways, into the Irish imagination. Reproductive rights activism in Ireland—from the 1971 Contraceptive Train to the 2014 Abortion Pill Train and the 2015 Abortion Pill Bus[33]—has repeatedly drawn on this migrant experience, highlighting the hypocrisy of enabling women to leave the state to access an abortion while criminalizing the same activity if done within the borders of the Irish State. These themes of mobility, exile, diaspora, and state hypocrisy have been central to women's reproductive rights activism. Medb Ruane writes, "Irish women's journeys have been part of Irish life for centuries. Mapping their stories engages the present with histories and biographies Ireland used to find it easier to ignore. Women travelled as domestic servants, nuns, farm workers, planters, breeding stock. Women today travel out of Ireland in search of an outcome their society refuses to face. The experience of abortion represents modern Ireland's hidden Diaspora."[34] By invoking these themes, activists hope to engage with the history of Ireland's other forced journeys and enable a confrontation with the reality of Ireland's anti-abortion regime.

The 1971 Contraceptive Train has become a model for much abortion rights activism in Ireland. Considered a failure by many of the activists who participated in the action at the time, it has, over time, acquired a significant place in the popular imagination and is now regarded as a key event in the history of reproductive rights struggle in Ireland and recently inspired a successful work of "political musical theatre," *The Train*, presented during the 2015 Dublin Theatre Festival.[35] The Contraceptive Train was organized originally by members of the IWLM who, following a packed meeting in Dublin's Mansion House in April 1971, identified access to contraceptives as a central issue for women's liberation.[36] Subsequently, the IWLM, supported by other women, staged the Contraceptive Train on May 22, 1971, by traveling via train to Belfast in order to purchase contraceptives, the sale, import, and advertisement of which was banned in Ireland since 1935. Upon their return to Connolly Train Station in Dublin, they collectively marched past Irish customs officers, chanting and waving banners. The protest created enormous media attention, both nationally and internationally, putting the issue of contraception firmly on the political agenda.[37]

However, this form of direct action, then and now, was not without controversy, creating a divide within the women's movement that is present today. In her work on the Irish women's movement, Linda Connolly suggests: "The direct action tactics of the movement had both a positive and negative effect. . . . A core faction subsequently diverted their energies and mobilized direct action through the provision of services for women. Others were more political and maintained their radical commitments through involvement specific campaigns. . . . In the process, however, more moderate activists both within the original group [IWLM] and in women's rights organizations were alienated."[38] Nevertheless, this form of action inspired several generations of activists who continue to invoke the specter of the Contraceptive Train in their actions. In October 2014, activists organized the Abortion Pill Train, this time traveling to Belfast in Northern Ireland to obtain abortion pills.[39] Activists returned to Connolly Train Station, where they recreated the 1971 iconic image of women marching through the station, chanting, this time waving packets of abortion pills. A small number of activists then took the abortion pills, a criminal offense carrying a prison sentence of up to 14 years, challenging the Irish State to prosecute them.[40] While the abortion pill is illegal, its availability through websites such as womenonweb.org and womenhelp.org has been a major step forward for women, allowing them to challenge mobility restrictions and have medical rather than surgical abortions within Ireland. Increasingly, medical abortion is where abortion activists worldwide are putting their emphasis. It is a much safer, simpler, and less invasive procedure, physically similar to miscarriage. More importantly, it removes control from the medical profession and the lawmakers, who all too frequently act as gatekeepers, and instead returns management of the process to women themselves. The Abortion Pill Train also served to highlight the difficulties that women living in Northern Ireland experience. The 1967 Abortion Act has never been extended to Northern Ireland, forcing women in the North to travel to Britain to access abortions. In June 2017, the British government agreed to fund women from Northern Ireland to access abortions in Britain via the NHS.[41] This is an important step forward, although it fails to address the financial and travel burdens that women living in the North experience.

Abortion activists have also frequently recreated the journeys that Irish women make to abortion services in Britain, drawing on the symbolic value of this journey of enforced temporary exile. In the months following the X case of 1992, more than 200 women under the auspices of the Women's Coalition Group took the boat from Dún Laoghaire to Holyhead in Wales and back, on the main sea route between Ireland and Britain. Their stated aim was to "stand with the women who make the lonely and often fearful decision to take the boat" to get an abortion in Britain.[42] The journey deliberately invoked the spirit of the 1971 Contraceptive Train, with women returning with the names, addresses, and telephone numbers of British abortion clinics, information then illegal under Irish abortion law. They released, upon their return from Holyhead, balloons with the number of an Irish helpline that would give women information about abortion clinics in Britain. The action was also designed to highlight the injunction issued by the Irish State against Ms. X to prevent her traveling out of Ireland to access an abortion. Ursula Barry, one of the coalition's spokespeople, said that women must "show our determination that never again will any woman be held against her will on this island because she is pregnant."[43]

During the 2002 referendum campaign, activists staged a number of silent protests across the city and outside Leinster House, the Irish Parliament, with participants wearing white T-shirts imprinted with a black letter *X*, black eye masks, and black mouth gags in memory of Ms. X and the thousands of anonymous Irish women who travel for abortions.[44] These themes have been taken up again, more recently, through the work of the Abortion Rights Campaign (ARC), which has consistently highlighted the necessity of women's mobility, should they need to access abortion services.[45] In their publicity during the run-up to the 2014 annual March for Choice, the ARC requested members of the public to bring a wheelie suitcase to the march to signify "the 12 women who travel from Ireland for abortions each day."[46] The suitcases made a strong audiovisual impact as the participants rolled them along the streets and roads of Dublin's city center. This mobility theme was extended into a postmarch event held in Filmbase in Dublin's Temple Bar. Following the march, participants could avail of a "baggage drop" for their suitcase and then proceed to the "check-in desk," where they were invited to "register" by signing a petition calling for the repeal of the Eighth Amendment. A sign marked "Departures" listed the typical destinations that pregnant women travel to access abortion services outside Ireland, such as London and Liverpool. Actors dressed as customs officials "patrolled" the event, and attendees were encouraged to enter into the "baggage scanner," or print workshop. In the workshop, participants could make cards in the shape of suitcases, which were then displayed in a gallery made to resemble an airport luggage belt.[47]

A 1992 referendum gave women a constitutional right to travel abroad for an abortion, and the introduction of the Regulation of Information Act (1995) eased, without fully eliminating, restrictions on abortion information. The 1995 act allows doctors, advisory agencies, and individual counselors to give information on abortion services abroad, should a woman request it.[48] These changes allowed abortion activists to shift focus and concentrate on questions of access. One of the most ambitious activities undertaken by Irish abortion rights campaigners was the 2001 "Abortion Ship." It would highlight the hypocrisy of the Irish abortion situation, build coalitions for legislative reform, and catalyze efforts to liberalize the abortion law. In the summer of 2000, Dublin-based abortion activists and the Cork Women's Right to Choose group invited the Dutch charity Women on Waves (WOW) to bring its ship to Ireland. WOW has also been active in Poland, as Ewelina Ciaputa indicates in this volume. Reproductive health services, including the abortion pill, would be provided on the ship. The ship would travel to Dublin and Cork, meet women from Ireland, and then sail outside Ireland's territorial waters, where Dutch law would apply (medical and surgical abortions are legal in the Netherlands) and medical abortions would be provided. More than 300 women contacted the ship's hotline, including women who had been raped, teenagers who could not find a feasible excuse to travel to Britain for a couple of days, mothers who could not pay for childcare during their journey, and asylum seekers who did not have the necessary papers to travel.[49] While the ship was unable to offer abortions after the Dutch authorities denied the ship a license on its way to Ireland, the journey was a success, not least because it highlighted the extensive class differences between women able to access abortion abroad and those who lack the ability and financial means to travel.

A similar event was organized by the feminist group ROSA in conjunction with Women on Web in October 2015, this time using a bus to travel to Galway, Cork, and Dublin to help women access the abortion pill.[50] This action helped more than 30 women directly and distributed illegal information about the availability of the abortion pill across the country.[51] While the state has shown little willingness to confront the illegality of these actions and prosecute activists, the threat of criminalization continues to produce, in the words of the European Court of Human Rights, a "chilling effect" on women and doctors. These illegal or quasi-legal acts, which have formed the basis of women's activism in

Ireland, have played a significant role in abortion rights activism in Ireland, not only because they explicitly challenge and break anti-abortion laws but because, as Mairéad Enright argues, they reveal the "spaces in which they are already broken: in which they are porous, not enforced, practically or politically unenforceable, or just about surmountable if you have the resources, the courage, the knowledge and the time."[52]

The London-based direct action, feminist performance, and protest group Speaking of IMELDA also references earlier forms of abortion activism but adopts a more mocking, satirical, and provocative tone. The group's name IMELDA—Ireland Making England the Legal Destination for Abortion—was a code word for abortion used by the 1980s Irish Women's Abortion Support Group (IWASG). The IWASG provided practical support for women traveling to access abortion services, work that is continued today by the Abortion Support Network.[53] The code word was necessary to protect women's confidentiality in the 1980s, when access to abortion information was restricted.[54] Speaking of IMELDA weaves the experiences of women's reproductive mobility into bold pieces of performance art, such as wheeling suitcases through the crowds at the 2014 St. Patrick's Day parade in London, asking members of the public for directions to an abortion clinic, or chanting "twelve women a day" when presenting a pair of women's underpants to Taoiseach Enda Kenny at a 2013 formal dinner celebrating Irish emigrants based in London. Similar to Irish women's early activism on contraception, these kinds of political protest engage in direct actions that challenge or disrupt the political status quo and the government's official discourse of abortion law reform.

The political effectiveness of these forms of activism highlighting the political and social hypocrisy that make women's reproductive mobility necessary was confirmed by the political process[55] that led to the Irish government's announcement in January 2018 that a referendum would be held in the summer of 2018 to remove Ireland's constitutional prohibition on abortion and allow for the introduction of legislation permitting more liberal abortion access, including abortion on request up to 12 weeks.[56] What was most notable about the political processes that led to this announcement was the inclusion of women's narratives of reproductive mobility within the mainstream discussion. This represented a marked contrast to previous abortion debates in Ireland, all of which may be characterized by a failure to include the voices of women who have traveled in order to access abortion care. When the Irish Parliament debated, in January 2018, the recommendation by the All-Party Oireachtas (Parliamentary) Committee that abortion reform was urgently required, many of the politicians who spoke during the debate described how hearing the stories of women who had traveled abroad for abortion care caused them to rethink their opposition to abortion reform in Ireland. Taoiseach Leo Varadkar, the first openly gay prime minister in Irish history, who supported a successful 2015 referendum to legalize gay marriage, had previously declared himself against abortion. However, when calling for a 2018 referendum to repeal the Eighth Amendment, he described his own change of views and concluded his public statement with the following remarks: "In recent weeks many people, mainly men, have spoken about the personal journeys they have been on. But we should remember that the saddest and loneliest journey is made by the Irish women who travel to other countries in their thousands to end their pregnancies. These journeys do not have to happen, and that can change. That's now in our hands."[57] This was the first time in the history of the Irish State that a prime minister had publicly supported the need for abortion access within Ireland and self-consciously attributed his change of position as a direct result of listening to women. In the subsequent campaign leading up to the referendum on May 25, 2018, the issue of travel was central. Together for Yes, the coalition group established to mobilize for a "Yes" vote in the referendum, emphasized the importance of women having access to healthcare in Ireland as a key campaign message. More directly, campaign posters from the left-wing Workers' Party starkly said, "End Forced Travel." The implications of the referendum for abortion travel concerning women from Ireland and Northern Ireland are explored further by Niklas Barke in his contribution to this volume.

Conclusion

In this chapter, we have argued that the concept of reproductive mobility, which includes travel to access abortion and other reproduction-related services, travel for the purposes of giving birth, and efforts to restrict such travel, offers a better insight into the experience that is described as "abortion tourism" elsewhere. As shown through the example of Ireland, reproductive mobility exposes the wider ideological issues associated with women's bodies and fertility as well as with travel and movement. Abortion, as one form of reproductive mobility, illustrates this clearly. As abortion is illegal in Ireland in almost all circumstances, except where there is a risk to the life of the pregnant woman, repro-ductive mobility is used as a way of managing unwanted pregnancy and, occasionally, problematic pregnancy (e.g., pregnancies that pose serious health risks or cases of fatal fetal anomalies). However, despite the de-monstrable need for this reproductive mobility, the Irish State has re-peatedly sought to control this mobility by restricting not only access to abortion services but also access to abortion information and, on oc-casion, to the right to travel. We argue that reproductive mobility for the purposes of accessing abortion services must be understood as part of a longer historical practice in Ireland. Historical forms of reproduc-tive mobility included the enforced mobility of pregnant women to religious-run mother and baby homes or Magdalene asylums, or the more voluntary mobility of temporary exile to Britain for the purposes of giving birth. In contemporary Ireland, the Irish State intervenes to restrict reproductive mobility by trying to control abortion information or travel, or by imposing immigration restrictions to protect pregnant women and fetal life.

The regulation of reproductive mobility has a deep resonance with contemporary attempts to fix mobility, such that the mobility of certain people is constructed as a problem that must be contained. This involves the control not just of territorial borders but also of the borders between citizen and migrant, "them" and "us." However, we equally show that reproductive mobility is also a contested space; it is a site of conflict, action, and potential political transformation. Irish abortion activists and campaigners have long exploited the political potentialities inher-ent in reproductive mobility, highlighting the hypocrisies and vulnera-bilities inherent in the various attempts by the Irish State to regulate and control women's fertility and mobility. We explored the various forms of activism that campaigners have engaged in over the past 40 years, arguing that the connections they have exploited between Irish narra-tives of migration and reproductive mobility reveal the limits and double standards inherent in reproductive mobility and attempts to control it. The regulation of reproductive mobility occurs at international, national, and local scales, from legislation with national or international reach to the embodied and everyday practices of individual women. Our empha-sis on reproductive mobility—which is material and symbolic, individual and collective—shows the double movement involved in fixing women's fertility and the activist spaces that open up for change and transformation. These spaces came into sharp focus with the result of the most recent referendum, when 66.4 percent voted to remove the Eighth Amendment from the Irish Constitution, thus creating the possibility of legislating for the provision of abortion care in Ireland. Until legislation is passed, women in Ireland continue to require reproductive mobility in order to access abortion services, and the nature of their future access—and potential limits to that access—remains unclear.

Notes

1. Christina Finn, "Pro Life Groups Call BPAS Advert in Irish Newspaper Today 'Disgusting' and 'Callous,'" *thejournal.ie*, November 2, 2013, http://www .thejournal.ie/pro-life-campain-irish-times-advert-abortion-bpas-1158046 -Nov2013/.

2. Sven Bergmann, "Fertility Tourism: Circumventive Routes That Enable Access to Reproductive Technologies and Substances," *Signs* 36, no. 2 (2011): 280–89.

3. Thomas Faist, "The Mobility Turn: A New Paradigm for the Social Sciences?," *Ethnic and Racial Studies* 36, no. 11 (2013): 1637–46.

4. Tim Cresswell, "Mobilities II: Still," *Progress in Human Geography* 36, no. 5 (2012): 649–50.

5. Dermot Keogh, "The Catholic Church and the Writing of the 1937 Constitution," *History Ireland* 13, no. 3 (2005): http://www.historyireland.com /20th-century-contemporary-history/the-catholic-church-and-the-writing-of-the -1937-constitution/.

6. Úna Crowley and Rob Kitchin, "Producing 'Decent Girls': Governmentality and the Moral Geographies of Sexual Conduct in Ireland (1922–1937)," *Gender, Place and Culture* 15, no. 4 (2008): 364.

7. Crowley and Kitchin, "Producing 'Decent Girls,'" 367.

8. Moira J. Maguire, "Foreign Adoptions and the Evolution of Irish Adoption Policy, 1945–52," *Journal of Social History* 36, no. 2 (2002): 387.

9. Mike Milotte, *Banished Babies: The Secret History of Ireland's Baby Export Business*, 2nd ed. (Dublin: New Island Books, 2012), 7.

10. The work of the Mother and Baby Homes Commission of Investigation remains ongoing. Its final report is due to be delivered on February 17, 2019. See the commission's website for more information: http://www.mbhcoi.ie/.

11. Lindsey Earner-Byrne, "'Moral Repatriation': The Response to Irish Unmarried Mothers in Britain, 1920s-1960s," in *To and from Ireland: Planned Migration Schemes c.1600–2000*, ed. Patrick J. Duffy (Dublin: Geography Publications, 2004), 155.

12. Mary E. Daly, *The Slow Failure: Population Decline and Independent Ireland, 1920–1973* (Madison: University of Wisconsin Press, 2006), 288; Paul Michael Garrett, "The Hidden History of the PFIs: The Repatriation of Unmarried Mothers and Their Children from England to Ireland in the 1950s and 1960s," *Immigrants and Minorities* 19, no. 3 (2000): 26.

13. Garrett, "The Hidden History"; Earner-Byrne, "Moral Repatriation."

14. Sandra McAvoy, "Before Cadden: Abortion in Mid-Twentieth-Century Ireland," in *The Lost Decade: Ireland in the 1950s*, ed. Dermot Keogh, Finbarr O'Shea, and Carmel Quinlan (Cork: Mercier, 2004), 147–63.

15. Diane Munday, Colin Francome, and Wendy Savage, "Twenty One Years of Legal Abortion," *British Medical Journal* 298, no. 6682 (May 1989): 1231.

16. "Abortion in Ireland: Statistics," Irish Family Planning Association, accessed October 31, 2015, https://www.ifpa.ie/Hot-Topics/Abortion/Statistics.

17. Ruth Fletcher, "Silences: Irish Women and Abortion," *Feminist Review* 50, no. 1 (1995): 44–66; Aideen Quilty, Sinéad Kennedy, and Catherine Conlon, eds., *The Abortion Papers Ireland, Volume II* (Cork: Cork University Press, 2015).

18. Sunniva McDonagh, *The Attorney General v. X and Others: Judgments of the High Court and Supreme Court. Legal Submissions Made to the Supreme Court* (Dublin: Dublin Incorporated Council of Law Reporting for Ireland, 1992).

19. James Kingston, *The Need for Abortion Reform in Ireland: The Case against the Twenty-Fifth Amendment of the Constitution Bill, 2001* (Dublin: Irish Council for Civil Liberties, 2001), 31.

20. Siobhán Mullally, "Debating Reproductive Rights in Ireland," *Human Rights Quarterly* 27, no. 1 (February 2005): 93.

21. Sinéad Kennedy and Mary Gilmartin, "Mobility, Migrants and Abortion in Ireland," in *Troubled Waters: Abortion in Ireland, Northern Ireland and Prince Edward Island*, ed. Colleen MacQuarrie, Claire Pierson, Shannon Stettner, and Fiona Bloomer (Charlottetown, PEI: Island Studies Press, 2018.

22. Kitty Holland, "Timeline of Ms Y Case," *Irish Times*, October 4, 2014, https://www.irishtimes.com/news/social-affairs/timeline-of-ms-y-case-1 .1951699.

23. Ronit Lentin, "After Savita: Migrant M/others and the Politics of Birth in Ireland," in *The Abortion Papers Ireland, Volume 2*, ed. Aideen Quilty, Sinéad Kennedy, and Catherine Conlon (Cork: Cork University Press, 2015), 179–89.

24. Ronit Lentin, "Strangers and Strollers: Feminist Notes on Researching Migrant M/others," *Women's Studies International Forum* 27, no. 4 (2004): 301–14.

25. Mary Gilmartin, *Ireland and Migration in the Twenty-First Century* (Manchester: Manchester University Press, 2015), 133.

26. Chrystel Hug, *The Politics of Sexual Morality in Ireland* (London: Macmillan, 1999), 158.

27. Under the Censorship of Publications Act (1967), books can be banned for two different reasons in Ireland: for being indecent or obscene, or for advocating the procurement of abortion or miscarriage (or the use of any method, treatment, or appliance for the purpose of procuring an abortion). As of the time of this writing, only one book has been banned for being indecent or obscene (Jean Martin's *The Raped Little Runaway* was banned in March 2016 for its graphic description of child rape), and eight books have been banned in Ireland for providing information on how to procure an abortion. Three of the books are explicitly about abortion: *Abortion Internationally* (banned since 1983), *Abortion: Our Struggle for Control* (also banned in 1983), and *Abor-*

tion: Right or Wrong (banned since 1942). Four of the banned books are sex guides: *How to Drive Your Man Wild in Bed* (banned since 1985) and *The Complete Guide to Sex* (banned since 1990) are prohibited because they appear to contain information about the procurement of abortion. *Make It Happy: What Sex Is All About*, *The Book of Love*, and the slightly more medical *The Love Diseases* have all been banned since the early 1980s. While the majority of banned books are reviewed after 12 years, this time limit does not apply to books banned for advocating the procurement of abortion.

28. Mullally, "Debating Reproductive Rights," 93.

29. See Linda Connolly, *The Irish Women's Movement: From Revolution to Devolution* (Dublin: Lilliput Press, 2003); Ann Rossiter, *Ireland's Hidden Diaspora: The 'Abortion Trail' and the Making of the London-Irish Underground, 1980–2000* (London: Iasc Publishing, 2009); Mary Muldowney, "Breaking the Silence on Abortion: The 1983 Referendum Campaign," *History Ireland* 21, no. 2 (2013), http://www.historyireland.com/20th-century -contemporary-history/breaking-the-silence-on-abortionthe-1983-referendum -campaign-2/; Mary Muldowney, "Breaking the Silence: Pro-Choice Activism in Ireland since 1983," in *Sexual Politics in Modern Ireland*, ed. Jennifer Redmond, Sonja Tiernan, Sandra McAvoy, and Mary McAuliffe (Dublin: Irish Academic Press, 2015); Mairéad Enright, "Meeting Mrs. McGee: Reflections on Feminist Judgment as Critical Legal Practice," Northern/Irish Feminist Judgments Project, January 22, 2015, http://www.feministjudging.ie/?p=1002; Mairéad Enright, "The Importance of Women-y Fringe-y Excesses of Irish Pro-Choice Activism," *Human Rights in Ireland* (blog), November 13, 2015, http://humanrights.ie /gender-sexuality-and-the-law/the-importance-of-the-women-y-fringe-y-excesses -of-irish-pro-choice-activism/.

30. The *Women to Blame* exhibition was researched and designed by Therese Caherty, journalist; Pauline Conroy, social researcher; Emma Loughran, photographer; Adam May, graphic designer, and Clio Meldon, graphic designer. It features visuals from the *Irish Times* and the work of photographers Clodagh Boyd, Rose Comiskey, Paula Geraghty, Emma Loughran, and Derek Speirs. Film director Cathal Black has provided interviews with leading lights in the women's movement, as has filmmaker Ruth Jacob. Reproductions of leaflets, posters, cartoons, magazines, and news cuttings give an overview of a major struggle in modern Irish history. The exhibition "Women to Blame" by Therese Caherty et al. occurred in Dublin, November 7–16, 2014. See http://filmbase.ie /women-to-blame-exhibition/#.W84rZafMyYU. Its title comes from an account of Joanne Hayes and the Kerry Babies Tribunal. See Nell McCafferty, *A Woman to Blame: The Kerry Babies Case* (Cork, Ireland: Attic Press, 1985).

31. Cited in Therese Caherty, "Women to Blame," *Look Left*, May 11, 2015, http://www.lookleftonline.org/2015/05/women-to-blame/.

32. Caherty, "Women to Blame."

33. The 1971 Contraceptive Train was a landmark moment in the Irish women's movement. Members of the newly formed Irish Women's Liberation Movement traveled to Belfast in Northern Ireland by train to buy contraceptives in protest against the law in Ireland prohibiting the importation and sale of contraceptives. See RTÉ News, "Contraceptive Train," directed by RTÉ, aired

May 22, 1971, on RTÉ ONE, http://www.rte.ie/archives/exhibitions/1666
-women-and-society/370226-contraceptive-train/.

34. Medb Ruane, "Introduction," in *The Irish Journey: Women's Stories of
Abortion*, ed. Irish Family Planning Association (Dublin: Irish Family Planning
Association, 2010), 10.

35. Anthea McTeirnan, "The 'Contraceptive Train' Spawns a Musical," *Irish
Times*, September 21, 2015, https://www.irishtimes.com/life-and-style/people/the
-contraceptive-train-spawns-a-musical-1.2357022.

36. Hug, *The Politics of Sexual Morality in Ireland*, 89.

37. Connolly, *The Irish Women's Movement*, 120–21, 126.

38. Connolly, *The Irish Women's Movement*, 121.

39. Abortion is also illegal in Northern Ireland, as the 1967 Abortion Act
was never extended to that region. However, while Irish customs began seizing
abortion pills in 2011, the pills are managing to make it through customs in
Northern Ireland. Through a series of underground and unofficial networks,
women needing to access the abortion pill have the pills sent to addresses in the
North.

40. Despite the presence of the Gardaí (Irish police force) at the train station
and the widespread media coverage of the action, there were no prosecutions or
even threats of prosecutions. Whackala, dir., "#AbortionPillTrain," aired on
October 31, 2014, on Vimeo, https://vimeo.com/110596301.

41. Jessica Elgot and Henry McDonald, "Northern Irish Women Win Access
to Free Abortions as May Averts Rebellion," *Guardian*, June 29, 2017, https://
www.theguardian.com/world/2017/jun/29/rebel-tories-could-back-northern
-ireland-abortion-amendment.

42. Padraig O'Morain, "Women Travel to Holyhead for Data," *Irish Times*,
May 7, 1992, 8.

43. Ursula Barry, cited in O'Morain, "Women Travel to Holyhead for Data," 8.

44. Catherine Nagi, "Reflections on a Successful Campaign, or When We
Brought the Country to Its Senses, or When We Avoided Overcrowding Irish
Jails," *Voices of Women: The Cork Women's Political Association. Special Issue
on the Eighth Amendment* (September 2003): 22.

45. The Abortion Rights Campaign was established in December 2012. For
an account of the origins and establishment of the campaign, see Cathie
Doherty and Sinéad Redmond, "The Radicalisation of a New Generation of
Abortion Rights Activists," in *The Abortion Papers*, ed. Aideen Quilty, Sinéad
Kennedy, and Julie Hornibrook (Cork: Cork University Press, 2015), 270–74,
and Alison Spillane, "The Impact of the Crisis on Irish Women," in *Ireland
under Austerity: Neoliberal Crisis, Neoliberal Solutions*, ed. Colin Coulter and
Angela Nagle (Manchester: Manchester University Press, 2015).

46. Abortion Rights Campaign, "Our Annual Report for 2014," accessed
2014, http://www.abortionrightscampaign.ie/2015/09/19/our-annual-report-for
-2014/.

47. Abortion Rights Campaign, "Our Annual Report for 2014."

48. The Information Act requires any information on abortion services to be
provided along with information on parenting and adoption, and may only be
given within the context of one-on-one counseling. The act also prohibits
doctors from making an appointment for an abortion on behalf of their patient,

which can have serious health consequences for women traveling abroad to obtain an abortion due to health problems.

49. "Ireland 2001," Women on Waves, accessed November 12, 2015, https://www.womenonwaves.org/en/page/769/in-collection/2582/ireland-2001.

50. "Abortion Pill Bus 2015," ROSA, accessed June 11, 2018, http://rosa.ie /abortion-pill-bus-2015/.

51. Misoprostol is legal in Ireland and is commonly used to treat ulcers, but it is not labeled for use as an abortifacient (abortion-inducer). Mifepristone is effectively banned in Ireland. A woman who uses these drugs to induce an abortion would be liable to fourteen years' imprisonment under the Protection of Life during Pregnancy Act (2013).

52. Enright, "The Importance of Women-y Fringe-y Excesses."

53. See Rossiter, *Ireland's Hidden Diaspora*, and "About ASN's Clients," Abortion Support Network, accessed November 13, 2015, https://www .abortionsupport.org.uk/about-the-women-we-help/.

54. McTeirnan, "The Contraceptive Train."

55. In September 2016, the Irish government established a Citizens' Assembly to consider a number of key political questions including that of abortion. The Citizens' Assembly was tasked with producing a report that was then considered by an All-Party Oireachtas (parlimentary committee), which reported in December 2017.

56. Marie O'Halloran, "Abortion Now in the Hands of the Electorate, Says Taoiseach," *Irish Times*, January 30, 2018, https://www.irishtimes.com/news /politics/oireachtas/abortion-now-in-the-hands-of-irish-electorate-says-taoiseach -1.3373887.

57. Leo Varadkar, "'Safe, Legal and Rare': Full Text of Taoiseach's Abortion Speech," *Irish Times*, January 30, 2018, https://www.irishtimes.com/news/social -affairs/safe-legal-and-rare-full-text-of-taoiseach-s-abortion-speech-1.3373468.

[6]

Tales of Mobility

Women's Travel and Abortion Services in a Globalized Australia

BARBARA BAIRD

THE RESEARCH literature about abortion in Australia in the post-war period is dotted with references to women's travel across long distances to access abortion services. But only a small number of studies have focused on this phenomenon, and these discuss only some states and only for certain periods of time.[1] The largeness of the Australian continent and the concentration of its population and health services in urban centers, most of which are located around the coastline, make the problem of access to abortion services for women in rural, regional, and remote areas potentially acute and widespread. This chapter creates a more comprehensive picture of women's travel to access abortion services in Australia since the 1970s, when the law and the provision of abortion was liberalized. In some cases, this refers to journeys across land and sea that stretch many hundreds and even thousands of kilometers.

The contemporary politics and provision of abortion in Australia, a country of nearly 25 million people at the time of writing, can be contextualized by the movement of capital, technologies, service providers, ideas, information, and imaginaries, although this movement is uneven and sometimes obstructed. That is, abortion in Australia is shaped by the process known as "globalization."[2] But while all women who seek abortions in Australia do so in conditions shaped by the intensified mobilities of globalization, in this chapter I argue that those who must travel to access abortion services are marginalized by the current globalized structure and culture of abortion provision.

The case of Australia allows for the investigation of the provision of abortion services at the intersections of liberal, indeed liberal feminist, views on abortion and its liberal provision, the ascendancy of neoliberalism as social and economic policy, and, lately, a resurgence of moral conservatism, in an affluent Western country of vast distances. The focus on the phenomenon of women who have had to travel to access abortion services and their stories offers a critique of the popular story of the liberalization of abortion in Australia and any celebratory narratives of globalization.

After proposing a theoretical and historical framework that locates abortion in Australia in a global context, I provide a state-by-state account of women's travel to access abortion services since the 1970s. The chapter concludes with the observation that while the intensified mobilities of globalization have the potential to reshape the provision of abortion in Australia in ways advantageous to women, they are not currently dismantling the disadvantages that have historically required, and still require, many women to travel. The attention to the micro- and macro-level features of the need of some women to travel for an abortion speaks to experiences of suffering and disadvantage, as well as to determination and imagination, that are the effect of gendered structural inequalities lived out in a global context.

Australia in the Global Present

Saskia Sassen argues that globalization is best understood "not simply in terms of interdependence and global institutions." Globalization can also describe processes located within a nation-state whose similarity to processes or formations in other locations might be, according to Sassen, "a localization of the global."[3] She includes local political struggles that have a global agenda, worldviews that are recognizably common across multiple localities, and the presence of similar economic policies in her definition of such processes. The sharing of social and economic policies among separate locations is particularly evident in the global dominance of "the so-called neoliberal consensus." This notion refers to the hegemony of "the political movement championing economic or free-market liberalism with minimal state intervention as a means of promoting economic development."[4] It also refers to the capture of formerly ideologically progressive notions. In their global survey of women's reproductive health in the period since the 1994 International Conference on Population and Development held in Cairo, Mohan Rao and Sarah Sexton describe growing global inequalities. These are accompanied by the hollowing out of formerly progressive notions such as "self-determination" or "women decide," which "now mesh well with neo-liberal individualism."[5] This is the backdrop to the discussion of the provision of Australian abortion services that follows.

The implication of Australian abortion law and medical practice in an international context did not, of course, begin with the current period of globalization. Until legal liberalization in Australia in the 1970s, abortion took place in the context of its criminalization by law that, as an artifact of colonialism, followed the pre-1967 British legislation, which, as Gayle Davis et al. suggest in this volume, was deeply problematic. Furthermore, chapters authored by Lena Lennerhed, Christabelle Sethna, and Hayley Brown demonstrate that women's international travel to access abortion services did not begin with the current period of globalization dating to the 1990s, a point reinforced in this volume by the work of Agata Ignaciuk and Anna Bogic. Davis et al. highlight the fact that domestic travel to access abortion services within Britain was an unintended consequence of the passage of the 1967 Abortion Act. In the case of Australia, it is apparent that some, mostly middle-class, women from South Australia (SA), Queensland (Qld), Tasmania, Western Australia (WA), and the neighboring country of New Zealand—the latter of these examined in this collection by Hayley Brown—traveled to both Sydney and Melbourne (Australia's two largest cities) seeking abortions from at least the 1940s onward.[6]

The liberalization of law and practice in Australia during the 1970s was part of a global trend. Liberalization unfolded distinctly in each of Australia's six states and two territories. British abortion law reform was literally the basis of law reform in South Australia in 1969 and then the Northern Territory in 1973. The Menhennitt ruling, in a Supreme Court case in the state of Victoria in 1969 in which a doctor was acquitted on abortion charges, set a precedent that was followed by the jurisdictions that did not have legislative reform, either in their own court rulings or as an accepted precedent. The 1973 *Roe v. Wade* ruling in the US Supreme Court was widely reported, and Australian abortion-providing doctors made contact with US and British counterparts from the early 1970s.[7] This was a period of progressive social change in Australia, and Australian public support for women's right to choose grew during this time, and has continued to be the clear majority view.[8] The ability to claim a rebate for the cost of an abortion after 1974, from the then new national universal health insurance scheme Medibank (later Medicare), made the procedure when performed privately, typically in a clinic, significantly more affordable from that time onward.

The system of the provision of abortion services in Australia that was established by 1980 has prevailed since. Law regarding abortion is a state or territory matter. Provision is predominantly in private sector (for-profit) clinics where women must pay.[9] The federally provided Medicare rebate continues to underwrite the affordability of privately provided abortion but is increasingly inadequate. Although prices vary from clinic to clinic, the rebate currently covers only about half the cost of both medical and surgical abortions, and the "gap" amount is usually required to be paid up front.[10] There are currently about 35 private clinics in Australia, most located in capital cities and mostly along the coastline; most provide medical and surgical abortion.[11] Provision in public hospitals, the domain of state governments, where abortion is provided at little or no cost, is limited except in the smaller jurisdictions of SA and the NT, where it predominates.[12] The medical workforce that enables the provision of abortion services is based in the mainland capital cities. The provision of services in private clinics outside these locations has relied on "fly-in-fly-out" doctors.[13] This phenomenon is evidence not only of small town conservatism but also of the small number of doctors who are prepared to specialize in performing abortions.[14] Incidentally, it is a sign of the mobile workforces that increasingly characterize the global economy.[15] Doctors and others involved in provision also travel overseas to attend conferences and visit or work with abortion providers, and refer to international benchmarks as horizons for their own local practice.[16] Together, they constitute a "diasporic public sphere" of health professionals.[17]

While the anti-abortion movement in Australia is an irritant more than a major force, it is enlivened by regular contact between local and US activists.[18] On the other side of the political divide, cross-border travel in people and ideas has, on occasion, been restricted. In 1999, immigration authorities attempted to obstruct visiting American abortion providers from attending an abortion conference in Australia. This was symptomatic of the influence of anti-abortionists in the Liberal Party (Australia's politically conservative party), which held power in the federal sphere in the period 1996–2007.[19] Increasingly, however, abortion provision and pro-choice abortion activist and advocacy organizations have sophisticated website presences, which give information and challenge anti-abortion ideas. Older forms of popular culture are also sites of contest. This includes positive representations of abortion in the United States of America (USA), Britain, and in locally produced documentary films, feature films and television series, and women's magazines.[20] The overwhelmingly pro-choice views of the Australian public are reflected in the twenty-first-century trend toward decriminalization. Five of eight jurisdictions have now removed abortion from the criminal law; a long-held goal of pro-choice and feminist politics is being realized, although this has not necessarily improved abortion access.[21]

The localizing of the global is exemplified in the Australian story of mifepristone, the medication that, when taken with misoprostol, induces early medical abortion (EMA).[22] After signs that Australian health and medical communities were preparing for mifepristone when this medication was first becoming available, including participation in a World Health Organization international trial in the early 1990s, in 1996 the Liberal federal government effectively banned its importation. In 2006, legislation overturning the ban was successfully introduced by a cross-party group of female senators. Individual doctors were then able to become "authorized providers" and, in the absence of its availability in Australia, import mifepristone from New Zealand. The availability of EMA grew slowly from this time. Its wider availability, however, awaited a sponsor of the commercial importation of this drug and its generalized approval for clinical use. Marie Stopes International (Australia) (MSIA) became involved. This organization, owned by the London-based sexual and reproductive health–providing nongovernmental organization Marie Stopes International, first invested in the Australian abortion market in 2000 and has grown to provide about one-third of all abortions in Australia at the time of writing. In 2012, MSIA's subsidiary, MS Health, received approval from the Therapeutic Goods Administration (TGA), the national body that regulates pharmaceutical drugs, to distribute mifepristone and misoprostol, packaged as MS-2 Step, for use up to seven weeks of pregnancy (subsequently extended to nine weeks). MS Health imports mifepristone from France. In 2013, MS-2 Step was listed on the national Pharmaceutical Benefits Scheme, making it available at a heavily subsidized rate. The availability of EMA grew steadily from 2013 onward.[23]

The TGA requires an arguably unnecessary and unduly onerous regime of mandatory training for prescribing doctors and pharmacists, 24-hour access to an information service, and follow-up medical care. An ultrasound to confirm pregnancy is recommended. Ideally the second medication (misoprostol) is taken 24 to 48 hours after the first (mifepristone).[24] Despite early hopes that the availability of EMA, if provided by local general practitioners (GPs), would solve the problems of access for rural and remote Australian women, EMA has not yet been widely taken up by doctors beyond those in clinics, and some public hospitals, that already provide surgical abortions. And it is not necessarily any cheaper than surgical abortion.[25] In 2015, two organizations began to offer home-based EMA via telehealth, although women in SA cannot access this form of abortion provision because the law in this jurisdiction requires that abortion be provided in a hospital. Within its first year, the Tabbot Foundation, the larger of the two telehealth organizations, grew to provide about 1 percent of all abortions in Australia.[26] About one-third of the abortions provided by MSIA clinics at the time of writing are via EMA; the proportion of surgical and medical abortion across Australia is not known.[27] Lastly, access to mifepristone via the internet, or via friends or family in other countries, means that extralegal and extramedical means can also be a source of access to abortion.[28] As one scholar of reproductive tourism notes: "In the age of globalization, the actions of citizens may sometimes supersede the regulatory arm of the state."[29]

From here on, this chapter draws on information from existing historical and sociological studies of abortion, reports from government and nongovernment organizations, and media sources to construct an overall account of abortion travel in a globally contextualized Australia.

The Need to Travel

Access to abortion services improved in the 1970s, although it has continued to be uneven in each Australian jurisdiction. In 1996, a landmark study into the adequacy of abortion services commissioned by the National Health and Medical Research Council (NHMRC) reported:

> While the accessibility of all health services varies according to place of residence, and people in rural communities are generally disadvantaged, this pattern is exaggerated in the case of access to TOP [termination of pregnancy] services. This is partly due to the general undersupply of services in the public sector. Also, while rural residents who are required to travel to capital cities for other surgical procedures are generally

eligible for assistance with the necessary costs, most women who travel for TOP services are not eligible. This arises because payments are restricted to services provided by medical specialists on referral, and the majority of TOPS are provided by general practitioners.[30]

Among other recommendations, the report called for state governments to take responsibility for the adequacy of abortion services. By the time the NHMRC report was completed, the aforementioned conservative federal Liberal Party government had been elected, and, amid significant controversy, the report was withdrawn by the minister for health shortly after its release.[31] Its recommendations have not been systematically implemented. More recent reports and research show that the problem of geographic disadvantage has not gone away.[32] When services are not available locally, cost and the distance to travel are the most cited obstacles to access, and may in some cases be too much to overcome.[33] Conservative rural communities and unhelpful local doctors, the need for privacy, poor access to information, the need for personal support, and logistical challenges when making arrangements are also cited as obstacles.[34] Young women are overrepresented among those who travel and bear disproportionate burdens when they do.[35] The disadvantage of living outside metropolitan centers is intensified not only for Indigenous women but also for rural refugee women and other recently arrived migrants, those with mental illness, and those in violent relationships. One Victorian rural health worker worries about "the anxiety associated with or the experience of coming to the big smoke [large city]."[36] Most recently, research into the experience of 2,326 women who had abortions at clinics run by Marie Stopes Australia across five jurisdictions conducted over a six-month period during 2014–2015 found that approximately 4 percent had traveled interstate to access the service. Over 11 percent of women had needed to stay overnight, presumably because of the need for long-distance intrastate as well as interstate travel.[37] These findings are hardly unique. Many of the women studied in this volume by contributors Lori A. Brown; Cathrine Chambers, Colleen MacQuarrie, and Jo-Ann MacDonald; and Mary Gilmartin and Sinéad Kennedy have experienced similar circumstances in the American state of Texas, the Canadian province of Prince Edward Island (PEI), and the country of Ireland, respectively.

Only SA and WA collect statistical information about abortion, so the following state-by-state account of women's travel for abortion starts with these jurisdictions. For the benefit of non-Australian readers, the geographic size and population of each jurisdiction is stated, and estimated greatest distances from the capital cities are included.[38] These numbers are given, somewhat monotonously, to emphasize the scale of geographic separation from access to healthcare experienced by some women in rural, regional, and remote locations in Australia.

South Australia

SA has a population of 1.7 million people. It incorporates a little less than one million square kilometers, about five times the size of Britain (209,000 sq km). Travel to the capital city of Adelaide could involve one-way distances of up to approximately 770 kilometers from the west, 450 kilometers from the southeast border, or more than 1,000 kilometers from the far north of the state. The SA criminal law was reformed in 1969, and free public hospital provision in Adelaide has dominated services from this time. The numbers of abortions being performed in SA increased dramatically each year until the end of the 1970s, suggesting that SA women had stopped traveling interstate by this time. By the mid 1980s, however, waiting times were increasing in Adelaide hospitals due to fewer staff offering abortion provision. In 1988, it was announced that abortion provision in the second trimester in SA had closed, meaning that between 1988 and 1991, women needing this service went to Sydney and Melbourne. After a government inquiry, and significant political battle, the Pregnancy Advisory Centre (PAC), a freestanding public abortion-providing clinic attached to a public hospital, the only one of its kind in the country, was opened in the capital city Adelaide in 1992.[39] The PAC has grown to perform more than half of all SA abortions, with other public hospitals performing the rest. Alongside securing this excellent public service in Adelaide, there has been a decline not only in private hospital provision (to almost zero) but also in the number of abortions performed in other public hospitals, most significantly those in rural areas, in the years since its opening. In 1990, 8.6 percent of all abortions were performed in rural hospitals, whereas 17.3 percent of women who had abortions were from rural areas.[40] In 2014, the percentage of women from rural areas who were having abortions was similar (18.9 percent), but the percentage performed in rural hospitals was down to 1.6 percent.[41] That is, since the early 1990s rural hospitals have increasingly limited or withdrawn from providing these services. The combination of the lack of provision in rural areas and the legal requirement in SA that all abortions be performed in hospitals has resulted in distressing experiences, over and above the burden of travel, for nonmetropolitan women seeking EMA. Although in other jurisdictions women are given the second medication to take at home, in SA the law has been interpreted to require that women be given each medication, taken 24 hours apart, in the hospital clinic. In some cases, this has led to the medication taking effect during the journey home, resulting in women being in significant pain and trying to manage bleeding en route.[42]

Western Australia

About 2.5 million people live in WA. It is the largest state in terms of land mass, more than 2.5 million square kilometers, about fifteen times the size of Britain. The one-way distance from the far north to Perth, WA's capital city located in the southwest corner, is more than 3,200 kilometers; from WA's southeastern border to Perth, it is 1,430 kilometers. From the mid 1970s, abortions have been provided predominantly by two private clinics in Perth, with some public hospital provision.[43] A third clinic operated through the 2000s. Law reform in 1998 mandated, among other things, the collection of statistics. These show that the provision of abortions outside Perth has declined in the years since law reform. The report for 2010–12 found that, "similar to previous years, approximately 95% of induced abortions in WA occurred in the metropolitan area with 85% of women having abortions living in the metropolitan area. Almost 80% of WA women of reproductive age live in the metropolitan area."[44] That is, since 1998, and no doubt before, many rural women have traveled to the capital city of WA to have abortions, *and* the abortion rate is lower for women living outside the metropolitan area. The report also shows that the proportion of abortions performed in the public health system has declined during this time. The sheer size of WA, and the remoteness of some cities and towns, including many Indigenous communities, makes any need to travel especially costly and time-consuming. In 2006, doctors from WA's remote Kimberley area stated: "[Women] are often required to wait several weeks for the procedure to be performed locally or when unable to be accommodated on our limited surgical lists, required to travel up to 3000 km to Perth. If performed locally, the procedure is subsidized by the public hospital system but if in Perth, although a woman may be given her airfare by the [state government-funded] Patient Assisted Travel Scheme, she is liable for the costs of the procedure herself as well as any accommodation, living expenses or local transport required."[45] Indigenous people comprise about 40 percent of the population in the Kimberley area and are typically socioeconomically disadvantaged, so the burden described here would have weighed most heavily on Indigenous women.

Queensland

This scale of distance, and remoteness, also applies to Qld, although it is not as vast as WA—only about 1.7 million kilometers in area, or eight times the size of Britain. Nearly five million people live in the state. A single pioneering clinic that opened in 1976 in the capital Brisbane, in the southeast corner of the state, and two other clinics nearby, just over the border in northern NSW, were the only providers for Qld women until the mid-1980s. Thus, many Qld women continued to travel to Sydney. The distance to the southeast from the north of the state or from the inland "outback" could be as much as 1,800 kilometers. In a 1986 court case following a politically motivated police raid on the state's only abortion clinic, a ruling similar to the Victorian Menhennitt judgment clarified the conditions under which abortion could be performed lawfully. This paved the way for three more clinics to open: a second in Brisbane and one each in the mid-north coastal regional centers of Rockhampton and Townsville.[46] The number of Qld women traveling interstate declined in the decade after the court ruling as the new clinics expanded access geographically and with respect to capacity.[47] More private clinics as well as general practice (GP) and obstetrics and gynecology (O&G) practices that included abortion provision subsequently opened in Brisbane and the nearby Gold Coast to the south and on the Sunshine Coast to the north, and in Mackay and Cairns in the far north, stretching along 1,700 kilometers of coastline. As a result, women along the coast are served reasonably well, but this is not the case in smaller towns or the more remote parts of Qld.[48] In 2016, the only private practitioner offering surgical abortion in Cairns retired. He had performed 500 procedures per year for "a vast catchment reaching to the far-flung indigenous communities of Cape York Peninsula," and his retirement left those women without a service, meaning that the public hospital had to send women as far south as Sydney.[49]

Apart from the small public sexual health clinic in Cairns, the farthest north of these locations, which began to offer EMA for free in 2005,[50] there has never been any significant public (hospital) provision of abortion in Qld, and the very small number of abortions that have been performed are most likely done for reasons of severe fetal anomaly or medically diagnosed threats to the woman's life. Given that there are some private clinics along the Qld coast, one example of current travel distance will suffice. The closest clinic for a woman in the inland mining city of Mount Isa (of more than 22,000 people) is more than 900 kilometers away, in Townsville.

An article published in the Royal Australian and New Zealand College of Obstetricians and Gynaecologists' magazine in 2005, which told the story of a pregnant woman's repeated travel from a remote Queensland community, initially to seek an abortion, illustrated the cruel and Kafkaesque nature of the Qld public health system.[51] On her first trip to a hospital in the closest small town, a sympathetic doctor explained that an abortion would involve further travel and significant expense; this was beyond her means, and she returned home. At 18 weeks pregnant and "found to be hypertensive," she made a second trip to town. This time, she was sent "by air via the Royal Flying Doctor Service to the public hospital in the [larger] town where she might have had a termination." Her illness was treated, but abortion was not considered; even maternal ill health does not guarantee an abortion in the public health system in Qld. The woman eventually discharged herself to return to her children. At 26 weeks of gestation, she became severely ill and was again flown to the same hospital in the larger town, this time to have an emergency caesarean, after which the baby died and the woman spent several days requiring high-level hospital care. That is, the failure of the Qld health system to respond meaningfully to this woman's unwanted pregnancy the first time around led to her serious ill health, her repeated travel and time away from family, and her delivery of a premature baby that died (and to avoidable deployment of health resources and funds).

New South Wales

The state of NSW is about 800,000 square kilometers in area, not quite four times the size of Britain. It has the largest population in the country, with more than 7.5 million people. The Levine court ruling of

1971 clarified the conditions under which abortions could be performed lawfully in NSW. Private clinics are scattered along the heavily populated coastline.[52] A clinic in Albury, a major regional city in the mid-south on the border with Victoria, which opened in the early 2000s, is the exception.[53] The maximum one-way trip from outback NSW to an east coast clinic would be about 800 kilometers. In 1990, public hospitals in this state performed only 9 percent of all abortions.[54] A study of abortion provision in NSW in that same year reported that in some regions, about two-thirds of women who had had abortions traveled to access a private service; that is, public hospitals in rural NSW were significantly underproviding abortion services.[55] More than 20 years later, a small qualitative study of the difficulties facing women in rural NSW who were seeking an abortion found a continuing shortage of abortion providers in rural areas and multiple barriers to accessing an abortion. The women who were interviewed reported that they traveled anywhere from two to nine hours one way to get to a clinic.[56]

Victoria

Just over six million people live in Victoria, in an area about 230,000 square kilometers, a bit bigger than the size of Britain. In the wake of the Menhennitt court ruling in 1969, abortions have been provided predominantly by private clinics. All these clinics and the most significant public hospital providers, which perform about 20 percent of all abortions in Victoria, are in the capital city of Melbourne. The greatest distance a woman may travel to an abortion clinic in Melbourne would be about 500 kilometers, although since the early 2000s, women in the central-north of the state could make a much shorter journey across the border into NSW to Albury (see previous paragraph). Since 2015, a non-profit primary healthcare clinic in Wodonga, near Albury on the Victorian side of the border, has provided EMA at very low cost.[57] Interviews with health service providers in rural western Victoria in the late 2000s showed that it is "not clear or widely advertised which hospitals in Victorian regional centers perform terminations."[58] Consequently, referring women to Melbourne was a widespread practice.[59] The capacity of the Melbourne public hospitals is, however, limited compared to the demands made on them. Thus, many women who travel must resort to private clinics.[60] While some rural public hospitals provide abortion services but do not promote or disclose their practice, and so offer only limited access, some do so in a more transparent way.[61] A newly appointed senior medical manager at the Bendigo Hospital, 150 kilometers northwest of Melbourne, introduced an abortion service there in the mid-to-late 2000s. At the time of his appointment, approximately 70 percent of all women having abortions traveled out of the region, presumably most to Melbourne.[62] The service closed in early 2012, when there was no longer a doctor willing to perform abortions, but reopened in August 2013, illustrating the fragility of regional services and their vulnerability to the movement of key abortion providers.[63] In 2017, the minister for health in the progressive Australian Labor Party government announced a new policy on women's sexual and reproductive health, the first such policy in the nation, and a modest budget for its implementation. Improving access to abortion for rural women was a priority.[64] At the time of writing, the impact of this government commitment is unknown.

Tasmania

Tasmania is an island to the south of southeast Australia. At nearly 70,000 square kilometers, it is the smallest state, about one-third the size of Britain. Tasmania has a population of 520,000 people and is Australia's poorest state. It bears a striking resemblance to Canada's smallest province, PEI, in terms of access difficulties on and off the island, as Cathrine Chambers, Colleen MacQuarrie, and Jo-Ann MacDonald show in their contribution to this volume. Some public hospitals provided abortions from the 1970s onward, but in 1985 the annual report from Family Planning Tasmania stated that Royal Hobart Hospital, located in the capital city of Hobart, was particularly reluctant to do so. It was found that approximately half of all women who were seeking abortions from Hobart had traveled to clinics in Melbourne.[65] Public hospitals were performing about only one-third of abortions overall for Tasmanian women at this time, and doctors operating in private hospitals also provided the service.[66] This story from one Tasmanian woman—23 years old with one child, recently separated from her husband, and who borrowed money to go to Melbourne for an abortion in 1985—captures many aspects of the experience of women living in the island state: "I sort of worked out it was going to be cheaper if I went by boat [to Melbourne], and came back by plane. It ended up costing me a hell of a lot though, because I had to go by boat on the Tuesday, but the abortion in Melbourne wasn't going to happen until the Thursday. So I had to pay for somewhere to stay. I had my son with me. He was about 18 months old. So it ended up costing an enormous amount."[67]

The problem persisted until a group of feminist women opened the Women's Health Foundation (WHF) private clinic in Hobart in 1991.[68] The need to travel to Melbourne was thus partially addressed, although at the end of the decade more than 25 percent of abortions performed on Tasmanian women were still provided in interstate facilities.[69] Even for those women who did not have to travel interstate, the WHF clinic's protocol meant that rural women had to undergo "two long day trips or stop in Hobart overnight for two separate appointments. For single parents from remote areas on a pension, for example, this can create a logistical nightmare."[70] The WHF clinic closed in 2001, and, coincidentally, a police investigation threatened the arrest of doctors at the Royal Hobart Hospital later that year. Parliamentary reform legislated the conditions under which abortion could be performed lawfully and resolved this political, legal, and health care crisis.[71] Early in the following year, a mainland-owned private business opened a fortnightly clinic in Hobart and then in Launceston, the island's other main city, to be followed shortly by a second private clinic that operated in the alternate week in Hobart. The second Hobart clinic service closed in 2014, and the Launceston clinic closed two years later. In both cases, the owners cited the unsustainable nature of the business, caused in part by women's choice to access EMA via telehealth. In 2018, the only remaining clinic in Tasmania closed; lack of viability was again the reason given. The minister for health in the conservative Liberal government, known to be opposed to abortion, announced that there would be no change to the public hospitals' practice of providing abortions only for women with medically diagnosed health conditions, or in the case of fetal anomaly, but the government's travel assistance scheme could be accessed for women who needed to travel. Women who cannot access EMA via telehealth—those over nine weeks pregnant or who wish to have a surgical abortion—are back where they were before 1991; they must fly to Melbourne or pay AUD$2,500 for a private gynecologist to perform the abortion. The Australian Labor Party opposition announced that if elected in March 2018, the party would enable some public provision of abortion services, but the Liberal government was reelected and the situation did not improve. The size of the market in

Tasmania, its still conservative medical community, and the need to fly in medical practitioners mean that the financial viability of private clinics has always been marginal; in 2013, Tasmania's public hospital system was performing less than 10 percent of Tasmanian women's abortions.[72]

Australian Capital Territory

The ACT is a very small territory existing entirely within NSW with a population of nearly 400,000 people, most of whom reside in the national capital of Canberra. In 1992, following a liberal law reform, an independent nonprofit clinic opened.[73] Before this time, abortions were performed in a public hospital, where there were often long waiting lists and the hospital required that women appear before a committee "to establish eligibility or otherwise."[74] To avoid the lengthy wait times, many women chose to travel interstate instead, most to Sydney, roughly 300 kilometers away. There are currently two clinics servicing the ACT, but women who are more than 16 weeks pregnant who are seeking abortions for so-called social reasons, that is, reasons determined by the woman and not by a medical diagnosis, still need to travel.[75]

Northern Territory

This territory covers a large area, 1.35 million square kilometers, more than six times the size of Britain. It has, however, only 245,000 people, 30 percent of whom are Indigenous. Whereas in other states travel from rural and remote locations by car, train, or plane to larger cities for abortion services is practically easy for women seeking an abortion (should they be able to afford the journey and make the personal arrangements), here the difficulty distance poses to some women who must travel for access is compounded by the poor conditions of some roads across desert country in the center and by the impact of tropical monsoon climate conditions on the roads across the river floodplains of the Top End. (These qualifications on travel also apply in northern Qld and WA.) In any case, many communities, particularly remote Indigenous communities where people live on their traditional land, are more than 800 kilometers from the two main NT centers, Alice Springs and Darwin. Most abortions are provided in the public hospitals in these cities. Since the 1990s, a small number have also been done in the Darwin Private

Hospital.[76] It is likely that about the same number again have been performed outside of the territory.[77] In 2015, it was reported that the main abortion-providing doctor at the public hospital in Darwin, the capital of the NT, had resigned and the public hospital in Alice Springs, 1,500 kilometers away, was now the only public provider in the territory.[78] This illustrated once again how the NT's "reproductive health services are fraught with access problems due to remoteness and disadvantage," especially for Indigenous women.[79]

Second- and Third-Trimester Services

In addition to those marginalized by location, four particular groups of women experience the need to travel to access abortion services. Women with pregnancies beyond the first trimester are a small percentage of all women who have abortions in Australia, but they have regularly faced the need to travel, whatever the local availability of first-trimester services. Travel costs aggravate the increased cost of a second-trimester abortion; the price in a private clinic rises for every week after 12 weeks. The complete cessation of second-trimester services in SA in the late 1980s, which caused SA women to travel to Sydney and Melbourne, is noted earlier in this chapter.[80] In 2005, David Ellwood reported that late-term abortions were performed in all jurisdictions except in Queensland and Tasmania, where abortions after 22 weeks were generally unavailable, but even in metropolitan Sydney, access to late-term procedures was then "restricted to a small number of the larger hospitals."[81]

After law reform in WA in 1998, women wanting an abortion who were more than 20 weeks pregnant needed to make a case to a ministerially appointed panel of doctors based at the King Edward Memorial Hospital in Perth, and such abortions could only be performed at that hospital. A review of all such abortions performed in the five-and-a-half-year period after law reform showed that all were permitted for reasons of severe fetal anomaly. A small number of applications based on "psychosocial reasons" (and some based on less severe fetal anomalies) were declined. Some WA women whose applications were denied then traveled interstate.[82]

Research about Victoria published in 2016 confirmed "the lack of availability of abortion for women over 20 weeks pregnant."[83] The cultural distinction between abortions for so-called medical reasons, which includes diagnoses of fetal anomaly and severe threats to the woman's physical health, and so-called social (or psycho-social) reasons applies across all jurisdictions, and it is likely that access to second-trimester abortions for the latter has reduced since Ellwood's assessment in 2005. As of 2017, only one private clinic in Australia performs abortions for women over 20 weeks pregnant where the woman's request is based on "social reasons." This Melbourne clinic performs abortions up to 24 weeks, as does the public clinic in SA (which is, however, only accessible to SA women).[84] There is no research to date that tracks the fate of women whose requests for second- or third-trimester abortions are denied, or of women who cannot afford the procedure. There is anecdotal evidence of women traveling to the USA, but presumably most women continue the pregnancy.

Indigenous Women

A study of the general healthcare experiences of Indigenous women in regional Queensland conducted by Indigenous researcher Bronwyn Fredericks identifies the assumption of whiteness and racism in mainstream healthcare services and also in services designed for women.[85] It is reasonable to assume that this may apply to many mainstream sexual health and abortion services, although there is very little published research about Indigenous women's experience of abortion. Another Indigenous researcher, Kerry Arabena, has argued that "the policies that have allowed non-Indigenous women to access services that positively resolve pregnancies since the mid 1960s have not been realized for remote area living Aboriginal and Torres Strait Islander women, particularly those who are young, living in poverty, unable to access education and who are vulnerable to violence."[86] She asserts that "many [Aboriginal and Torres Strait Islander] adolescents would need second trimester abortions or end up having the child, because not having the child is too hard."[87] While many Indigenous people live in urban and inner regional areas, they are much more likely than non-Indigenous people to live in outer regional, remote, and very remote areas, and so disproportionately experience geographic disadvantage in relation to access to healthcare as well as socioeconomic disadvantage.[88] Lori A. Brown makes similar observations about poor, rural women and undocumented migrants from Mexico in her contribution to this volume.

Not surprisingly, the small number of studies that have provided data about Indigenous women's experiences of abortion show or suggest that they are disproportionately represented among those who had to travel long distances.[89] Furthermore, they may lack resources and support to negotiate travel to the city.[90] Whether poor access is a factor in WA Indigenous women's lower rate of abortion when compared to non-Indigenous women in that state is unknown.[91] Elsewhere, figures suggest that Indigenous women have abortions at roughly the same rate as non-Indigenous women.[92] A recent study about healthcare for Indigenous people living in SA rural and remote areas concludes: "the seemingly inevitable disconnect between health care, transport and support systems further complicates already complex and challenging journeys."[93]

Temporary Disruptions

In WA in 1998, Tasmania in 2001, and Qld in 2009, unexpected police interventions into the practice of abortion resulted in short-term cessations of some abortion services.[94] These ostensibly anachronistic, one-off legal-political healthcare crises also contributed to Australian women's need to travel to seek an abortion. The relevant state parliaments reformed the law in each case to enable the resumption of the status quo, but this process took several weeks, if not months. In the meantime, some women needing an abortion had to travel. In WA and Qld, women seeking late-term abortions were most disadvantaged.[95] During the Qld crisis, approximately 100 women traveled to NSW, Victoria, and ACT to seek the service and a smaller number with existing family connections "found it easier" to go to New Zealand, the United Kingdom and India.[96] Sometimes abortion services in regional areas have ceased when the medical provider upon whom the service relied has left the hospital, or the area, and there is no replacement doctor; women must then travel. These local crises can also be understood as political insofar as they illustrate the ongoing stigma attached to abortion and the lack of government and/or institutional attention to workforce issues.[97]

Asylum-Seeking Women

Since the early 1990s, large numbers of asylum seekers, many who gain formal refugee status, have been held in mandatory immigration detention in Australia. An unknown number of asylum-seeking women have had abortions. From 2013 onward, asylum seekers who arrive in Australia by boat have been mandatorily sent to two offshore detention centers, one in Papua New Guinea and the other on the Pacific Island nation of Nauru, 3,000 kilometers from Australia. All female asylum seekers are in Nauru, where abortion is illegal. At the time of writing, there are over 900 refugees on Nauru; this includes single women and family groups, mostly from Iran and surrounding countries. Women who request an abortion can be sent to Australia; in 2016, they were being taken to Papua New Guinea, even though abortion is illegal in that country.[98] These women are "stateless and without rights," facing "arbitrary and indefinite detention," and consequently experiencing "vulnerability to sexual assault, and to pregnancy as a result of such assaults." Social worker Patricia Hayes identifies their circumstances as "state-based reproductive coercion" and argues that it is impossible for them to give informed consent to an abortion, or to motherhood.[99] The violation of their human rights, including the poor quality of healthcare that is available to them, includes much more than lack of easy access to abortion, but nonetheless they have a place in this chapter. The precarious status of asylum seekers is also raised by Mary Gilmartin and Sinéad Kennedy in this volume when considering restrictions on reproductive mobility in Ireland.

Notwithstanding the injustice and suffering of all the women described in this chapter, the diversity and resourcefulness of such women should also be noted. One study of Victorian women notes that "not all rural people felt that access to reproductive health services was difficult."[100] The Tasmanian woman who needed to travel across the sea to Melbourne in the 1980s, whose story is quoted earlier in the chapter, faced significant hardship. But her experience of the procedure was easy and provided a new horizon of possibility, which some characterize as an upside of globalization: "It was really quick, it was really easy, and there was no trouble with it. And it had been made to be such a big deal here [Tasmania]."[101]

The reflections of one rural NSW woman who traveled to Qld for an abortion referred to the thousands of Irish women who travel to Britain for abortion services annually: "in that car driving over the [state] border I felt like the women in Ireland,"[102] illustrating the "link to be found between the work of the imagination and the emergence of a postnational political world."[103] Similarly, in relation to the young woman who was arrested along with her Ukrainian boyfriend in Cairns, Qld, in 2009 for illegally taking abortion pills that her boyfriend's sister had imported, the case that led to the crisis in Qld referred to previously, Kate Gleeson argues that it was not only the connection with Ukraine that enabled her actions. A global, feminist, and neoliberal discourse of women's right to choose was apparent in her explanation of her actions when questioned by police. The young woman was quoted saying "It wasn't really that much of a big deal. . . . [I] just decided that I wasn't ready for a child."[104] Both young people were acquitted by a jury 18 months after being arrested.[105]

Conclusion

On the one hand, the liberalization of abortion law and practice as well as doctors' willingness to travel to nonmetropolitan clinics has diminished Australian women's need to travel since the 1970s. Most women living in the capital cities and in some of the larger regional centers will be able to access an abortion without the need to travel. The recitation of numbers in this chapter, however, stands in for the untold stories of women who must travel—the number of weeks pregnant, kilometers to traverse, hours or days away from home, dollars spent, and the rates of abortion that differ between urban and rural women. These numbers are the calculus of disadvantage, injustice, and suffering.

In the period after liberalization, the need for intrastate travel has become the most significant sign of geographical disadvantage faced by Australian women seeking abortions, although interstate travel has not disappeared, particularly for women who seek second- or third-trimester abortions for "social reasons." The provision of EMA by telehealth and by rural and regional GPs is only just beginning to make a dent in the problems of access faced by women in these areas. It is too soon to tell how this solution will develop and whether it will be at the cost of the provision of surgical abortions. This seems to be the local outcome of the closure of the Tasmanian clinics.

While reliable statistics are available only for SA and WA, it seems that at least 10 percent of women who have abortions have had to travel to access the services since liberalization in every jurisdiction. At different times in the smaller jurisdictions of Tasmania and the NT, this figure has been as high as 50 percent, even if only for short periods. The period of time from early 2018 onward, during which Tasmanian women will have to travel to seek a surgical service, is unknown. Of all women in rural and remote locations, it seems that between 50 and 100 percent in each jurisdiction examined here have had to travel. Women in rural and remote WA, Qld, and NT will travel the greatest distances. Tasmanian women will have to cross the sea, as will women in immigration detention on Nauru. The disproportionate socioeconomic disadvantage, especially in relation to healthcare, of rural and remote populations in Australia is compounded by the geographic disadvantage of all in these areas. Similarly, Indigenous women's disproportionate residence in remote locations and their disproportionate poverty means that they bear an undue burden of cost and travel only to find services that may be culturally inappropriate. Women who travel to Adelaide in SA and Darwin and Alice Springs in the NT, where the public hospitals provide all or most abortions, and some lucky Victorian women who travel to Melbourne and are able to secure an appointment at a public hospital will at least not have to pay for the procedure. But most women in Victoria and nearly all in NSW, Qld, WA, NT, Tasmania, and the ACT who travel will end up in a private clinic. Women in SA and Victoria who seek an abortion after 20 weeks of pregnancy for "social reasons" can access the service in their capital city and in SA for free. All other women currently must travel to Melbourne.

These experiences of Australian women who travel long distances to have an abortion mirror those of women from similar countries. As Christabelle Sethna and Marion Doull argue for Canada, "the journeys of women seeking access to abortion services in a timely fashion signal how profoundly gendered structural constraints and globally stratified inequities can shape women's reproductive lives."[106] There is more research to be done in Australia on the historical and contemporary incidence of women who travel to seek abortions, including in relation to varying abortion rates among different groups of women. There should also be research into the conditions that currently do and potentially might make abortion services accessible in rural, regional, and remote settings in Australia, so that these can be identified, assessed, and disseminated. Furthermore, the experiences of women in Australia who have had to travel to access abortion services, often at a significant cost, must be kept at the forefront of any picture of abortion in Australia. This is true too for advocacy and activism. We must call for an end to the mandatory detention of women in immigration detention at the same time as we call for their reproductive healthcare needs when so detained. Calls for governments to take responsibility for adequate access to abortion for all women challenge the neoliberal norms of government policy, and they must continue.[107]

Women are not passive subjects in the process of seeking access to abortion, even when their desires are unjustly thwarted. New means of abortion provision such as medical abortion in the form of abortion pills do not necessarily solve old inequalities. Border crossing of all sorts can traverse some traditional lines of advantage and disadvantage, but it remains a sign of marginalization. There are no women in Australia who are untouched by global forces, even if it is in the re-creation of preexisting inequalities that prevent access to what transnational flows may otherwise promise. Women who must travel long distances to access abortion services are not left out of globalization. They are its othered subjects.

Notes

1. Carolyn Nickson, Julia Shelley, and Anthony Smith, "Use of Interstate Services for the Termination of Pregnancy in Australia," *Australian and New Zealand Journal of Public Health* 26, no. 5 (2002): 421–25; Carolyn Nickson, Anthony Smith, and Julia Shelley, "Travel Undertaken by Women Accessing Private Victorian Pregnancy Termination Services," *Australian and New Zealand Journal of Public Health* 30, no. 4 (2006): 329–33; Frances Doran and Julie Hornibrook, "Rural New South Wales Women's Access to Abortion Services: Highlights from an Exploratory Qualitative Study," *Australian Journal of Rural Health* 22, no. 3 (2014): 121–26.

2. Arjun Appadurai, *Modernity at Large: Cultural Dimensions of Globalization* (Minneapolis: University of Minnesota Press, 1996); Saskia Sassen, *A Sociology of Globalization* (New York: W. W. Norton, 2007).

3. Sassen, *A Sociology of Globalization*, 4.

4. Mohan Rao and Sarah Sexton, "Introduction: Population, Health, and Gender in a Neo-Liberal Times," in *Markets and Malthus: Population, Health, and Gender in a Neo-Liberal Times*, ed. Mohan Rao and Sarah Sexton (New Delhi: SAGE, 2010), 8.

5. Rao and Sexton, "Introduction," 19.

6. Barbara Baird, "*I Had One Too . . .": An Oral History of Abortion in South Australia before 1970* (Adelaide: Women's Studies Unit, Flinders University of SA, 1990); Stefania Siedlecky and Diana Wyndam, *Populate and Perish: Australian Women's Fight for Birth Control* (Sydney: Allen and Unwin, 1990); Suellen Murray, "Breaking the Rules: Abortion in Western Australia, 1920–1950," in *Sexuality and Gender in History*, ed. P. Hetherington and P. Maddern (Perth: Centre for WA History at UWA, 1993), 223–41; Caroline De Costa, *Never, Ever, Again . . .* (Brisbane: Boolarong Press, 2010), 75; Allison McCulloch, *Fighting to*

Choose: The Abortion Rights Struggle in New Zealand (Wellington: Victoria University Press, 2013).

7. Siedlecky and Wyndam, *Populate and Perish*, 78–89.

8. Katharine Betts, "Attitudes to Abortion: Australia and Queensland in the Twenty-First Century," *People and Place* 17, no. 3 (2009): 25–39.

9. National Health and Medical Research Council (NHMRC), *An Information Paper on Termination of Pregnancy in Australia* (Canberra: Australian Government Publishing Service, 1996).

10. Mridula Shankar et al., "Access, Equity and Costs of Induced Abortion Services in Australia: A Cross-sectional Study," *Australian and New Zealand Journal of Public Health* 41, no. 3 (2017): 309–14.

11. "Interstate Abortion Providers," *Children By Choice*, accessed May 6, 2017, https://www.childrenbychoice.org.au/forwomen/abortion/clinicsinterstate.

12. National Health and Medical Research Council, *An Information Paper on Termination of Pregnancy*, 4.

13. This information is obtained from oral history interviews that I have conducted from 2013 to 2017 as part of a research project about the provision of abortion services in Australia since 1990. The project has been funded by Flinders University, and I am the principal investigator.

14. National Health and Medical Research Council, *An Information Paper on Termination of Pregnancy*, 19–20.

15. Graeme Hugo, "Temporary Migration and the Labour Market in Australia," *Australian Geographer* 37, no. 2 (August 2006): 211–31.

16. Key Centre for Women's Health in Society et al., *Abortion in Victoria: The Melbourne Declaration*, November 2007, http://whwest.org.au/wp-content/uploads/2012/03/melb_declaration2007.pdf (page no longer available).

17. Appadurai, *Modernity at Large*.

18. Donna Wyatt and Katie Hughes, "When Discourse Defies Belief: Anti-abortionists in Contemporary Australia," *Sociology* 45, no. 3 (2009): 235–53; Barbara Baird, "Abortion Politics during the Howard Years: Beyond Liberalisation," *Australian Historical Studies* 44, no. 2 (2013): 245–61; Jeremy Roberts, "Kenyon Hosts US 'Pro-Life' Legislator," *In Daily*, April 30, 2013, http://indaily.com.au/news/2013/08/30/kenyon-hosts-us-pro-life-legislator/.

19. Baird, "Abortion Politics," 251.

20. Barbara Baird and Erica Millar, "More Than Stigma: Interrogating Counter Narratives of Abortion," *Sexualities* (forthcoming).

21. Barbara Baird, "Decriminalization and Women's Access to Abortion in Australia," *Health and Human Rights Journal* 19, no. 1 (2017): 197–208.

22. Barbara Baird, "Medical Abortion in Australia: A Short History," *Reproductive Health Matters* 23, no. 46 (2015): 169–76.

23. Baird, "Medical Abortion in Australia."

24. Baird, "Medical Abortion in Australia."

25. Shankar et al., "Access, Equity and Costs," 5.

26. Paul Hyland and E. Mulligan, "The Advent of Telemedicine Abortion Has Had a Broad Impact on Australian Abortion Services" (Presentation at International Federation of Professional Abortion and Contraception Associates Conference, Lisbon, 2016).

27. Shankar et al., "Access, Equity and Costs," 5.

28. Baird, "Medical Abortion," 171–72.

29. Lauren Jade Martin, "Reproductive Tourism in the Age of Globalization," *Globalizations* 6, no. 2 (2009): 257.

30. National Health and Medical Research Council, *An Information Paper on Termination of Pregnancy*, 7.

31. Baird, "Abortion Politics."

32. Talina Drabsch, *Abortion and the Law in New South Wales*, Briefing Paper 9/05, NSW Parliamentary Library Research Service (2005), 50; Key Centre for Women's Health in Society et al., *Abortion in Victoria*, 21, 25; Victorian Law Reform Commission, *Law of Abortion: Final Report* (Melbourne: Victorian Law Reform Commission, 2008); L. A. Keogh et al., "Intended and Unintended Consequences of Abortion Law Reform: Perspectives of Abortion Experts in Victoria, Australia," *Journal of Family Planning and Reproductive Health Care* 43, no. 1 (2016): 18–24; Shankar et al., "Access, Equity and Costs."

33. P. L. Adelson, M. S. Frommer, and E. A. Weisberg, "A Survey of Women Seeking Termination of Pregnancy in New South Wales," *Medical Journal of Australia* 163, no. 8 (1995): 419–22; Caroline De Costa, "Rural Women's Access to Termination of Pregnancy: The View from Far North Queensland," *O&G Magazine* 7, no. 1 (2005): 58–60; Julie Kruss, "'Country Women are Resilient but . . .': Family Planning Access in Rural Victoria" (unpublished PhD diss., Victoria University, 2012); Shankar et al., "Access, Equity and Costs."

34. De Costa, "Rural Women's Access to Termination"; Kruss, "Country Women Are Resilient"; Doran and Hornibrook, "Rural New South Wales."

35. Adelson, Frommer, and Weisberg, "A Survey of Women"; Nickson, "Travel Undertaken by Women"; Kruss, "Country Women Are Resilient."

36. Kruss, "Country Women Are Resilient," 119.

37. Shankar et al., "Access, Equity and Costs," 3.

38. "3101.0—Australian Demographic Statistics, Mar 2018," Australian Bureau of Statistics, accessed October 3, 2018, http://www.abs.gov.au/ausstats /abs@.nsf/mf/3101.0; "Area of Australia—States and Territories," Geoscience Australia, accessed October 3, 2018, http://www.ga.gov.au/scientific-topics /national-location-information/dimensions/area-of-australia-states-and -territories. Distances are calculated using Google Maps, accessed August 15, 2017, https://www.google.com.au/maps.

39. Abortion Rights Network of Australia, *Abortion: Legal Right, Women's Right, Human Right* (West End, Qld: Women's Abortion Campaign, 1993), 39; Lyndall Ryan, Margie Ripper, and Barbara Buttfield, *We Women Decide: Women's Experience of Seeking Abortion in Queensland, South Australia and Tasmania 1985–1992* (Adelaide: Women's Studies Unit, Flinders University, 1994), 71, 78.

40. A. Chan, J. Scott, and K. McCaul, *Pregnancy Outcome in South Australia 1990* (Adelaide: Pregnancy Outcome Unit, SA Health Commission, 1992), 33–34.

41. Wendy Scheil et al., *Pregnancy Outcome in South Australia 2014* (Adelaide: Pregnancy Outcome Unit, SA Health, Government of South Australia, 2016), 54.

42. "Fact sheet 9," SA Abortion Action Coalition, accessed August 15, 2017, https://saabortionactioncoalition.com/.

43. Stephanie Grayston, "Changing Attitudes and Services: Abortion in Western Australia, 1970–1990," in *Sexuality and Gender in History*, ed. Penelope Hetherington and Philippa C. Maddern (Perth: Centre for WA History at UWA, 1993), 242–54.

44. M. Hutchinson, A. Joyce, and M. Cheong, *Induced Abortions in Western Australia 2010–2012, 4th Report of the Western Australian Abortion Notification System* (Perth: Department of Health, Western Australia, 2013), 2.

45. A. Cawley (Broome Regional Aboriginal Medical Service), Submission to the Inquiry into Therapeutic Goods Amendment (Repeal of Ministerial Responsibility for Approval of RU486), Bill 2005. No. 606, (n.d.).

46. Ryan, Ripper, and Buttfield, *We Women Decide*, 23.

47. Carolyn Nickson, Julia Shelley, and Anthony Smith, "Use of Interstate Services for the Termination of Pregnancy in Australia," *Australian and New Zealand Journal of Public Health* 26, no. 5 (2002): 423.

48. De Costa, "Rural Women's Access to Termination," 58.

49. Gina Rushton, "Women Are Flying Interstate for Surgical Abortions Because One Doctor Retired," *BuzzFeedNews*, March 24, 2018, https://www.buzzfeed.com/ginarushton/women-are-flying-interstate-for-surgical-abortions-because?utm_term=.kdJOon5565#.aqOwgazz6z.

50. Caroline De Costa et al., "Introducing Early Medical Abortion in Australia: There Is a Need to Update Abortion Laws," *Sexual Health* 4, no. 4 (2007): 223–26.

51. De Costa, "Rural Women's Access to Termination," 58.

52. Children by Choice, "Interstate Abortion Providers."

53. Melissa Davey, "Albury's Only Abortion Clinic: Protests 'Push Women to Self-Harm,'" *Guardian*, December 9, 2014, https://www.theguardian.com/world/2014/dec/09/women-seeking-abortions-harassed-by-protesters-to-point-of-suicide.

54. National Health and Medical Research Council, *An Information Paper on Termination of Pregnancy*, 4.

55. Adelson, Frommer, and Weisberg, "A Survey of Women."

56. Doran and Hornibrook, "Rural New South Wales," 123.

57. L. Coelli, A. Davidson, and C. Orr, "Increasing Access to Medical Termination of Pregnancy through Nurse-Led Models of Care" (Presentation at Australian Sexual Health Medicine Conference, n.p., 2016).

58. Kruss, "Country Women Are Resilient," 18.

59. Women's Health Victoria, *Victorian Rural Women's Access to Family Planning Services: Survey Report August 2012* (Ballarat, Victoria: Rural Services of the Women's Health Association of Victoria, 2012), 54–75.

60. Kirsten Black, Jane Fisher, and Sonia Grover, "Public Hospital Pregnancy Termination Services: Are We Meeting Demand?" *Australian and New Zealand Journal of Public Health* 23, no. 5 (1999): 525–27; Nickson, Smith, and Shelley, "Travel Undertaken by Women," 329–33.

61. Key Centre for Women's Health in Society et al., *Abortion in Victoria*, 31–36.

62. Key Centre for Women's Health in Society et al., *Abortion in Victoria*, 32.

63. Dianne Dempsey, "Abortion Clinic Back in Bendigo," *Bendigo Weekly*, August 16, 2013, http://bendigoweekly.designexperts.com.au/news/abortion-clinic-back-in-bendigo.

64. State of Victoria Department of Health and Human Services, *Women's Sexual and Reproductive Health: Key Priorities 2017–2020* (Melbourne: Victorian Government, 2017).

65. Ryan, Ripper, and Buttfield, *We Women Decide*, 45.

66. National Health and Medical Research Council, *An Information Paper on Termination of Pregnancy*, 4.

67. Ryan, Ripper, and Buttfield, *We Women Decide*, 117.

68. Abortion Rights Network of Australia, *Abortion*, 43–45.

69. Nickson, Shelley, and Smith, "Use of Interstate Services," 423.

70. Abortion Rights Network of Australia, *Abortion*, 44–45.

71. Barbara Baird, "The Futures of Abortion," in *Feminist Temporalities*, ed. Elizabeth McMahon and Brigitta Olubas (Perth: University of Western Australia Press, 2006), 128–29.

72. Matt Smith, "Fears Raised as Abortion Clinic Closes," *Mercury*, July 19, 2014, 2; Emily Baker, "Launceston Abortion Centre to Close," *Examiner*, May 10, 2016, http://www.examiner.com.au/story/3899702/ab ortion-centre-to-close/; Rhiana Whitson, "Tasmanian Election: Liberals Stand by Plan to Send Women Interstate for Abortions," *ABC News*, February 1, 2018, http://www.abc.net.au/news/2018-01-31/tas-abortion-policies-revealed/9378756.

73. Abortion Rights Network of Australia, *Abortion*, 33–34.

74. Gwendolyn Gray Jamieson, *Reaching for Health: The Australian Women's Health Movement and Public Policy* (Canberra: Australian National University E Press, 2012), 203.

75. *Children by Choice*, "Interstate Abortion Providers."

76. Suzanne Belton and Karen Dempsey, "Termination of Pregnancy: Trends, Women's Characteristics, Implications for Public Health Planning in the Northern Territory" (unpublished report, 2016).

77. Nickson, Shelley, and Smith, "Use of Interstate Services," 422.

78. Cate Swannell, "Medical Abortion Access Extended," *Medical Journal of Australia, InSight* 27, no. 2 (January 2015): https://www.mja.com.au/insight/2015/2/medical-abortion-access-extended.

79. Suzanne Belton, Caroline De Costa, and Andrea Whittaker, "Termination of Pregnancy: A Long Way to Go in the Northern Territory," *Medical Journal of Australia* 202, no. 3 (February 2015): 130–31.

80. Abortion Rights Network of Australia, *Abortion*, 39.

81. David Ellwood, "Late Terminations of Pregnancy—An Obstetrician's Perspective," *Australian Health Review* 29, no. 2 (2005): 139–42.

82. Jan E. Dickinson, "Late Pregnancy Termination within a Legislated Medical Environment," *Australian and New Zealand Journal of Obstetrics and Gynaecology* 44, no. 4 (2004): 337–41; Caroline De Costa, "Abortion Law,

Abortion Realities" (Mayo Lecture, James Cook University, Townsville, September 3, 2008).

83. Keogh et al., "Intended and Unintended Consequences," 22.

84. "Late Term Abortion," Marie Stopes Australia, https://www.mariestopes.org.au/abortion/late-term-abortion/.

85. Bronwyn Fredericks, "How the Whiteness Embodied in Health Services Impacts on the Health and Well-Being of Indigenous peoples," in *The Racial Politics of Bodies, Nations and Knowledges*, ed. Barbara Baird and Damien Riggs (Newcastle upon Tyne: Cambridge Scholars Publishing, 2009), 11–27.

86. Kerry Arabena, "Preachers, Policies and Power: The Reproductive Health of Aboriginal and Torres Strait Islander Peoples in Australia," *Health Promotion Journal of Australia* 17, no. 2 (2006): 85–90.

87. Kerry Arabena, "Preachers, Policies and Power," 88.

88. Australian Institute of Health and Welfare, *The Health and Welfare of Australia's Aboriginal and Torres Strait Islander Peoples 2015* (Canberra: Australian Institute of Health and Welfare, 2015).

89. Nickson, Shelley, and Smith, "Use of Interstate Services"; Shankar et al., "Access, Equity and Costs."

90. Kruss, "Country Women Are Resilient"; De Costa, "Rural Women's Access to Termination."

91. Hutchinson, "Induced Abortions," 3.

92. Belton, *Termination of Pregnancy*, 7–8.

93. Janet Kelly et al., "Travelling to the City for Hospital Care: Access Factors in Country Aboriginal Patient Journeys," *Australian Journal of Rural Health* 22, no. 3 (2014): 109–13.

94. Baird, "The Futures of Abortion"; De Costa, *Never, Ever, Again . . .*, 110–12.

95. Cheryl Davenport, "Achieving Abortion Law Reform in Western Australia," *Australian Feminist Studies* 13, no. 28 (1998): 300; De Costa, *Never, Ever, Again . . .*, 113.

96. De Costa, *Never, Ever, Again . . .*, 113.

97. Key Centre for Women's Health in Society et al., *Abortion in Victoria*; Dempsey, "Abortion Clinic Back"; Swannell, "Medical Abortion Access."

98. Wendy Bacon et al., *Protection Denied, Abuse Condoned: Women on Nauru at Risk* (Potts Point, NSW: Australian Women in Support of Women on Nauru, 2016), 6–7, 50.

99. Patricia Hayes, "Reproductive Coercion and the Australian State: A New Chapter?," *Australian Community Psychologist*, 28, no. 1 (2016): 90–100.

100. Maggie Kirkman et al., "Abortion Is a Difficult Solution to a Problem: A Discursive Analysis of Interviews with Women Considering or Undergoing Abortion in Australia," *Women's Studies International Forum* 34, no. 2 (2011): 124.

101. Ryan, Ripper, and Buttfield, *We Women Decide*, 117.

102. Doran and Hornibrook, "Rural New South Wales," 125.

103. Appadurai, *Modernity at Large*, 22.

104. Kate Gleeson, "The Limits of 'Choice': Abortion and Entrepreneurialism," in *Reframing Reproduction: Sociological Perspectives on the Intersection between Gender, Sexuality and Reproduction in Late Modernity*, ed. Meredith Nash (London: Palgrave, 2009), 69–83.

105. Cosima Marriner, "Abortion Couple Not Aware They Broke Law," *Sydney Morning Herald*, September 19, 2009, www.smh.com.au/national /abortion-couple-not-aware-they-broke-the-law-20090918-fvcg.html.

106. Christabelle Sethna and Marion Doull, "Accidental Tourists: Canadian Women, Abortion Tourism and Travel," *Women's Studies* 4, no. 4 (2012): 471.

107. In October 2018, the Qld government's bill to remove abortion from the criminal law and make it available on request up to 22 weeks, and with the approval of two doctors after that point, passed with a comfortable majority. See Ben Smee, "Queensland Parliament Votes to Legalise Abortion," *Guardian*, October 17, 2018, https://www.theguardian.com/australia-news/2018/oct/17/ queensland-parliament-votes-to-legalise-abortion. This change will not, however, lead to any automatic improvement in access for women in rural, regional, and remote areas but *may* encourage doctors to offer EMA and public hospitals to offer abortion services.

[7]

Don't Mess with Texas

Abortion Policy, Texas Style

LORI A. BROWN

ACCORDING TO PUBLIC health officials, there is a public health threat to women living in Texas, in the United States of America (USA). Due to the Texas state legislature's anti-abortion policies in 2013 and 2014, almost half of all clinics providing abortion services have closed across the state.[1] As Kinsey Hasstedt has written in the Guttmacher Institute Spring 2014 *Policy Review*, not only do one-quarter of all Texas adult women live below the federal level of poverty, but Texas also has the highest proportion of adult women in the country who do not have health insurance.[2] There are limited contraceptive services available, although Texas has the highest percentage of women needing publicly funded contraception. There are also high rates of unintended pregnancies, teen pregnancies, and sexually transmitted illnesses (STIs).[3]

The state's sex education curriculum is "abstinence only."[4] Abstinence is promoted as a prophylactic against unintended pregnancy and STIs, as described in both the middle school and high school downloadable curriculum overview from the Texas Education Agency's "Texas Essential Knowledge and Skills for Health Education." The curriculum supports "abstinence from sexual activity [a]s the preferred choice of behavior in relation to all sexual activity for unmarried persons of school age."[5] The only difference between middle and high school curricula is that a high school education requires discussion about health choices and their impact on fetal development in order for students to understand better the influence their individual health behaviors have on pre- and postnatal outcomes.[6]

Hasstedt claims ominously, "Texas stands as a warning sign for the rest of the nation."[7] Anti-abortion successes in reducing abortion access across the state demonstrate how precarious women's reproductive healthcare actually is in the USA. Similar trends are also evident in other states such as Louisiana, Mississippi, South Dakota, North Dakota, Kentucky, and Alabama.[8] Texas represents what happens when abortion is legal on paper yet inaccessible for a large population segment due to state restrictions that have produced massive clinic closures.[9] As a result, what was once considered typical travel to access reproductive healthcare within the state has become a difficult endeavor for many Texas women. Because some of the most stringent abortion laws in the country were passed by the Texas legislature during 2013 and 2014, and signed into law by Governor Rick Perry, only 19 clinics providing abortion services remained in operation in the second most populous and the second-largest state in the country after California.[10]

It is important to point out that the math does not add up. Texan women of reproductive age simply do not have an adequate number of clinics statewide to fulfill patient demand for reproductive healthcare. And they face a similar problem that Barbara Baird, in her contribution to this volume, identifies in regard to Australian women. Because Texas, like individual states in Australia, is geographically so vast, it is now not uncommon for a woman living in Texas to have to travel several hours in order to reach an abortion clinic that remains open within the state. This situation was created by the Texas legislature's incremental erosion of a woman's federally guaranteed right to abortion from the 1973 United States Supreme Court decision *Roe v. Wade* onward. Due to the continually changing political climate in Texas, and more broadly throughout the country, this chapter examines the time period between 2013 and 2015, when the Texas legislature passed a series of anti-abortion laws and phased in their implementation, resulting in significant fluctuations in access to abortion across the state.

Demographics, Texas Style

Texas is the second-largest state by square miles and the second most populous state in the country after California.[11] The 2017 census data estimates that the Texas state population was more than 28 million, with 50.4 percent recorded as female. The state poverty rate is 15.6 percent[12] compared to the national average of 12.7 percent.[13] Of the ten most populous counties in the USA, Texas claims two: Harris County is the third most populous and Dallas County is the ninth.[14] Of the ten most populated cities in the country, Texas boasts three: Houston is fourth with more than two million people, San Antonio is seventh with more than 1.4 million people, and Dallas is ninth with more than 1.3 million people.[15]

During the three-year time period this chapter examines, and of the 19 clinics providing abortion services that remained open in Texas, 15 were located in the three most populous Texan cities. The Dallas–Fort Worth metropolitan area had a combined six clinics—Dallas had four clinics, and Fort Worth had two. Houston had six clinics, and San Antonio had three.[16] It is difficult to fathom that these 19 clinics could have handled the needs of not only their immediate population but also the enormous influx of women from the western part of the state, where only one clinic in the city of El Paso and one clinic in the city of McAllen remained open.[17] On the one hand, it is sensible to have clinics concentrated in the most populous cities in Texas. On the other hand, what is nonsensical is to presume that 19 clinics alone can serve the entire state due to its large population and geographic enormity.

Figure 7.1 contextualizes the location of clinics within the state in 2015. Neighboring state clinics are also included because sizeable areas of the state no longer have providers. Figure 7.2 illustrates the extensive gaps throughout the states that had no access to an abortion provider in 2015.[18]

Population Diversity

Sharing a border with Mexico, Texas has significantly large Hispanic and Latinx populations. According to the 2016 census data, 39.1 percent of the Texas population is either of Hispanic or Latinx origin, compared to 17.8 percent of Americans nationally.[19] At that time, Texas had the second-greatest Hispanic population only after California. The average age of the Hispanic population in Texas is 28 years, and the poverty rate of Hispanics 17 years of age and younger is 34 percent, compared to 10 percent for non-Hispanic whites and 33 percent for non-Hispanic blacks in the same age range. The rate of medically uninsured Hispanics is 31 percent compared with 11 percent of non-Hispanic whites and 17 percent of non-Hispanic blacks. Additionally, Hispanics and Latinxs comprise 48 percent of all students from kindergarten to grade 12.[20] According to the Pew Research Center, Hispanic and Latinx popula-

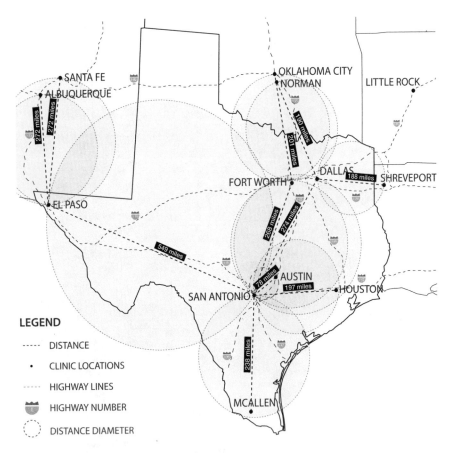

Figure 7.1. Texas abortion clinic locations.

tions are predicted to become the majority in Texas, increasing in numbers more quickly than any other census-identified population.[21]

Although Hispanics and Latinxs comprise a growing percentage of the state's population, the Texas government did not support the efforts of former president Barack Obama's administration to create a path to their legal citizenship. In February 2015, Texas District Court Judge Andrew Hanen issued an injunction preventing the Obama administration from moving forward with its Deferred Action for Childhood Arrivals (DACA) and the new Deferred Action for Parental Accountability (DAPA), which would have allowed approximately 4.9 million undocumented migrants to receive a work permit and avoid deportation. Led by Texas, 26 states filed a lawsuit against DACA and DAPA in

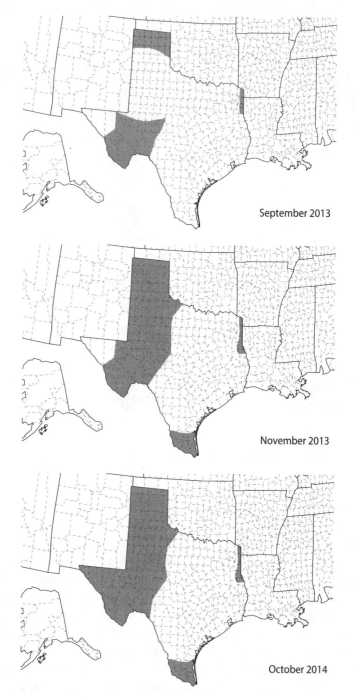

September 2013

November 2013

October 2014

Figure 7.2. Regions (shaded) of Texas, USA, that lack abortion providers.

order to hinder this legislation from being enacted.[22] The June 2016 Supreme Court's split decision of *United States v. Texas* denied these programs from going into effect, thereby reinforcing the legal precarity of undocumented Hispanics and Latinxs living in the USA. In September 2017, the Republican-dominated administration of President Donald Trump, fulfilling its tough-on-immigration policies, officially ended the DACA program, setting the stage for congressional battles and lawsuits.[23] These battles continued, as demonstrated by the legislative impasse that shuttered the federal government for three days in January 2018. Thereafter, the future of DACA remained uncertain, despite the promise of subsequent rounds of negotiations.[24] Even more controversy erupted later that same year after the Trump administration announced a "zero tolerance policy" for illegal border crossings. It began detaining undocumented migrants from Central and South America who were streaming into Texas and other border states, separating parents from their children and housing both in cage-like structures.[25]

According to the Guttmacher Institute, the largest proportion of abortion patients in the USA who seek abortion services at greater rates are the most economically disadvantaged.[26] And, as lawyer Madeline Gomez has observed, various and "intersecting oppressions result in disproportionate harm to women and communities of color, resulting in outcomes far beyond a lack of access to abortion."[27] In fact, data from Jenna Jerman, Rachel K. Jones, and Tsuyoshi Onda show that the majority of women seeking abortion pay for the procedure out of pocket, and that Medicaid coverage was the second most common form of payment. As is discussed later, due to the high rates of medically uninsured women in Texas and the state's refusal to allow Medicaid to cover abortion, Medicaid coverage was not an option, thereby reducing even further a poor woman's ability to pay for medical care. Additionally, Jerman, Jones, and Onda cite Guttmacher's director of public policy Heather Boonstra, who confirmed that the increases in state abortion restrictions disproportionally affect the most economically disadvantaged.[28] Based on medical and legal research, one can extrapolate that during the time period under investigation, the geographic size of Texas, combined with its demographics—high rates of poverty, a lack of medical insurance, the rise in the numbers of Hispanic and Latinx youths, and their shaky legal status—meant that young Hispanic and Latinx women were among the most vulnerable to the already-inadequate access to abortion services in the state.

Guns, Crime, and Punishment

According to the Law Center to Prevent Gun Violence, in 2014 Texas stood 29th in both gun law rank, with extremely weak gun laws, and gun death rank, and in 2016, the state exported the third largest number of crime guns among all states.[29] Seventy percent of guns recovered from crimes scenes in the neighboring country of Mexico were traced to their sale in Texas since 2009.[30] Texas also has the highest rate of incarceration in the country, with 24 percent more prisoners than California. Whites comprise 45 percent of the Texas population and 33 percent of the prison population, while African Americans comprise just 12 percent of the Texas population yet as much as 32 percent of the prison population. Latinxs comprise 38 percent of the Texas population and 32 percent of the prison population.[31] In 2014, Texas had more imprisoned noncitizens than any other state.[32] Death row numbers for 2016 reveal that Texas ranks third in the country, with 254 such inmates. Only two other states exceed these statistics: Florida is second with 396 prisoners on death row, and California is first with 741.[33] Since the United States Supreme Court affirmed capital punishment's constitutionality in 1976, Texas has executed more prisoners than any other state.[34] As Texas governor between 2000 and 2015, Perry actively supported state executions and oversaw more executions than any other governor in the country.[35]

Critics of Texan abortion policies see a great philosophical dissonance between a pro-life abortion position taken by a pro-gun, pro-incarceration, pro-death penalty state that also enforces aggressive deportation policies targeting undocumented migrants.[36] Moreover, the Texas government, which strongly supports gun rights and refuses to impose strict gun control regulations on its populace, has systemically increased its control over abortion, making it almost unacceptable for a woman to determine her own reproductive autonomy. Indeed, by Texan law, a woman is required to wait 24 hours to access abortion services, longer than is needed legally to purchase a gun in Texas.[37]

Social Services

As noted earlier, Texas remains at the forefront of the country's incarceration, execution, and deportation rates. The state also leads the way in gutting state-provided social services. This has been years in the making, and former governor Perry, now secretary of energy in the Trump administration, was particularly invested in ensuring it happened. He adamantly opposed the passage of the Affordable Care Act (ACA), which provided health insurance to millions of previously uninsured Americans and became the signature domestic accomplishment of the Obama administration, and is now popularly known as "Obamacare." Perry asserted, "Obamacare is bad for the economy, bad for health care, bad for freedom." In response to the United States Supreme Court's upholding of the ACA, he wrote a letter to Kathleen Sebelius, former secretary of the federal Department of Health and Human Services, expressing his opinion that the expansion of Medicaid[38] and the creation of state insurance exchanges were "a brazen intrusion into the sovereignty of our state [of Texas] . . . and would not help create better 'patient protection' or . . . more 'affordable care.'"[39] Yet in an interview with television's Fox News on the very same day his letter was sent to Sebelius, Perry offered no proposals to counter the ACA, leveling only criticism, even though the television correspondent cited data that ranked Texas last in the nation in health services for Texans, with 25 percent of the population medically uninsured.[40] Perry's arguments against the ACA have been taken up by the Trump administration and Republican-led congressional efforts to repeal and replace the ACA. Thus far, the Republicans have been unsuccessful in their efforts, even though an estimated 20 million Americans would become uninsured if either the House or Senate's plans should become law. Much of the American public, anxious, angry, and vocal about the drastic and devastating changes being proposed, await the outcome of the ACA.[41]

Perry's publicized "Texas Miracle" of low taxes, low services, and low regulations was one created by reliance on federal stimulus monies; in fact, Texas relied more heavily on these than any other state in 2010. It has been estimated that the stimulus filled 97 percent of the state's budgetary gap; however, there was a 25 percent child poverty rate in the state.[42] In 2011, with a major revenue shortfall, Perry was willing to reduce services for children by US$10 billion over two years to fill the gap.[43] As one perceives, right-wing conservative politics play out in Texas in a variety of ways and have been used to reconfigure and drastically reduce the social safety net for the middle and lower classes. Texas is both an American anomaly and a clear demonstration of the power of the right-wing conservative branch of the Republican Party and their continued efforts to decrease, even decimate, state support for the underserved. Although there are greater numbers of the Texas population in need, they receive less and less support.

Church and State

It is important to highlight that Texas is a state with many extremes. Easily distinguished from other conservative states, Texas brash extremism is said to be a badge of honor for most Texans, and the state views itself as a model for the rest of the country to follow.[44] Religion plays an integral role in the state's identity, with a significant number of Texans religiously active and self-identifying as Christian. According to the *Texas Almanac*, at least 59–60 percent of the Texas population practices Christianity compared to the national average of 48.8 percent. The five largest religious groups in Texas are Catholics with 18.59 percent of the state population, Southern Baptists with 14.8 percent, nondenominational Christians with 6.15 percent, United Methodists with 4.46 percent, and Muslims with 1.68 percent.[45]

Given these social and political complexities, it is not surprising to discover the strong influence of Christianity in civic life, a factor that Mary Gilmartin and Sinéad Kennedy also explore in this volume in their discussion about abortion access in Ireland, as do Cathrine Chambers, Colleen MacQuarrie, and Jo-Ann MacDonald in their research on Prince Edward Island, Canada. Agata Ignaciuk's chapter on Spain and Ewelina Ciaputa's chapter on Poland share similar findings. Texas Right to Life is an active group that has demonstrated quite the political acumen in advancing its antichoice agenda. The push for antichoice abortion legislation can be directly connected to this group. Another avenue of religious influence is through crisis pregnancy centers (CPCs), essentially fake clinics providing free ultrasounds and misinformation to pregnant women in hopes of influencing them not to have an abortion. In 2005, the Texas state budget contained a rider that, as of 2011, moved US$18 million from preventative women's health and family planning services to an "alternatives to abortion" program. This program provides no recommended health services but instead gives taxpayer money to the primary contractor, Texas Pregnancy Care Network. These type of facilities comprise up to 70 percent of this network. These groups have no confidentiality agreements or state oversight.[46] However, Texas has laws supporting CPCs, it funds CPCs, and it deliberately refers pregnant women seeking possible abortion services to CPCs.[47]

Reproductive Access in Texas

The slogan "Don't Mess with Texas" marked an anti-litter campaign for highways introduced by the Department of Transportation in the 1980s, only to become the state's boastful marketing mantra. Critics agree that the state's behavior toward its most vulnerable residents is arrogant, and it has wreaked havoc upon millions of reproductive-age women. As many healthcare providers have highlighted, Texas women continue to face extraordinary obstacles in accessing reproductive healthcare because of the increase of state abortion restrictions, combined with fewer functioning clinics. Consequently, Texas remains an urgent and necessary case study due to the state's vast geography, its anti-abortion policies, and the impact of those policies on accessing reproductive healthcare in the wider USA.

Between 2013 and 2015, when numerous clinics were closed due to Texas House Bill 2 (HB2), women needing access to abortion services were left with far fewer abortion providers across the state. This lack further escalated the expenses involved and the time taken for the procedure, including follow-up care. Prior to the passage of HB2, there were 41 medical practices licensed to provide abortions in Texas. Two years after HB2 was signed into law, only 19 remained open. As lawyer Madeline Gomez has noted, in 2011 the Texas legislature drastically restructured state funding for family planning centers (ones that do not provide abortion services) and reproductive health clinics (ones that do provide abortions) by cutting two-thirds of the family planning budget. The budget dropped from US$111 million to US$37.9 million. The restructuring prioritized clinics that provided other services in addition to family planning. Secondly, Texas ceased funding any Planned Parenthood affiliates due to their connections with abortion providers. This decision affected more than half of all Texas women who had previously received family planning care through the state's Women's Health Program (now consolidated with the Expanded Primary Health Care for Women program to create a Healthy Texas Women program). Not only did those women no longer receive family planning services, but because federal Medicaid matching funds are dependent on state designation, clinics were no longer able to receive these Medicaid funds, resulting in many clinic closures throughout the state. These changes greatly impacted women across Texas but even more so those living along the Rio Grande Valley because of the additional burden of the region's lower numbers of primary healthcare providers and limited access to healthcare.[48]

As stated previously, Texas HB2 refers to the law that regulates "abortion procedures, providers, and facilities"; provides penalties; and was approved on July 18, 2013, by Governor Perry. This law created some of the most draconian abortion regulations in the country, according to many physicians and medical and public health researchers. Included in the law were what are referred to as four "supply-side abortion restrictions": the banning of abortions after 20 weeks; hospital admitting privileges only for physicians within a 30-mile area of the facility; medical abortions required to follow a more inflexible FDA dosage schedule,[49] with up to four trips to the same doctor's office;[50] and clinic building codes for abortion facility standards that had to be "equivalent to the minimum standards . . . for ambulatory surgical centers [ASCs]."[51] The latter HB2 requirement essentially required clinics providing abortion services to renovate their facilities at their own cost to become similar to outpatient hospital–like centers. Many healthcare professionals expressed concern that such requirements would result in an increase in self-induced abortions, as well as in the numbers of women traveling to nearby Mexico for both medical and surgical abortions.[52]

Over a 17-month period, there was significant fluctuation in clinic accessibility. Daniel Grossman et al., a group of researchers and physicians from the Bixby Center for Global Reproductive Health at the University California–San Francisco, the School of Public Health at the University of Alabama–Birmingham, and the Population Research Center at the University of Texas–Austin, did remarkable research in providing as close to a temporal analysis of the abortion legislation changes and their on-the-ground impact as possible as HB2 was phased into implementation. Highlighting their data illustrates how access to abortion services shifted dramatically in geographical terms during this time period. Six months before the passage of HB2, and before the situation began to change drastically, 41 facilities provided abortions between November 1, 2012, and April 30, 2013. At this point, approximately 10,000 women lived less than 200 miles from a Texas clinic. However, between May 1, 2013, and October 31, 2013, HB2 was publicly debated and passed, but not yet enforced. Thirty-three clinics provided care and eight closed. Then, between November 1, 2013, and April 30, 2014, all provisions except the ASC requirement were enforced. Twenty-two facilities provided care and 11 closed or stopped providing abortions. Five clinics providing abortion services reopened once their doctors were finally granted hospital admitting privileges, but another five closed due to doctors losing these privileges, or for other reasons. It was also estimated that approximately 290,000 women now lived more than 200 miles from a Texas clinic. In between the two aforementioned time periods, regions outside metropolitan areas were most affected, with 11 out of 13 clinics closed.[53]

The changes legally required of clinics, as described by Texas state officials, were created to "protect women's health."[54] Ironically, they produced a situation in which more than 900,000 reproductive-age women ended up living more than 150 miles from the nearest abortion provider, an almost 10.5 percent increase from earlier statistics that showed that 86,000 women lived more than 150 miles from a clinic.[55] As a result of the United States Supreme Court's October 2014 order blocking a Texas law that had previously shuttered 33 clinics, there would no longer be clinics operating in the western and lower Rio Grande Valley regions of the state. Grossman et al. found that within just the first year after implementation, the laws significantly reduced the number of abortions in Texas by 46 percent, such that "vast swaths of the state were left without a provider and the number of women required to travel great distances to reach a provider increased dramatically."[56]

Although the official rationale of needing to protect women's health was reiterated often, physician organizations argued quite differently. Not only did the American Congress of Obstetricians and Gynecologists (ACOG) and the Texas Medical Association (TMA) disagree with the waves of restrictions on abortion services, but the Texas Hospital Association (THA) also opposed the requirement of hospital admitting privileges for physicians providing clinic abortions. The ACOG and the TMA were concerned about the state's direct encroachment into medical practice. The THA countered that "any women needing emergency care can already receive such care at the hospital,"[57] and that admitting privileges for doctors did "nothing to protect women's health."[58] In opposition to HB2, the THA held that the Texas Medical Board (TMB) "is the appropriate agency to address whether physicians are delivering appropriate care to patients, as the TMB regulates all physicians.

Hospitals should not be required to assume responsibility for the qualifications of physicians who do not practice in the hospital."[59] Grossman et al. concurred, stating that the legislation "represents a stunning incursion into the physician's exam room, allowing state representatives to dictate how doctors should practice medicine" and was "in blatant contradiction to evidence-based medicine."[60]

On the ground, women were having great difficulty in accessing abortion services, adding significantly more stress to the process of locating an appointment in a timely manner. Affordability, although an obstacle on an individual level, was not the primary issue in Texas—geographic availability was. More and more clinics were being forced to close. Two of the most prevalent legislative acts that precipitated clinic closures across the country were abortion doctors unable to receive hospital admitting privileges *and* clinics providing abortion services that were unable to afford the renovations to meet ambulatory building code requirements. To have a clinic become ambulatory compliant varies from state to state but may include an array of changes that, on the surface, appear to be minor alterations. However, spatial changes such as increasing door and hallway widths, building additional closets for medical supplies, and increasing dimensions of patient rooms, and entire clinic changes that include installing sprinkler systems or even sophisticated air-quality control systems are costly. These renovations may cost up to millions of dollars per clinic, rendering change unaffordable to most independent abortion providers. Life and safety concerns, the primary focus of building codes, were not improved by these restrictions.[61]

As a result of clinics being unable to employ doctors who had not been granted hospital admitting privileges or being unable to afford renovation expenses, clinics continued to close, as noted by several feminist groups. As fewer and fewer clinics remained open, one was required to ask: How far is too far to travel for medical services? What are the ramifications of distance, time, and expense on a patient? What happens when a clinic is no longer a short distance away but located hundreds of miles from communities in need or when reproductive healthcare is no longer readily available? In response, one must acknowledge that laws in Texas were manipulated solely for political gain.

The great rural regions of Texas pose yet another extreme layer of difficulty for women seeking to access abortion services. Lisa Pruitt, lawyer and legal scholar, argues that the complicated and multilayered dimensions of rural women's lives are often ignored in regard to the law. She notes that there are many economic and spatial disadvantages for those living in rural areas and that the "law often fails to appreciate the influence of structural barriers that constrain rural women's choices."[62] She provides examples where courts have considered these barriers relative to insurance payments for home healthcare services, transportation costs for medical treatments, and even medical devices for the home when these services are too far away to access. However, crucially, she suggests that judges do not exhibit the same degree of understanding when rural women confront abortion access hardships.[63]

It is also critical that women's lived experiences inform how courts consider the impact of legislation on patients. Pruitt and coauthor Marta Vanegas insist that when legal deliberations do not include discussion of the literal impact on access to health services and the sociospatial and economic limitations involved, women's agency is severely limited, especially in the case of rural women. The courts' failure "to recognize that the undue burden test is context specific"[64] is not just a philosophical or theoretical argument but a matter that has a devastating impact on women seeking abortion services. Pruitt and Vanegas contend that these laws "govern unevenly, as the regulations and their consequences are 'differently refracted through the social architecture of spatialities.' In short, the material spaces along the rural-urban continuum dictate how law happens or operates."[65] Not taking these aspects into consideration has even further disenfranchised millions of women from access to abortion services.

Women along the Rio Grande Valley, which borders Mexico, live this reality daily. More recently, because of the Trump administration's aggressive position on immigration, more Immigration and Customs Enforcement agents have been added to patrol within 100 miles of the USA border regions.[66] This heightened presence of border patrol creates ever more tenuous situations for undocumented migrants from Mexico. In addition to fixed checkpoints, "tactical checkpoints" have been added within this 100-mile range. The fear of being caught has produced a situation in which undocumented Latinxs and Hispanics are now "landlocked," making accessible healthcare difficult, if not impossible, for those living in these areas. The Texas Policy Evaluation Project, a University of Texas–Austin collaborative research group that evaluates the repercussions of legislation for reproductive healthcare in Texas, confirms that they have found fewer Latinxs and Hispanics seek abortion services in Texas clinics.[67]

Medical Tourism

When a woman has no other option but to travel hundreds of miles to access an abortion provider, she becomes a tourist within and outside her own state. I discovered in researching for my book *Contested Spaces: Abortion Clinics, Women's Shelters and Hospitals* (2013) that prior to the legalization of abortion in North America, abortion tourism was a common occurrence for American women of means. This could mean international or interstate travel. American women traveled to European countries and to Mexico to access abortion services. Although abortion was illegal in Mexico prior to the 1973 United States Supreme Court decision *Roe v. Wade*, which legalized abortion in the first trimester, it was not uncommon for women to travel to various cities in Mexico to terminate their pregnancies, creating a steady stream of patients.[68] At least one organization, the Clergy Consultation Service on Abortion, expanded across the USA in the late 1960s and early 1970s. It was instrumental in connecting women with doctors in the country and across the Mexican border who would provide abortions,[69] and it functioned as did many abortion referral agencies in facilitating access to abortion services, often over long distances, as Hayley Brown, Christabelle Sethna, and Agata Ignaciuk detail in their respective chapters in this volume.

In Canada, women were compelled to travel to access abortion services, and this remains the case for certain regions today. Christabelle Sethna found that Canadian women who could afford the costs traveled abroad for abortion services in the 1960s and 1970s.[70] Sethna and Marion Doull have researched more contemporary conditions, showing that some Canadian women are required to travel considerable distances to access abortion services because clinic access is actually quite uneven across the country. Similar to the USA, women who reside in larger cities have a greater degree of access than their rural counterparts.[71] In smaller and more remote communities, extralegal impediments can create delays in reaching providers located in larger cities such as Ottawa or Montreal. As they note, since the 1988 Canadian Supreme Court decision *R v. Morgentaler*, which struck down a restrictive abortion law passed in 1969, "marginalized populations of women—Aboriginal women, young women, women from the North, women from rural areas, and women from Atlantic Canada—have tended to travel farthest within Canada to access abortion services."[72]

Geography Matters and Spatial Ramifications

Although abortion is federally guaranteed in the USA, women residing in states like Texas have extraordinary difficulties accessing abortion in a timely manner. In Texas between 2013 and 2015, women faced circumstances that seemed at times to be shockingly similar to pre–*Roe v. Wade* scenarios. On this note, it is critical to understand and visualize relationships among clinic locations, cost of travel, Texas geography, and demographics, especially in relation to the spatial ramifications of HB2. Although the Guttmacher Institute stated that in 2014, 96 percent of counties in Texas had no provider and 43 percent of all women in Texas lived in these counties,[73] this statement did not adequately reflect the geographic reality of reproductive-age women seeking abortion services, especially if those women lived in the Rio Grande Valley.

Additionally, abortion clinics in states bordering Texas reported significant increases in new patients as a result of HB2 going into effect. A pattern of interstate and interprovincial travel to access abortion services is also noted in this volume by Barbara Baird and by Cathrine Chambers, Colleen MacQuarrie, and Jo-Ann MacDonald. Dr. Susan Robinson of Southwestern Women's Options in Albuquerque, New Mexico, told journalist Robin Marty: "We had a lot more calls, mostly about getting a medication abortion. Of course the answer is yes, but unfortunately, we are required to say 'You must come back for a follow-up.' We can't say, 'Oh, I know you traveled here for 10 hours; you can go see someone at home.' You have to tell them they must return for a follow-up and that discourages a lot of people." The owner of Hope Medical Group for Women in Shreveport, Louisiana, also mentioned an increase in patients: "We started to see an uptick with the original clinics closing in Texas. . . . With the continued enforcement of HB2 moving into the [ambulatory surgical center] ASC requirements, we've definitely seen more women from Texas and from other points beyond. Even though this is recent, there was enough of a change for us to notice."[74]

There are clinics in neighboring New Mexico, Louisiana, Oklahoma, Kansas, and Arkansas. However, state restrictions can differ dramatically and create stark inequalities of access from state to state. During the time period in question, there were no waiting periods for an abortion in New Mexico.[75] However, in Oklahoma the required waiting period was 24 hours, as was the case in Louisiana, Arkansas, and Kansas.[76] With no clinics between these large cities, there was an ever-increasing number of women trying to access care. The owner of the Shreveport Hope clinic remarked of the complicated travel involved: "What is happening is women would call from Oklahoma, they would call in to Dallas, and Dallas would say, 'We can't see you for another month.' So we have seen patients coming in from that far. They just keep heading down the highway."[77]

Travel within the state of Texas also posed problems because of the vast distances involved. Below are the compiled distances between several cities for one-way travel to provide better context of scale and distances:

Lubbock to Fort Worth: 314 miles; over 4.5 hours by car; by bus, 5 hours, 40 minutes (direct), ticket cost: US$49.00 (economy)

College Station to Austin: 107 miles; 2 hours by car; by bus, 3 hours, 55 minutes (1 transfer, 35-minute wait), ticket cost: US$43.00 (economy) (no bus from College Station, but there is a bus from the neighboring city of Bryan)

El Paso to Houston: 743 miles; over 10 hours by car; no clinics in between; by bus, 14 hours, 50 minutes (1 transfer), ticket cost: US$95.00 (economy) or 18 hours, 40 minutes (1 transfer with multiple stops), ticket cost: US$120.00 (economy)

Corpus Christi to San Antonio: 147 miles; 2 hours by car; by bus, 2 hours, 30 minutes (direct), ticket cost: US$34.00 (economy)

Odessa to El Paso: 280 miles; 3.75 hours by car; by bus, 5 hours, 20 minutes (direct), ticket cost: US$64.00 (economy)

Amarillo to Oklahoma City: 260 miles; 4 hours by car; by bus, 4 hours, 45 minutes (direct), ticket cost: US$75.00 (economy)

As journalist Olga Khazan has found, travel expenses, including gasoline if one had a car, or a ticket if using public transportation, significantly increased the total cost of the abortion. As she calculated, if a woman traveled from the southernmost tip of Texas, the closest clinic meant a 1,000-mile round-trip and more than US$150 in gas, compared to a woman living in central Texas, who would have to make a round-trip of 400 miles and spend about US$50 in gas. Due to Texas's 24-hour mandatory delay for an abortion, one must add lodging to the travel expenses, because of the need to spend the night near a clinic. Finally, there was the cost of the procedure itself, which could range anywhere from US$400 to US$950.[78] The Texas Policy Evaluation Project, a three-year study at the University of Texas–Austin, examined the impact of reduced family planning coverage by Texas since 2011 on five areas of the state where clinics did not meet ambulatory surgical center requirements. Researchers surmised that if the two clinics providing abortion services in the Rio Grande Valley were required to meet the ambulatory surgical center code standards, which they would be unable to do due to expensive renovation costs, women would then have to make two long-distance round-trips to San Antonio clinics that did meet these code requirements. These journeys increased the costs associated with the abortion. And the longer a woman waits or is delayed in scheduling the abortion, the more expensive the procedure becomes because late-term abortions cost much more.[79]

As I have previously written, from a spatial and geographical perspective, it is vitally important to discover ways to increase abortion access through considering alternative places to provide abortions.[80] Local hospitals are an obvious choice, but, as Cathrine Chambers, Colleen MacQuarrie, and Jo-Ann Macdonald show in this volume, hospitals can become battlegrounds for antichoice activism. Texas hospital participation in providing abortion services would dramatically and immediately increase abortion access, especially since these are ambulatory facilities. If this were the case, then Texas could have gone from a state with 19 facilities to 469 facilities that could provide abortion services.[81]

Figure 7.3 locates all the hospitals throughout the state. If all hospitals were required to provide the full spectrum of women's reproductive healthcare including abortion, then there would be exponentially greater access for women across almost the entire state.

Never Ending, Always Changing

Abortion may be federally guaranteed since *Roe v. Wade*, but it is not always state accessible.[82] In this case study of Texas between 2013 and 2015, antichoice policies on the part of the state government created

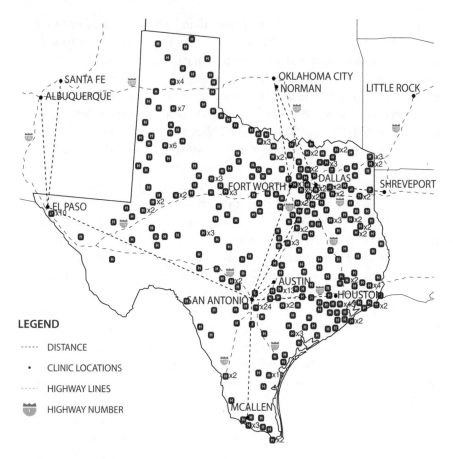

Figure 7.3. Hospital locations in Texas, USA.

major obstacles to access abortion services, especially if women lived outside urban centers. On June 27, 2016, the United States Supreme Court ruled 5-3 in *Whole Woman's Health v. Hellerstedt* that Texas abortion restrictions created through HB2 generated an undue burden for women seeking abortion access.[83] In Justice Stephen Breyer's opinion, neither the provisions of admitting privileges nor ambulatory surgical center requirements offered "medical benefits sufficient to justify the burdens upon access that each imposes. Each [provision] places a substantial obstacle in the path of women seeking pre-viability abortion, each constitutes an undue burden on abortion access . . . and each violates the Federal Constitution." The Supreme Court agreed with earlier district court findings that these two provisions "erect a particularly high barrier for poor, rural, or disadvantaged women."[84]

Although this decision was a significant win for women's reproductive access, Fund Texas Choice, a reproductive justice nonprofit group, reports that as of March 2017, only 14 clinics remain across the state, even fewer than during the peak HB2 turmoil.[85] It is unclear if some of the closed clinics will reopen. Madeline Gomez has remarked that the damage cannot be undone—the problem of abortion access remains. It may possibly take years for clinic numbers to return to pre-2013 levels, if they ever will. And the women most dramatically impacted are rural, poor, and Latinx and Hispanic migrants.[86]

Texas continues to create cumbersome and degrading new abortion restrictions for women. Within the past six months, the state legislature proposed a series of bills further restricting access. These include making it legal for doctors to misrepresent the health of a woman's pregnancy—in effect, permitting doctors to lie to her to prevent her from having an abortion.[87] Such bills further dictate how medicine should be practiced, for example, requiring abortion facilities to bury fetal remains rather than landfilling biological medical waste, as is the medical norm and is typically practiced,[88] and to categorize abortion (with no exceptions for rape or fetal abnormalities) as a felony for women and abortion providers.[89] And in retaliation for the United States Supreme Court decision in *Whole Woman's Health v. Hellerstedt*, the Texas state legislature sought to ban a common second-trimester dilation and evacuation surgical abortion procedure, charge doctors with a felony for performing the procedure, and stop the sale or donation of fetal tissue.[90]

Conclusion

Currently, the Trump administration is demonstrating a great propensity to create devasting effects for women and their reproductive healthcare. First, Trump appointed Charmaine Yoest, the former president of the anti-abortion organization Americans United for Life, to become the assistant secretary of public affairs for the Department of Health and Human Services.[91] More recently, Trump has stated that he wants to revive the Ronald Reagan–era "Global Gag Rule" and deploy it domestically. It would require a complete separation between facilities for family planning and those for abortion in the USA, making it that much more difficult for women to access comprehensive reproductive healthcare within the same physical space.[92] How would the return to duplication of clinic support services such as telephones, staff, and accounting systems actually serve anyone but a certain ideology that is antiwomen?[93] A reproductive justice framework for change is critical in light of the ever-expanding curtailment of women's ability for personal autonomy of her own body. As Laura Briggs argues in her most recent book, *How All Politics Became Reproductive Politics*, until the USA actually addresses all aspects of reproductive policies, from childcare, to family assistance programs, domestic support, and reproductive services, the crisis in the country will only continue to worsen.[94]

Where does this state of affairs leave women seeking abortions in Texas? Long-distance travel to abortion providers inside and outside the state will remain the norm for women. However, this is mainly true for women who are financially able to travel. Although Fund Texas Choice[95] and the Lilith Fund,[96] another reproductive justice nonprofit group, were established to help provide financial support for women who cannot otherwise afford an abortion, a normal and routine medical procedure such as abortion should not be relegated only to women of means or through charity. Additionally, due to the hard-line stance on immigration taken by Texas and the Trump administration, undocumented migrant women remain in the crosshairs. The consequences are disturbing, especially for those living in the Rio Grande Valley region who, due to their precarious immigration status, fear traveling through border control checkpoints and thus have extreme difficulty in accessing reproductive healthcare, if at all. In January 2018, the Trump administration even attempted to deny abortions to four detained migrant women from Mexico, including an undocumented minor.[97] However, in March, a federal judge ruled that the government could block access to abortion for detained teens in immigration custody, and to do so is unconstitutional.[98]

Texas demonstrates that the state is willing to drastically eliminate women's access to reproductive healthcare with little to no regard for the consequences it has on millions of women's lives. Texas anti-abortion policies are copied by the states of Missouri and Iowa, and the Trump administration is working to expand similar policies internationally by refusing to provide American aid to any international organization that discusses abortion.[99] Many other states are following their lead.[100] Texas serves as a frightening wake-up call to the rest of the country on so many levels: high rates of poverty, incarceration, immigration, deportation, and an extremely pro–gun rights state. The state's assault on social services and reproductive healthcare leaves many women with little choice but to travel long distances to access abortion services. Should the situation continue, it will go from very bad to much worse.[101]

Notes

1. Robert Barnes, "Supreme Court Blocks Texas Abortion Law," *Washington Post*, October 14, 2014, https://www.washingtonpost.com/politics/courts_law /supreme-court-blocks-texas-abortion-law/2014/10/14/a3c51252-53ad-11e4 -892e-602188e70e9c_story.html?utm_term=.9619f7342bfa.

2. Kinsey Hasstedt, "The State of Sexual and Reproductive Health and Rights in the State of Texas: A Cautionary Tale," *Guttmacher Policy Review* 17, no. 2 (Spring 2014), https://www.guttmacher.org/gpr/2014/03/state-sexual-and -reproductive-health-and-rights-state-texas-cautionary-tale [first published online March 14, 2014].

3. Hasstedt, "The State of Sexual and Reproductive Health," 15.

4. "Reproductive Rights," Texas Freedom Network, accessed May 20, 2018, http://tfn.org/issue/reproductive-rights/. See also Texas Department of State Health Services Abstinence-Centered Education Program, http://www .dshs.texas.gov/schoolhealth/pgtoc.shtm?terms=sexual%20education%20 for%20middle%20school (page no longer available). These issues have also found their way into Texas textbooks where Holt, a major publisher for high school textbooks, as well as two other publishers, did not include any information at all on family planning and disease prevention except through abstinence.

5. Texas Education Agency, Chapter 115 Texas Essential Knowledge and Skills for Health Education Subchapter B. Middle School, 115.23.B.5F.

6. Texas Education Agency, Chapter 115 Texas Essential Knowledge and Skills for Health Education Subchapter C. High School, 115.32.B.3.

7. Hasstedt, "The State of Sexual and Reproductive Health," 20.

8. Hasstedt, "The State of Sexual and Reproductive Health," 20.

9. For a recent update on state policies, see Elizabeth Nash et al., "Laws Affecting Reproductive Health and Rights: State Policy Trends in the First Quarter of 2017," Guttmacher Institute, April 12, 2017, https://www .guttmacher.org/article/2017/04/laws-affecting-reproductive-health-and-rights -state-policy-trends-first-quarter-2017.

10. Adam Liptak, "Supreme Court Allows Texas Abortion Clinics to Stay Open," *New York Times*, October 14, 2014, https://www.nytimes.com/2014/10 /15/us/supreme-court-allows-texas-abortion-clinics-to-stay-open.html?_r=1.

11. "Fast Facts Study Guide (State Areas)," US50, accessed November 29, 2014, http://www.theus50.com/fastfacts/area.php.

12. "State and County Quickfacts Texas," United States Census Bureau, accessed February 1, 2018, https://www.census.gov/quickfacts/fact/table/TX /PST045217.

13. "Income and Poverty in the United States: 2016," United States Census Bureau, accessed February 1, 2018, https://www.census.gov/library/publications /2017/demo/p60-259.html.

14. Paul Mackun and Steven Wilson, "Population Distribution and Change: 2000 to 2010," *United States Census Bureau*, March 2011, https://www.census .gov/prod/cen2010/briefs/c2010br-01.pdf.

15. "The 15 Most Populous Cities: July 1, 2016," United States Census Bureau, accessed February 5, 2018, https://www.census.gov/content/dam/Census /newsroom/releases/2017/cb17-81-table3-most-populous.pdf; and "State and County Quickfacts Texas," United States Census Bureau, https://www.census .gov/quickfacts/fact/table/TX/PST045217.

16. "Texas Abortion Clinic Map," Fund Texas Choice, accessed June 7, 2018, https://fundtexaschoice.org/index.php/about/.

17. "2010 Census: Population of Texas Cities, Arranged in Descending Order," Texas State Library and Archives Commission, accessed November 29, 2014, https://www.tsl.texas.gov/ref/abouttx/popcity32010.html.

18. This builds on the graphic analysis by Nadja Popovich, Kenton Powell, and Feilding Cage in the *Guardian*. See Lauren Gambino, "Appeals Court Allows Texas to Enforce Controversial Anti-Abortion Law," *Guardian*, October 2, 2014, https://www.theguardian.com/world/2014/oct/02/appeals-court -texas-abortion-law.

19. "Quick Facts Texas," United States Census Bureau, accessed February 28, 2015, https://www.census.gov/quickfacts/TX. As defined by the United States Census, Hispanic or Latinx refers to any person or their family ancestors from Spanish cultures or origins regardless of race. "Quick Facts United States," United States Census Bureau, accessed February 5, 2018, https://www.census .gov/quickfacts/fact/table/US/PST045217.

20. "Demographic Profile of Hispanics in Texas, 2014," Hispanic Trends, Pew Research Center, accessed March 24, 2017, http://www.pewhispanic.org /states/state/tx/.

21. Mark Hugo Lopez, "In 2014, Latinos Will Surpass Whites as Largest Racial/Ethnic Group in California," *Pew Research Center Fact Tank News*, January 24, 2015, http://www.pewresearch.org/fact-tank/2014/01/24/in-2014 -latinos-will-surpass-whites-as-largest-racialethnic-group-in-california/.

22. Michael Oleaga, "Immigration Executive Order Lawsuit: White House Gives Judge Andrew Hanen Deadline to Lift Injunction," *Latin Post*, March 6, 2015, http://www.latinpost.com/articles/41169/20150306/immigration -executive-order-lawsuit-white-house-gives-judge-andrew-hanen.htm. The other twenty-four states that have joined the Texas lawsuit include Arizona, Arkansas, Florida, Georgia, Idaho, Indiana, Kansas, Louisiana, Maine, Michigan, Mississippi, Montana, Nebraska, Nevada, North Carolina, North Dakota, Ohio, Oklahoma, South Carolina, South Dakota, Tennessee, Utah, West Virginia, and Wisconsin. Josh Gerstein, "Feds Act to Lift Hold on Obama Immigration Moves," *Politico*, February 23, 2015, https://www.politico.com/blogs/under-the -radar/2015/02/feds-act-to-lift-hold-on-obama-immigration-moves-202959.

23. Haeyoun Park and Alicia Parlapiano, "Supreme Court's Decision on Immigration Case Affects Millions of Unauthorized Immigrants," *New York*

Times, June 23, 2016, https://www.nytimes.com/interactive/2016/06/22/us/who -is-affected-by-supreme-court-decision-on-immigration.html. See also Priscilla Alvarez, "Immigration Hardliners Praise Trump for Ending DACA," *Atlantic*, September 5, 2017, https://www.theatlantic.com/politics/archive/2017/09 /immigration-hardliners-trump-daca/538602/.

24. "Stopgap Bill to End the Federal Government Shutdown Passes Congress," *New York Times*, January 22, 2018, https://www.nytimes.com/2018/01 /22/us/politics/government-shutdown.html.

25. "Trump Migrant Separation Policy: Children 'in Cages' in Texas," *BBC News*, June 18, 2018. https://www.bbc.com/news/world-us-canada-44518942.

26. Jenna Jerman, Rachel K. Jones, and Tsuyoshi Onda, "Characteristics of US Abortion Patients in 2014 and Changes Since 2008," Guttmacher Institute, May 2016, https://www.guttmacher.org/report/characteristics-us-abortion -patients-2014. See also Guttmacher Institute, "Abortion Patients More Likely to Be Poor in 2014 Than in 2008," Guttmacher Institute, May 10, 2016, https://www.guttmacher.org/news-release/2016/abortion-patients-more-likely-be -poor-2014-2008.

27. Madeline M. Gomez, "Intersections at the Border: Immigration Enforcement, Reproductive Oppression, and the Policing of Latina Bodies in the Rio Grande Valley," *Columbia Journal of Gender and Law* 84, no. 1 (2015): 116.

28. Jerman et al., "Characteristics," 11.

29. "Annual Gun Law State Scorecard 2014," Law Center to Prevent Gun Violence, accessed March 7, 2015, http://lawcenter.giffords.org/scorecard2014/; "Texas," Giffords Law Center to Prevent Gun Violence, accessed June 7, 2018, http://lawcenter.giffords.org/gun-laws/state-law/texas/.

30. John Lindsay-Poland, "America's Guns: Made in the US, Killing in Mexico," *Al Jazeera*, March 28, 2018, https://www.aljazeera.com/indepth /opinion/america-guns-killing-mexico-180328060253902.html.

31. "Whites Are Underrepresented in Texas Prisons and Jails," Prison Policy Initiative, accessed March 29, 2015, https://www.prisonpolicy.org/graphs /201opercent/TX_Whites_2010.html; and "Blacks Are Overrepresented in Texas Prisons and Jails," Prison Policy Initiative, accessed May 20, 2018, https://www .prisonpolicy.org/graphs/201opercent/TX_Blacks_2010.html; "Racial and Ethnic Disparities in Prisons and Jails in Texas," Prison Policy Initiative, accessed June 20, 2017, https://www.prisonpolicy.org/profiles/TX.html.

32. Emily DePrang, "More Prisoners, More Problems: Mass Incarceration Climbs Again," *Texas Observer*, September 17, 2014, https://www.texasobserver .org/prisoners-problems-mass-incarceration-climbs/.

33. "Death-Row Prisoners by State," Death Penalty Information Center, accessed March 22, 2017, https://deathpenaltyinfo.org/death-row-inmates-state -and-size-death-row-year.

34. Dave Jamieson, "Rick Perry on Clayton Lockett Execution: 'I Don't Know Whether It Was Inhumane Or Not,'" *Huffington Post*, May 4, 2014, http://www.huffingtonpost.ca/entry/rick-perry-executions_n_5263404.

35. Terri Langford, "The Perry Legacy: Criminal Justice Ushering in Reform by Stepping Aside," *Texas Tribune*, December 28, 2014, https://apps .texastribune.org/perry-legacy/criminal-justice/.

36. Texas has the highest number of deportation outcomes to date. See "Outcomes of Deportation Proceedings in Immigration Court by Nationality, State, Court, Hearing Location, and Type of Charge," Transactional Records Access Clearinghouse, accessed July 6, 2017, http://trac.syr.edu/phptools /immigration/court_backlog/deport_outcome_charge.php.

37. Dabney Bailey, "More States Require Wait for Abortion Than Wait for Guns," *Opposing Views*, June 20, 2013, https://www.opposingviews.com /category/more-states-require-wait-abortion-wait-guns.

38. "Eligibility," Centers for Medicare and Medicaid Services, accessed March 31, 2015, https://www.medicaid.gov/medicaid/eligibility/.

39. Melissa del Bosque, "Rick Perry's Refusal to Expand Texas' Medicaid Program Could Result in Thousands of Deaths," *Texas Observer*, January 2, 2013, http://www.texasobserver.org/rick-perrys-refusal-to-expand-texas -medicaid-program-could-result-in-thousands-of-deaths/.

40. "Medicare Program—General Information," Centers for Medicare and Medicaid Services, accessed March 31, 2015, https://www.cms.gov/Medicare /Medicare-General-Information/MedicareGenInfo/index.html. Medicare Program General Information, accessed March 31, 2015, https://www.cms.gov /Medicare/Medicare-General Information/MedicareGenInfo/index.html.

41. Robert Pear, Maggie Haberman, and Reed Abelson, "Trump to Scrap Health Care Subsidies, Hitting Obamacare Again," *New York Times*, October 12, 2017, https://www.nytimes.com/2017/10/12/us/politics/trump -obamacare-executive-order-health-insurance.html.

42. Josh Dorner, "Priorities? GOP Governors Shift Burden to Poor, Middle Class to Pay for Tax Breaks for Rich, Corporations," *ThinkProgress*, February 22, 2011, https://thinkprogress.org/priorities-gop-governors-shift-burden-to -poor-middle-class-to-pay-for-tax-breaks-for-rich-corporatio-5f572927fbd4/.

43. Pat Garofalo, "Child Poverty Hits 25 Percent in Texas, but Gov. Perry Still Proposing Deep Cuts to Child Service," *ThinkProgress*, February 4, 2011, https://thinkprogress.org/child-poverty-hits-25-percent-in-texas-but-gov-perry -still-proposing-deep-cuts-to-child-services-e836bf0f26a4/.

44. Joshua Blank and Bethany Albertson, "Polling Center: Texan First, American Second," *Texas Tribune*, April 3, 2014, https://www.texastribune.org /2014/04/03/polling-center-texan-first-american-second/.

45. "Religious Affiliation in Texas," Texas State Historical Association, accessed February 28, 2015, http://texasalmanac.com/topics/religion/religious -affiliation-texas.

46. NARAL Pro-Choice, *Crisis Pregnancy Centers Lie: The Insidious Threat to Reproductive Freedom* (Washington, DC: NARAL Pro-Choice America, 2015), 17.

47. Jennifer Ludden, "States Fund Pregnancy Centers That Discourage Abortion," *NPR*, March 9, 2015, https://www.npr.org/sections/health-shots /2015/03/09/391877614/states-fund-pregnancy-centers-that-discourage -abortion.

48. Gomez, "Intersections at the Border," 99–101. See also Wade Goodwyn, "Gov. Perry Cut Funds for Women's Health in Texas," *NPR*, September 20, 2011, https://www.npr.org/2011/09/20/140449957/gov-perry-cut-funds-for -womens-health-in-texas.

49. Daniel Grossman et al., "Change in Abortion Services after Implementation of a Restrictive Law in Texas," *Contraception* 90, no. 5 (November 2014): 496–97. Prior to HB2, most clinics providing medical abortions used an evidenced-based regime with more flexibility depending on how the woman responded to the first round of mifepristone. Reducing the gestational age from 63 days to 49, HB2 required women to make two additional office visits: once for the misoprostol plus a follow-up appointment. These new regulations created a total of four mandated office visits plus dictated a more expensive drug dosage than the evidence-based regime dosage.

50. "FAQ: New Abortion Laws in Texas," Lilith Fund, accessed March 31, 2015, https://www.lilithfund.org/new-laws/.

51. TX HB2 2013, 83rd Legislature 2nd Special Session, "Relating to the Regulation of Abortion Procedures, Providers, and Facilities; Providing Penalties," *LegiScan*, accessed November 27, 2014, http://legiscan.com/TX/text/HB2/2013/X2.

52. Grossman et al., "Change in Abortion," 73.

53. Grossman et al., "Change in Abortion," 497–99.

54. Liptak, "Supreme Court Allows Texas Abortion Clinics to Stay Open."

55. Liptak, "Supreme Court Allows Texas Abortion Clinics to Stay Open."

56. Daniel Grossman et al., "The Public Health Threat of Anti-Abortion Legislation," *Contraception* 89, no. 2 (February 2014): 500.

57. Hasstedt, "The State of Sexual and Reproductive Health," 19.

58. Hasstedt, "The State of Sexual and Reproductive Health," 19.

59. "Texas Hospital Association's Statement of Opposition to Section 2 of the Committee Substitute for Senate Bill 5 by Glenn Hegar Relating to the Regulation of Abortion Procedures, Providers, and Facilities; Providing Penalties" (Texas Hospital Association, 2013).

60. Grossman et al., "The Public Health Threat," 73.

61. Lori A. Brown, "Zoned Out: Buildings and Bodies," "Family Planning," *Harvard Design Magazine* #41, 2015.

62. Lisa R. Pruitt, "Toward a Feminist Theory of the Rural," *Utah Law Review* 2007, no. 2 (2007): 438, 441.

63. Pruitt, "Toward a Feminist," 477.

64. Planned Parenthood Ariz., Inc. v. Humble 753 F.3d 905, 914 (9th Cit. 2014), quoted in Lisa R. Pruitt and Marta R. Vanegas, "Urbanormativity, Spatial Privilege, Judicial Blind Spots in Abortion Law," *Berkeley Journal of Gender, Law and Justice* 30, no. 76 (Winter 2015): 141n355.

65. David Delaney, quoted in Pruitt and Vanegas, "Urbanormativity, Spatial Privilege, Judicial Blind Spots in Abortion Law," 151.

66. Telephone conversation with Customs and Border Patrol local affiliate, June 21, 2017.

67. Dania Y. Pulido, "When Giving Birth Becomes a Liability: The Intersection of Reproductive Oppression and the Motherhood Wage Penalty for Latinas in Texas," *Scholar* 19, no. 111 (2016): 126–27. For more information, see Joseph E. Potter, "Texas Policy Evaluation Project," University of Texas–Austin, Liberal Arts, accessed February 22, 2018, https://liberalarts.utexas.edu/txpep/.

68. Debbie Nathan, "Abortion Stories on the Border," in *Gender through the Prism of Difference*, 2nd ed., ed. Maxine Baca Zinn, Pierrette Hondagneu-Sotelo,

and Michael A. Messner (Boston: Allyn and Bacon, 2000), 123; and Leslie J. Reagan, "Crossing the Border for Abortions: California Activists, Mexican Clinics, and the Creation of a Feminist Health Agency in the 1960s," in *Women, Health, and Nation: Canada and the United States since 1945*, ed. Georgina Feldberg, Molly Ladd-Taylor, Alison Li, and Kathryn McPherson (Montreal: McGill-Queen's University Press, 2003), 355–78.

69. Lori A. Brown, "Case Studies and Spatial Awareness," *Contested Spaces: Abortion Clinics, Women's Shelters and Hospitals* (Surrey, England: Ashgate, 2013), 85.

70. Christabelle Sethna, "All Aboard? Canadian Women's Abortion Tourism, 1960–1980," in *Gender, Health and Popular Culture Historical Perspectives*, ed. Cheryl Krasnick Warsh (Waterloo, ON: Wilfrid Laurier University Press, 2011), 89–108.

71. Christabelle Sethna and Marion Doull, "Far from Home? A Pilot Study Tracking Women's Journeys to a Canadian Abortion Clinic," *Journal of Obstetrics and Gynaecology Canada* 29, no. 8 (August 2007): 640–45.

72. Christabelle Sethna and Marion Doull, "Accidental Tourists: Canadian Women, Abortion Tourism, and Travel," *Women's Studies: An Interdisciplinary Journal* 41, no. 4 (June 2012): 466–70. See also Sethna and Doull, "Far from Home?," 640–45; Christabelle Sethna and Marion Doull, "Journeys of Choice: Abortion, Travel, and Women's Autonomy," in *Critical Interventions in the Ethics of Healthcare: Challenging the Principle of Autonomy in Bioethics*, ed. Stuart J. Murray and Dave Holmes (Farnham, UK: Ashgate, 2009), 163–79; and Lori Brown, Shoshanna Ehrlich, and Colleen MacQuarrie, "Subverting the Constitution: Anti-Abortion Policies and Activism in the United States and Canada," in *Abortion History, Politics, and Reproductive Justice after Morgentaler*, ed. Shannon Stettner, Kristin Burnett, and Travis Hay (Vancouver: University of British Columbia Press, 2017), 239–61.

73. "State Facts about Abortion: Texas," Guttmacher Institute, updated January 2018, https://www.guttmacher.org/fact-sheet/state-facts-about-abortion -texas.

74. Robin Marty, "The Long Road to a Safe and Legal Abortion," *Slate DoubleX*, October 20, 2014, http://www.slate.com/articles/double_x/doublex /2014/10/abortion_clinic_crisis_women_of_texas_could_have_to_drive_up_to _600_miles.html.

75. "State Facts about Abortion: New Mexico," Guttmacher Institute, updated January 2018, https://www.guttmacher.org/fact-sheet/state-facts-about -abortion-new-mexico.

76. "State Facts about Abortion: Oklahoma," Guttmacher Institute, updated January 2018, https://www.guttmacher.org/fact-sheet/state-facts-about-abortion -oklahoma. The waiting period for Louisiana, Arkansas, and Kansas are also 24 hours. "State Facts about Abortion: Louisiana," Guttmacher Institute, updated January 2018, https://www.guttmacher.org/fact-sheet/state-facts-about-abortion -louisiana; State Facts about Abortion: Arkansas," Guttmacher Institute, updated January 2018, https://www.guttmacher.org/fact-sheet/state-facts-about -abortion-arkansas; "State Facts about Abortion: Kansas," Guttmacher Institute, updated January 2018, https://www.guttmacher.org/fact-sheet/state-facts-about -abortion-kansas.

77. Marty, "The Long Road to a Safe and Legal Abortion."

78. Olga Khazan, "The Cost of Driving to an Abortion," *Atlantic*, October 28, 2014, https://www.theatlantic.com/health/archive/2014/10/the-cost-of-driving-to-an-abortion/381985/.

79. Becca Aaronson and Shefali Luthra, "Texas Senators Reopen Debate on Abortion Regulations," *Texas Tribune*, July 8, 2013, https://www.texastribune.org/2013/07/08/texas-senators-reopen-debate-abortion-regulations/.

80. Lori A. Brown, *Contested Spaces: Abortion Clinics, Women's Shelters and Hospitals* (Surrey, England: Ashgate Publishing Limited, 2013), 193–210.

81. "Texas Abortion Clinic Map," Fund Texas Choice, accessed December 21, 2014, https://fundtexaschoice.org/index.php/about/.

82. "State Government: Texas," NARAL Pro-Choice America, accessed November 27, 2014, https://www.prochoiceamerica.org/state/texas/; and "AUL's 2018 Life List," Americans United for Life, accessed June 7, 2018, http://www.aul.org/auls-2018-life-list/.

83. Jessica Mason Pieklo, "The Court Strikes Texas Abortion Restrictions," *Rewire*, June 27, 2016, https://rewire.news/article/2016/06/27/supreme-court-strikes-texas-abortion-restrictions/.

84. 579 US Whole Woman's Health et al. v. Hellerstedt, No. 15–274, 2016, 2,6.

85. "Texas Abortion Clinic Map," Fund Texas Choice, accessed March 24, 2017, https://fundtexaschoice.org/index.php/about/.

86. Madeline M. Gomez, "More Than Mileage: The Preconditions of Travel and the Real Burdens of H.B.2," *Columbia Journal of Gender and Law* 33, no. 1 (2016): 50–51.

87. Jessica Valenti, "The Week of Patriarchy: Texas Doctors Fight for Right to Lie to Pregnant Women," *Guardian*, March 3, 2017, https://www.theguardian.com/world/commentisfree/2017/mar/03/the-week-in-patriarchy-texas-doctors-abortion-law.

88. Liam Stack, "Texas Will Require Burial of Aborted Fetuses," *New York Times*, November 30, 2016, https://www.nytimes.com/2016/11/30/us/texas-burial-aborted-fetuses.html.

89. Lyanne A. Guarecuco, "New Bill Aims to Make Abortion a Felony in Texas," *Texas Observer*, January 13, 2017, https://www.texasobserver.org/new-bill-aims-make-abortion-felony-texas/.

90. Associate Press, "Texas House Approves New Limits on Abortion," *New York Times*, May 20, 2017, https://www.nytimes.com/2017/05/20/us/politics/texas-house-approves-new-limits-on-abortion.html?_r=1.

91. Molly Redden, "Trump Picks Former Anti-abortion Leader for Health and Human Services Post," *Guardian*, Friday April 28, 2017, accessed June 7, 2018, https://www.theguardian.com/us-news/2017/apr/28/trump-health-human-services-anti-abortion-charmaine-yoest.

92. Sabrina Siddiqui, "Trump Administration to Revive Reagan-Era Abortion 'Gag' Rule," *Guardian*, Friday May 18, 2018, accessed June 7, 2018, https://www.theguardian.com/world/2018/may/18/trump-administration-abortion-gag-rule-reagan-era.

93. Joan Finn-McCracken, "I Helped Women Get Abortions for 28 Years, through Protests and Shifting Rules," *Washington Post*, May 25, 2018, https://

www.washingtonpost.com/outlook/i-helped-women-get-abortions-for-28
-years—through-protests-and-shifting-rules/2018/05/25/4f680826-5eb8-11e8
-a4a4-c070ef53f315_story.html?utm_term=.fbf982907o2d.

94. Lynne Segal, "How All Politics Became Reproductive Politics: From
Welfare Reform to Foreclosure to Trump, by Laura Briggs," *Times Higher
Education*, October 19, 2017, https://www.timeshighereducation.com/books
/review-how-all-politics-became-reproductive-politics-laura-briggs-university-of
-california-press.

95. See Fund Texas Choice's website at: https://fundtexaschoice.org/.

96. See Lilith Fund's website at: https://www.lilithfund.org/.

97. Brigitte Amiri, "A Fourth Young Immigrant Woman is Being Blocked by
the Trump Administration from Obtaining an Abortion," *ACLU Reproductive
Freedom Project*, January 11, 2018, https://www.aclu.org/blog/reproductive
-freedom/abortion/fourth-young-immigrant-woman-being-blocked-trump
-administration.

98. Ann E. Marimow, Spencer S. Hsu, and Maria Sacchetti, "U.S. Government Ordered to Allow Abortion Access to Detained Immigrant Teens,"
Washington Post, March 30, 2018, https://www.washingtonpost.com/local
/public-safety/us-judge-orders-government-to-allow-abortion-access-to-detained
-immigrant-teens/2018/03/30/19e9fcf8-3128-11e8-94fa-32d48460b955_story
.html?utm_term=.69567fa17682.

99. Editorial Board, "The Way Texas Treats Women," *New York Times*,
May 19, 2017, https://www.nytimes.com/2017/05/19/opinion/the-way-texas
-treats-women.html.

100. Lindy West, "To Save Abortion Rights, We Have to Think Beyond Roe,"
New York Times, April 11, 2018, https://www.nytimes.com/2018/04/11/opinion
/abortion-rights-access-roe.html?action=click&module=Associated&pgtype
=Article&region=Footer&contentCollection=Lindy%20West.

101. Lawrence Wright, "America's Future Is Texas," *New Yorker*, July 10 and
17, 2017, https://www.newyorker.com/magazine/2017/07/10/americas-future-is
-texas.

[8]

Trials and Trails

The Emergence of Canada's "Abortion Refugees" in
Prince Edward Island

CATHRINE CHAMBERS, COLLEEN MACQUARRIE,
AND JO-ANN MACDONALD

EXISTING RESEARCH highlights the relationship between the distance a woman must travel to secure a surgical abortion[1] and the
likelihood that she will obtain one.[2] Furthermore, women's mobility is
limited by socioeconomic factors, including geography, class, race, and
ability.[3] Some scholars argue that patients who cannot afford medical
treatment in their home community and must, therefore, travel to receive necessary medical services can be classified as "medical refugees."[4]
These patients are not choosing to travel for elective surgeries in exotic
locations. Rather, they are seeking essential and affordable medical care
that is simply not available at home.[5] To date, however, there has not
been a concerted exploration of the notion of women as "abortion refugees" embarking on either domestic or international travel in order to
obtain abortion services.

In this chapter, we argue that the concepts of medical tourism, health
tourism, or abortion tourism are insufficient to describe the plight of
women living in Prince Edward Island (PEI), Canada's smallest province, where abortions were unavailable from 1986 until early 2017, and
where current access is still fettered by ongoing issues of systemic and
structural oppression. The geographical variability of abortion provision even where abortion is legal is also addressed by Gayle Davis et al.
in this volume in regard to Britain. The term "abortion refugees" more
accurately reflects the urgency and lack of options experienced by PEI
women who have sought abortions off island and exposes the persecution they have faced in various aspects of their lives as they have attempted to obtain safe and legal abortions. Importantly, persecution is
a key factor in determining who constitutes a refugee.[6] We review in

detail the experiences of PEI women seeking abortions through an analysis of the results of a participatory action research project we called "Understanding for a Change: Exploring 20 Years of Denying PEI Women Access to an Abortion."[7] Themes of persecution and resiliency are revealed throughout this chapter as we explore the meanings of direct quotations from our research participants and analyze the significance of their lived experiences of abortion access. In order to demonstrate the role persecution has played in the evolution of PEI's abortion refugees, we discuss the three main findings of the project: (1) the unique PEI context, notably its political conservatism and religious traditionalism; (2) the barriers to abortion access; and (3) the politics of island women's resilience.

The PEI Context

Access to abortion is strongly influenced by time, place, culture, and geography, and remains highly contested.[8] The broad picture in PEI shows that economic equality for women lags behind other provinces in the country. Recent studies point toward a trend whereby full-time, full-year employed women earn approximately 82 percent of what their male counterparts make.[9] More than 95 percent of the population is affiliated with Canada's majority religions (Protestant and Catholic), both of which promote traditional heterosexual gender roles for women that validate women as wives and mothers, a tendency that is strongly apparent in the Irish context, as described by Mary Gilmartin and Sinéad Kennedy, by Ewelina Ciaputa in relation to Polish society, and by Agata Ignaciuk in her discussion of Spain in this volume. Similarly, individuals in the Atlantic provinces express more conservative opinions when asked about the importance of "family values" in comparison to other provinces, due in part to the existence of patriarchal religious institutions and the strength of religious beliefs.[10] Atlantic Canada, which encompasses PEI, as well as the neighboring provinces of New Brunswick, Nova Scotia, and Newfoundland and Labrador, has the highest level of religious commitment and antichoice activism of any region in the country, and has been labeled Canada's "Bible Belt."[11]

The oppressive circumstances at play in PEI that contribute to women's loss of choice have not been adequately addressed.[12] There are several factors unique to PEI that reinforce barriers to accessing abortion. Islands can be conservative places steeped in a sense of tradition, and inhabitants can be uncomfortable with social phenomena that challenge their cultural sense of island identity.[13] Even the Confederation Bridge, a structure that connects PEI to the mainland, was hotly contested. Voted on in 1988, coincidentally the same year in which abortion was banished from PEI, construction of the bridge was opposed on the grounds that it would forever alter islanders' sense of themselves and would impact the preservation of the island's "moral landscape."[14] In fact, the bridge itself has been theorized as a physical representation of the alienation, stigma, and lack of protection women face in PEI because they need to traverse it to obtain an abortion in another province.[15] Lori A. Brown, in her contribution to this volume, notes that Texas, the second-largest state in the United States of America (USA), markets itself brashly. In contrast, tiny PEI has been dubbed "The Gentle Island" by its tourism industry. It is often branded as a place that is separate, self-contained, and disconnected from the rest of the world, where the stresses of everyday life evaporate upon arrival. This depiction of the island as a place where tourists can escape the difficult realities of everyday life and travel back to simpler times makes it more likely that issues surrounding access to abortion will be excluded from notions of what is important about life on the island. However, as in the case of Texas, abortion rights are decidedly not part of PEI's brand.

Historically, religious traditionalism was instrumental in the spread of antichoice ideology,[16] a feature pertinent to the state of Texas and also to countries such as the Republic of Ireland, Poland, and Spain, as evoked powerfully by Lori A. Brown, Mary Gilmartin and Sinéad Kennedy, Ewelina Ciaputa, and Agata Ignaciuk, respectively, in this volume. Specifically, during the 1980s, the antichoice movement[17] in PEI relied on the support of the Catholic Sisters of Saint Martha during the critical period of time when abortion was restricted on the island. By exerting their influence from within the hospitals, the sisters were able to ensure that no abortions would take place; that is, they advocated for "medical and religious care in accordance with natural law and Catholic morality."[18] The antichoice movement has since attempted to block women's access to abortion through the use of several strategies, including putting pressure on local politicians, members of the community, healthcare administrators, and members of provincial and local parliaments; extensive letter-writing campaigns; and hindering the delivery of abortion services through aggressive picketing, obstructing entrances to abortion clinics, and various other forms of harassment.[19] While there were, and continue to be, pro-choice activists on the island, the relentless maligning of those in favor of access by the antichoice movement has left many fearful of the repercussions of advocating openly for access to abortion.[20]

Legislators in PEI have also worked in many ways to restrict local access. The delivery of medical services in PEI is governed by a public act, and at the time of the Canadian Supreme Court's *R. v. Morgentaler* decision in 1988, the PEI Hospital and Health Services Commission was vested under public law to determine what types of care and procedures qualified as fundable Medicare services as stipulated in the Health Services Payment (HSP) Act Regulations of PEI.[21] However, individual hospitals acting through their elected boards have the authority to determine which specific services they will provide. It was at the level of these individual hospital boards that the PEI Right to Life Association celebrated a major success in the early 1980s, when the Catholic hospital refused to establish a Therapeutic Abortion Committee (TAC) within their hospital.[22] After Canada reformed its abortion laws in 1969, only hospital-based TACs could approve or deny a woman's request for a legal abortion based on the threat the pregnancy posed to her life or health. Feminist groups throughout the country disliked TACs, arguing that they demeaned women. No hospital was obliged to establish a TAC, but the Protestant hospital board on the Island did. However, the construction of a new, single, large hospital in PEI's capital city of Charlottetown resulted in the amalgamation of the Catholic and Protestant hospital boards. A long public battle over the provision of abortion services then took place, in which antichoice lobbyists threatened to withhold financial support for the equipment drive at the new hospital if their demands were not met.[23]

Following a successful campaign to shut down abortion access in the new hospital, the island's antichoice movement targeted the last remaining TAC in the province, at the Protestant Prince County Hospital in the city of Summerside.[24] A board membership drive and intense lobbying by church representatives resulted in the removal of the TAC at the Prince County Hospital and effectively ended access to safe surgical abortions in 1986.[25] The provincial government refused to get involved with health service delivery at the hospital board level, stating that the independence of the hospital boards took precedence.[26] Thus, while the rest of Canada was extending access to abortion in the 1980s, PEI became the only province in Canada where women had to travel to another province to secure access to safe, legal abortions. Not much changed in PEI after the Morgentaler decision, a landmark Supreme Court case that was centered in the struggles of Dr. Henry Morgentaler, a Montreal physician who provided clinic abortions that were technically illegal.[27] The antichoice movement took advantage of the heightened rhetoric and emotions sweeping across the province and succeeded in branding PEI as a "life sanctuary" for fetuses.[28] By the time the Morgentaler decision was delivered, island politicians were united in their resistance to it.[29]

In 1995, the PEI government negotiated an agreement to refer women to the Queen Elizabeth II Hospital (QEII) in the city of Halifax, the capital of the neighboring province of Nova Scotia. Under the new rules, women had to be referred by a PEI physician to a physician in the Termination Pregnancy Unit (TPU) at the QEII. The gestational limit was set at 15 weeks, the pregnant woman had to have an ultrasound, and she could not have had more than one referral for an abortion, a stipulation that penalized women who had undergone more than one procedure.[30] While some women were able to travel to Halifax to obtain an abortion, access depended on several factors, including the ability to make the four-hour trip by ferry or a three-hour journey by car or bus across the Confederation Bridge. Travel costs were not covered by the government. Thus, women had to absorb the cost of transportation, accommodation, meals, and other expenses themselves,[31] a burden common to many who have traveled domestically or internationally for abortion services, as several chapters in this volume make apparent.

In the event a woman's pregnancy was beyond the 15-week gestational limit, she had to come up with the funds to travel to a private clinic, possibly in the USA, that offered late-term abortions. If a woman had undergone a previous abortion, she had to come up with the money to fund the abortion at an out-of-province private clinic. Some women traveled by plane to the Morgentaler abortion clinic in Montreal, Quebec, if they did not meet the criteria for abortion services set by the QEII in Halifax.[32] The agreement with the QEII was a small victory for the pro-choice lobby but was kept hushed. The provincial government refused to educate its citizens about it.[33] It was not until 2011, when the PEI Reproductive Rights Organization (PRRO), a young feminist pro-choice activist group, orchestrated a series of media interviews, garnered national attention, and held the first public pro-choice rally in more than 20 years, that the province finally relented.[34] Finally, in December 2011 the PEI government included access to abortion information on its website.[35]

Between 2011 and 2015, members of PRRO, along with academic feminists and local pro-choice activists, formed the PEI Abortion Rights Network and began to lobby for local access to abortion services. Due in part to their unyielding activism and a change in political leadership at both the provincial and federal levels, the PEI government announced its new policy on June 2, 2015, permitting PEI women to access abortions somewhat closer to home in the publicly funded hospital in Moncton, a city in New Brunswick, a provincial neighbor.[36] In this volume, Barbara Baird and Lori A. Brown have each raised the importance of neighboring regions that offer abortion services to women living in jurisdictions where they are unavailable, illegal, or inaccessible. However, the Abortion Rights Network argued that this new policy was insufficient as it did not support the necessary aftercare following a surgical abortion off island. Nor did it address the barriers to medical abortions on PEI or include funding for travel to Moncton. Furthermore, continuing to require women to travel off island for an abortion at a public hospital meant that concerns about confidentiality, time off work, childcare, and travel difficulties during inclement weather remained.[37]

On June 16, 2015, Peter Bevan-Baker, a member of the Legislative Assembly in PEI, tabled a petition with more than 1,000 signatures calling for local access to abortion, yet nothing was done to change the existing policy over the following weeks and months.[38] In the meantime, Abortion Access Now PEI, formed to pursue legal action, joined with Nijhawan McMillan Barristers of Halifax and the Women's Legal Education and Action Fund (LEAF), and prepared to seek full and unrestricted access to local, publicly funded abortion services for PEI women.[39] On January 5, 2016, Abortion Access Now PEI filed a Notice of Application in the Supreme Court of PEI against the government of PEI (Minister of Health and Wellness).[40] Subsequently, on March 31, 2016, the PEI government announced that surgical abortions would be available in PEI by the end of the year. Wade MacLauchlan, the newly elected premier of PEI, acknowledged that it would have likely been impossible to defend the government's prohibitive legislation regarding access to abortion against the charge that the province's policies were in violation of the Canadian Charter of Rights and Freedoms.[41] Although this decision was celebrated by island women, funding for abortions in PEI is still restricted to surgical procedures completed in hospitals only, and prior to 12 weeks' gestation, while medical abortions are free of charge only when accessed through one clinic on the Island, the Women's Wellness Program in Summerside.[42] In the event a woman wishes to have a surgical abortion at a private clinic, or if the pregnancy is past 12 weeks of gestation, she continues to face significant barriers and might still have to travel off island to secure access. If she wishes to access a medical abortion outside the Women's Wellness Program (e.g., through her family doctor), she must pay out of pocket approximately C$300 for the treatment. These remaining barriers continue to be challenged by pro-choice advocates in PEI.[43]

On April 4, 2017, New Brunswick health minister Victor Boudreau announced that his government would provide funding for women seeking a medical abortion by covering the drug Mifegymiso under the provincial health plan.[44] Since then, the provinces of Alberta, Ontario, Quebec, British Columbia, and Nova Scotia have followed suit.[45] However, the PEI government has not as yet introduced initiatives or programs aimed at training the necessary physicians and pharmacists to ensure that the administration of and follow-up for medical abortions is consistent and reliable throughout the medical system. As such, the notion of choice in PEI in terms of medical abortion remains troubled and complicated.[46]

Participants' Experiences

In the interviews conducted for our project and excerpted here verbatim, participants shared their experiences and reflections about PEI as a place that can be profoundly oppressive to women, particularly in regard to issues of abortion access. PEI emerges as a geo-politico-religious site that is steeped in patriarchal attitudes and approaches to abortion. As will be seen in the following sections, some PEI women seeking information and/or access to an abortion, and/or engaging in pro-choice activism were persecuted for their actions and choices when interacting with antichoice individuals, agencies, and organizations. Furthermore, many PEI women continue to be alienated from their home communities as a result of seeking and/or obtaining an abortion. Both the persecution of PEI women and their alienation are key factors in supporting the notion that PEI women are not simply medical tourists but abortion refugees.

The most significant barrier to access at the time of the research was a dearth of information about and the absence of access to local abortion services. Just five months before taking part in our project, one participant was unable to find any information about how to access an abortion in PEI, despite searching extensively. When she looked online, the only results that came up were antichoice, religiously funded crisis pregnancy centers. Additionally, participants reported that some island doctors did not know about the publicly funded arrangement through the QEII in Halifax and were, therefore, unable to provide patients with this information. For other women, the lack of money and means to travel to a clinic or hospital off island hampered their access to abortion services.

One of the most chilling consequences of the dearth of information about and the absence of access to local abortion services was the myth on the street that abortion is illegal in PEI. This myth is perpetuated by the mistreatment that women receive from some of their health professionals when they ask for help. One participant contacted her gynecologist for information about how to obtain an abortion, since he had cared for her during her previous pregnancies. When she questioned the receptionist about it, she was told: "we deliver babies, not kill them," leading her to assume that abortion was an illegal procedure in PEI. Another participant shared that her family physician walked out of her appointment without explanation after she asked for information about how to obtain an abortion, leaving her feeling confused and humiliated.

These experiences illustrate some of the ways in which the topic of abortion is surrounded by silence in PEI. This silence is one of the biggest obstacles PEI women must overcome and one of the factors that sustains women's persecution. The maintenance of this silence by government and community contribute to inadequate assistance, protection, and support for women seeking an abortion. The government's role in setting the tone for access to abortion was questioned by many participants in our project. Women even reported altering their actions, speech, and engagements in the community intentionally out of fear of alienation and retribution. Furthermore, they expressed a fear of persecution from antichoice forces in PEI. One participant active in her community shared the following with us during an interview:

Like, for example, would I come out and talk about this stuff openly, in public, in a group situation, to help further the cause [of abortion] now? Probably not. And you know why? It would be because I would be afraid that it might—I know there's so many people out there that are so judgmental, and I don't know who is in what camp, and I do a lot of fundraising for volunteer groups, and I wouldn't want it to influence anything I do in any of those groups. . . . We're reliant on many people, and key people in key organizations for money, and I would never do anything to jeopardize that. . . . They're very—these judgmental people, well then, it's fear. You hear about the shootings [of abortion providers], about all the danger that these doctors have been in, and they've been killed, and their practices, and their homes, and targeted, and the persecution because of people's judgment.[47] And that was in every walk of life. If it wasn't such a small place, if I wasn't involved in these other things, I don't think I would have the problem that I am saying I would have here.

Some women reported experiencing fear of rejection and alienation from their families and communities as a result of their choice to have an abortion. They reflected on PEI as a small and insular place with a profound lack of anonymity. Coupled with ideas about abortion steeped in political conservatism and religious traditionalism, participants expressed feeling terrified that they would be banished and their friends and families would no longer talk to them if the abortion were discovered. This silence has had an emotional impact on women, generating feelings of frustration, anger, shame, and isolation. Speaking about her own abortion, a participant explained:

It was clothed in secrecy and isolation, and it was a couple to a few years that I ever spoke of it afterwards, and when I did tell my sister, then she revealed to me that she had actually had an abortion within a couple of months of the time that I did, and both of us were shocked and saddened for each other that we couldn't—that we didn't—share and support each other at the time . . . that she did it in isolation and insularity and loneliness, and didn't reach out due to shame and fear, and . . . hmm. You know, the sense of wronging that you've done. Against God.

INTERVIEWER: And do you think that's what kept you isolated from each other?

PARTICIPANT: No, more the social taboo. And shame of being pregnant out of wedlock, and then to have an abortion. You know, it really wasn't looked upon very favorably.

Many women expressed a pervasive need to be secretive about the procedure, although they knew getting an abortion was the right decision for them. This secrecy appears to have been the direct result of the alienation women face as they seek access to abortions in PEI. One of the participants said: "Same old—I just can't tell anyone. I have to keep it in. Even my support, I'm very careful. Even my family. You know, if any of them found out they would probably . . . disown me, or at least blacklist me, and just not talk to me." This participant did everything primarily on her own, without protection from the psychological and emotional impacts of the antichoice movement. She was reluctant to involve her mother and only did so in order to secure childcare for her trip to Halifax, and felt her friends wouldn't "receive it [news of her abortion decision] well," resulting in further silencing.

Barriers to Access in PEI

Women's experiences obtaining an abortion reveal a maze of four intersecting pathways, or trails. Each has multiple barriers that threaten to block entirely access to a safe and legal abortion. As we explored and analyzed these trails, and the trials women endured as they traversed them, we began to ask ourselves if PEI women's experiences of having to travel to obtain an abortion fit the criteria for refugee status. The United Nation's Committee on Economic, Social, and Cultural Rights states that reproductive and sexual health, including access to abortion, should be universally available, accessible, and safe.[48] The PEI government's refusal to respect this fundamental right to health has resulted in the persecution of women seeking an abortion in PEI. The 1951 United Nations Convention Relating to the Status of Refugees and subsequent 1967 protocol define a refugee as a person who, "owing to a well-founded fear of being persecuted for reasons of race, religion, nationality, membership of a particular social group or political opinion, is outside the country of his nationality, and is unable to or, owing to such fear, is unwilling to avail himself of the protection of that country or return there because there is a fear of persecution."[49] This definition of refugeehood is predicated on the existence of a bond between the citizen and the state that implies trust, loyalty, protection, and assistance. Refugees come to exist as a result of the severing of this bond.[50] The sundering of this implicit contract results in the absence of protection for a citizen's basic needs. In other words, it results in persecution, whether or not international borders have been crossed.[51] Taking these factors into account, we argue that PEI women have become abortion refugees as a result of the government's inability to ensure their basic human rights. By exploring the following trails that women navigated as they sought access to abortion services, we reveal the importance of understanding their collective experiences in the context of refugeehood.

The surgical abortion through the public healthcare system trail (figure 8.1) outlines access to abortion for women in PEI in optimal circumstances, where resources were readily available. But as abortion refugees, women faced additional barriers and negative impacts as a result of having to travel to obtain this basic medical procedure, even when they had the resources to do so. When a woman discovered she was pregnant, she typically contacted her doctor for information about all of her options, including abortion. In some cases, women received this kind of support; however, it was not universal, consistent, or guaranteed. One participant described going to her doctor for information about access to abortion. She expressed being unsure about how he would respond, highlighting the uncertainty many women face when

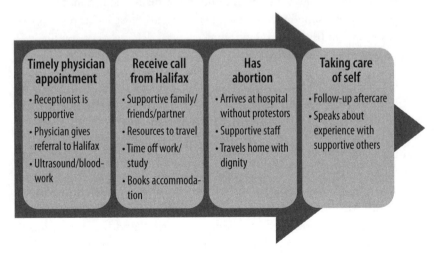

Figure 8.1. Trail 1: Surgical abortion through the public healthcare system in Prince Edward Island. Created by Colleen MacQuarrie; redrawn by Jenn Paulson.

approaching their primary care physicians in PEI. Although her doctor was helpful, he did not have the information she needed. Another participant booked an appointment for a pap smear, fearing her doctor would refuse to see her if she disclosed that she needed an appointment to discuss abortion options.

If a woman were able to receive information about how to access a surgical abortion via the public health route, she needed to have blood work and an ultrasound completed. Women's experiences varied, but in some cases, they encountered ultrasound technicians who used anti-choice tactics to influence their decisions. Mandated ultrasound procedures have become a political tool, effectively rendering pregnant women as the "gatekeepers to life," whereby the fetus becomes the focus of care and concern, and the pregnant woman's own experience is relegated to the background.[52] Thinking back to her appointment for an ultrasound, a participant shared:

> So, I don't know, the way she [ultrasound technician] asked me [about my pregnancy] I just felt like she was trying to make me feel something about it, but really, I'd done a lot of feeling already, you know? I didn't want—and it's personal. I don't know her. I don't—she doesn't need to see me and how I feel about this, because she's a professional. It's a professional situation. . . . What happened is that she started trying to, like, point out [the images appearing on screen], "Well, like, this is the head, and this is the . . ." yeah. . . . And she seemed—I still want to say sad, but, like, disappointed [in me]. Just seemed—"disgust" is probably too strong, but [the ultrasound technician was] definitely not comfortable with the situation.

Time delays at any point in the system caused women to need later-term abortions than would have been necessary. One participant described waiting ten days to get an appointment to see her doctor (who subsequently refused to provide her with a referral for a second abortion a couple years later). She was put on the waiting list for an ultrasound, which took several more days. When it came time for the necessary blood work, she was unable to have it completed at her family doctor's office for unexplained reasons and waited several weeks to have it done. These delays resulted in feelings of distress and fear about missing the 15-week gestational limit for a surgical abortion at the QEII in Halifax. Although she was able to secure the abortion eventually, she was several weeks further along in the pregnancy, resulting in a more invasive and painful abortion procedure. Another participant reported waiting six weeks for her ultrasound, at which point she was unsure how far along she was in her pregnancy, or whether she would be able to obtain the abortion. Still another participant, whose access was delayed because she did not have the financial means to cover the cost of the trip to Halifax, reported that the abortion procedure "was probably the most painful, aside from actual childbirth, experience that I've ever had. And then they said that was because it was so late."

Some participants also said that they felt profoundly stressed when planning for travel off island and when making the journey itself. Until they were called by the hospital in Halifax with a scheduled time for the procedure, women received no communication regarding the process, resulting in feelings of frustration and helplessness. The cost of funding the travel also caused delays, increasing levels of anxiety, and uncertainty. This situation was especially true for poor and marginalized women who often didn't have access to the necessary funds to travel. One participant recounted her experiences supporting women on income assistance when they asked their case workers at the Department of Family and Human Services for emergency money to travel for an abortion. She shared that women had to disclose the reasons for the request, which violated their privacy and left them feeling humiliated. Furthermore, access to emergency money was not guaranteed. It was up to each individual case worker to decide whether to approve the funds to travel for the abortion. While some women did receive the necessary financial support to travel to Halifax, others did not. Additionally, when money was provided, the process of having to make this "special request" often resulted in delays of several weeks.

In optimal circumstances, once a woman received a call to schedule an appointment with an abortion provider, she would make the necessary travel arrangements and have adequate resources to undertake the out-of-province trip. Upon arriving at the hospital or clinic, she would not encounter antichoice protesters, which would have added another layer of stress to her journey. The medical professionals would be helpful, nonjudgmental, and supportive. Once the abortion was completed, the woman would travel home safely and comfortably with the person who accompanied her, have adequate time to rest, and receive appropriate aftercare. This is the scenario that feminist groups and organizations attempted to arrange for New Zealand women traveling to Australia for abortion services, according to Hayley Brown's findings in this volume.

By contrast, many women reported experiences of their off-island abortion that robbed them of their dignity and self-worth. Even women who were not on a fixed income discussed the financial burden of traveling to obtain an abortion. Women also had to book their own accommodation, ensure they had someone to travel with them there and back, take time off work or school, and find adequate childcare, if warranted. These arrangements put women in the position of having to rely on the generosity and goodwill of others in the context of a highly stigmatized need. Furthermore, weather conditions in the region often deteriorated rapidly during winter, resulting in an additional barrier to travel. In just one exchange with an interviewer working on this research project, a participant, returning from an abortion at the QEII in Halifax, remembered:

PARTICIPANT: But it's just like it [the abortion procedure] hurt. Like, I'm on a shuttle back to PEI for five and a half hours, and I'm bleeding all over the place—you know what I mean? It's just Advil [mild over-the-counter pain medication] just ain't cutting it so . . .

INTERVIEWER: How were you able to keep from bleeding through onto your clothing?

PARTICIPANT: Well I wasn't. (laughs) I took a plastic bag to sit with me on the shuttle (laughing) 'cause, like, when I had went before I had bled all over my mom's new car 'cause I had fallen asleep in the car. And I had, like, those big hospital pads on, a couple of them just to . . ."

INTERVIEWER: Yeah, but you just bled through . . ."

PARTICIPANT: Yeah and you can't, you can't ask the driver to pull over [because] I need to use the bathroom. Yeah it's pretty—Oh there's blood, like I bled all over the bag, like, it was horrible. And it's like you gotta kind of hide it whenever you are getting out 'cause it's, and it [blood] didn't go on the seat, thank God, but it's like . . ."

INTERVIEWER: Did you take something to wrap around your bum when you stood up?

PARTICIPANT: A towel. Well I was wearing black sweatpants so it kind of covered a little bit, but you'd see, like, you know what I mean, like . . .

yeah, so it's just, it's so pathetic. We get out at the McDonald's [fast food restaurant] parking lot and, yeah. So, and then you're sore and it's just, I don't know. Kind of degrading a little bit, (laughing) I guess you could say. Instead of just going a couple miles and going home.

Once the abortion was over, the woman would ideally go on with her life. But even when the participants had the explicit support of friends and family, many talked about the negative impact of PEI's conservatism and traditionalism following their abortions, particularly when they felt silenced.

For women on a dead-end trail (figure 8.2), information and resource barriers resulted in an inability to travel off island to obtain an abortion. These women can also be considered abortion refugees, but they remained at home, trapped in an environment characterized by persecution and alienation. For these women, this oppressive environment resulted in carrying their unwanted pregnancies to term. One such participant, who was pregnant but unable to leave the island for an abortion, insisted: "They [pregnant women] need—if they have [a] choice, which we say they do, how can they have a choice if they don't have access to the information to make the choice? The information to make a choice, like I said, money, travel, support, counseling, if they don't have information about where those things are, then how are they making a good choice? Sometimes they're just not choosing because they don't have the information, and then they end up with something they didn't want." For another participant, carrying an unwanted pregnancy to term resulted in her being more deeply ensnared in an abusive relationship:

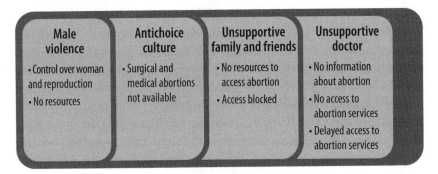

Figure 8.2. Trail 2: The dead end. Created by Colleen MacQuarrie; redrawn by Jenn Paulson.

Well I was still in school and I was living on my own, or with . . . with the father. And I didn't want to be pregnant at all. And he had already had a couple of kids that for whatever reason he wasn't looking after, so. It didn't . . . it didn't seem like it was going to be very good for me . . . but I didn't have any money at the time. Like at all. The only money I had was something called, like, minor living apart . . . so I . . . I didn't realize you could get them covered. And I didn't know about the morning-after pill. . . . I looked into abortion and seen how much it was going to cost and that I would need to find a way to Fredericton [capital of New Brunswick]. Or maybe it was Halifax at the time. Somewhere I couldn't find a way to without telling, like, my parents . . . "hey, can you take me here, cause I need to get an abortion." Like I didn't have my vehicle or my license or any money. So now I have a five-year-old! [laughter] . . . but I didn't have a choice. . . . I still would have had to find a way to get to the hospital, I guess it's in Halifax so you're— without telling a parent or, I don't know who else I could've told that it wouldn't—and they wouldn't have—my parents wouldn't have been for me doing it so. . . . And then, well [son's name] was born in December. . . . I love my son and it changed—he changed who I am to be the person that I am now. And that probably wouldn't have happened without him. But at the time I didn't want to have him and I didn't have a choice or that's—and no woman should have to do that. And unfortunately, I'm tied to his deadbeat, useless, like, abusive, harasses me whenever possible, father for the rest of my life. And there's nothing I can do about that.

In one instance, a participant who was on income assistance had been calling her case worker for several weeks, asking for financial assistance to go to Halifax for an abortion. She had no available means to support the necessary travel and no other option than to wait for her case worker to call her back. Eventually, it became clear that she would need a late-term abortion, which could not be done at a private clinic in Atlantic Canada or at the QEII in Halifax. Because she didn't have the money to fund an even longer trip to a clinic farther away, she was unable to have the abortion and carried the unwanted pregnancy to term. For another participant, a lack of information and resources resulted in engaging in an unwelcome adoption process after deciding to give up her child she brought to term. This failure of the government to provide

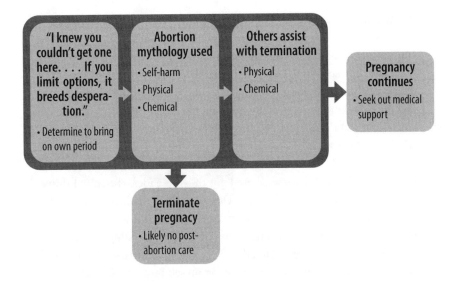

Figure 8.3. Trail 3: At home. Created by Colleen MacQuarrie; redrawn by Jenn Paulson.

basic health services resulted in a systematic denial of women's basic human rights, resulting in profound negative effects on women's physical and mental health.

For some participants, the lack of support, information, resources, and assistance from the government and community was so profound that it resulted in desperate attempts to self-induce an abortion. Participants taking the at-home trail (figure 8.3) reported that attempts often resulted in physical and emotional anguish, as well as violence and trauma. Some participants explained how the idea of bringing on their periods by subjecting their bodies to some kind of trauma was part of their access pathway. One participant, unsure about her options, recounted:

> I knew you couldn't get one [an abortion] here [in PEI]. Um, I don't know if I knew where you had to go but I know that you had to leave. Um, and how would I leave? Like, you know what I mean? Like, close friends would have been my age, with no car, no driver's license . . . Uh, th—I had—there was no money to leave and there was no car to leave, so I was stuck (laughs) so this—it really was, um, like, a decision, like, that, like . . . probably became my life for the next couple of weeks, was trying to self-induce. . . . I think everybody kind of knows the

throw-yourself-down-the-stairs thing. I think that's—however that got into our minds, or into our culture, or whatever, that's kind of been there. Um, so I tried that. Um, you can't do that sober because you—you break your own fall, so I think I got pretty drunk and tried that. Um, vinegar. I drank a substantial amount of vinegar. Um, something about ginger. Uh, and my grandmother was really into, uh, like, naturopathic medicine or something so I think I just dug through her herbs and I probably ate a whole bottle of whatever contained ginger. Um, and something about uh, a tampon. And I don't remember—like, parsley? Uh, and I—like, I—and I—like, I really wish I knew where I got th—these ideas, because I think that's really important, but I don't. Um, something made me really sick. Like, I don't know if it was—I can't remember what it was, but I can remember thinking "if someone comes home, I'm probably going to the hospital and I'm screwed." Um, that sick. But, uh, nobody came home so that was good (laughs). And, r—running myself into a table that was probably the—just the perfect height. And I did that for a wh—a while. Like, probably a couple [times]—'til the leg broke. Um, and if I had to guess, that's probably what induced my period but I don't remember the order that I tried these things in, and I don't remember—like, I don't think—it was probably a couple of weeks from after taking the test to bringing on a period. But, like, there was substantial bruising from the table. Um, I got suspended because I skipped gym so much. 'Cause I couldn't change. Like, substantial bruising, like, it was hard to lay down. Uh, yeah. It wasn't good. But, mission completed.

Some participants considered, and often implemented, even more desperate measures to rid themselves of an unwanted pregnancy. One participant thought about several dangerous possibilities: "Just things like—thinking about walking out into traffic, like, 'Maybe if I just cross onto this jaywalk, maybe I'll just get hit.' Or fall down the stairs in my house—I'm on the third floor of my apartment building. But I didn't want to hurt me. I just wanted to be out of the situation I was in (crying)."

Another participant actively tried to self-induce an abortion and even considered suicide: "I wasn't having a baby. Um, I wasn't. So, if it got to a point where it looked like that was probably happening, I guarantee that would have—I would have k—I, yeah. I wasn't emotionally stable at—enough at all to—to handle something progressing like that. It wouldn't—wouldn't have been good. I think the ways that I tried to induce probably would have gotten more risky to my health, um, and then, yeah. That's—suicide probably would have been a viable option at the end."

Other participants searched the internet for information about how to self-induce by chemical means. One mentioned her knowledge that "copious amounts of drinking" might bring on a miscarriage. Another tried taking 12 birth control pills at one time in the hope of provoking a miscarriage, and when that didn't work, she asked her boyfriend to punch her several times as hard as he could in her stomach. As their unwanted pregnancies progressed, the participants became more desperate. They regarded a self-induced abortion as their only solution, given the impossibility of traveling off island to access abortion services.

Participants on the self-referral surgical abortion outside the public healthcare system trail (figure 8.4) reported that their access to surgical abortions in the private fee-for-service healthcare system outside the province occurred through a physician, friend, or family member, or they sleuthed the information themselves. Some doctors did help participants use fee-for-service clinics prior to 1982, when TACs refused their requests for legal abortions. Between 1982 and 1995, there was no option other than to guide women to off-island abortion clinics. After 1995, when the public health system began paying for abortions off island, some doctors failed to inform their patients of this option or misinformed them to believe that their only option was a private clinic where they would have to pay for the procedure.

Participants spoke about being in a precarious position even when they had a doctor who was willing to help them. One recounted a conversation with her doctor in 1979, who was supportive of her decision

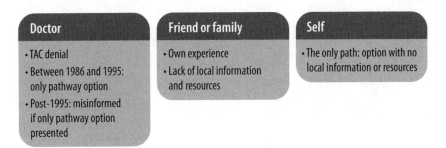

Doctor

- TAC denial
- Between 1986 and 1995: only pathway option
- Post-1995: misinformed if only pathway option presented

Friend or family

- Own experience
- Lack of local information and resources

Self

- The only path: option with no local information or resources

Figure 8.4. Trail 4: Self-referral surgical abortion outside the public healthcare system. Created by Colleen MacQuarrie; redrawn by Jenn Paulson.

but had no options to offer her. At that time, the doctor told her that unless she had a medical reason why she couldn't carry the child to term, she would have to travel to Montreal to access an abortion provider. In this case, she was able to fund-raise the money she needed to travel to the Morgentaler clinic in that city, but her boyfriend at the time, who was emotionally and physically abusive, insisted on making the trip with her since the clinic was so far away. For many participants, having a supportive doctor was necessary, but so was having a trusted family member or friend to count on. One participant remembered her experience of having to travel off island to a private clinic as "terrifying," given that her boyfriend at the time wasn't supportive. She didn't know how to drive and had to rely on her mother for transportation, despite the fact that her mother didn't like to travel. It resulted in a journey that was "very, very, very stressful" and resulted in her "shutting off from everything and everyone."

The Politics of Women's Resilience

Participants in our research project clearly articulated the lack of access to abortion services as a political issue that required them to seek out both internal and external resources, whether they wanted to or not. Much like refugees, who sometimes report that their harrowing experiences increase their sense of resilience,[53] participants exemplified profound strength, despite the numerous and significant barriers they faced as they sought to exercise their right to a safe and legal abortion. One participant expressed that she felt "weak" during the process of having to travel off island, but that the journey helped her feel like she could "get through anything" and that she was "definitely stronger for it now."

Nevertheless, several of the participants struggled with guilt, shame, and self-silencing. One participant described the slow process of healing emotionally after her abortion:

> It did take a long time for me to go from feeling sorry for myself and feeling guilty to feeling like, you know what? Maybe what I did wasn't wrong. And maybe I shouldn't have been made to feel that way by anybody else . . . like, yeah. I don't know. I don't know how else it changed me. We'll say it made me angry eventually. At first it didn't. At first it took a long time to get rid of the guilty feeling. I felt really guilty

I guess. And then I felt guilty for knowing that I wouldn't have changed it. It was like, "well you can't be feeling that guilty if you wouldn't go back and change it." And I'm like, but I feel guilty about that (laughter). You have to self-reflect, and things like this really make you—force you to self-reflect. And at the end of the day, I personally—I'm proud of my decision. Um, I mean, I'm good with me. And there's nobody that could change my mind on that at this point. Which is wonderful to say that I got to that point, and I wouldn't have gotten there without this, you know, without going through that experience. It's a part of me, and it's become a positive influence in my life.

All participants indicated how crucial they thought this participatory action research project was to improving access to safe abortions in PEI. Many reflected on a sense of catharsis, which emerged from the act of telling their own stories. Most of all, they reported that it is essential that women have unrestricted local access to abortions in the future. Participants demanded that the PEI government work toward greater local access to abortion services so that women have a full array of choices and an unfettered ability to act on them. During and following the research project, these demands took the form of local organizing, advocacy, and unprecedented pressure on the PEI government to change their policy on local access to abortions.[54] Born from stigma and silencing, one such initiative saw pro-choice activists in PEI transform the iconic image of Anne of Green Gables from a symbol of innocence, insularity, and traditionalism to a revolutionary figure complete with a Zapatista bandana and hashtags such as #AccessNow and #TrustIsland-Women in a poster campaign across the island.[55] Despite their harrowing experiences, PEI women have demonstrated not only their resilience and agency in the face of persecution but the ability to change laws and policies through their activism.

Conclusion

Women's basic health needs and citizenship rights have been hampered by the PEI government's long-standing antichoice policies and practices surrounding access to abortion. Despite the claim that women could travel for an abortion, this option was limited by antichoice doctors, medical professionals, government agencies, individuals, and community organizations. As such, any discussion of the participants' individual decision making regarding the trails they traversed must necessarily be understood as taking place within the social, economic, and political island landscape in which they are embedded. Human rights framed as "choices" were simply not available to PEI women seeking an abortion, particularly when they were marginalized or lacking the privilege of mobility. The freedom to choose is not simply an individual right or an independent act of autonomy. In order to freely choose, access to both economic and social resources is necessary—a fact that is glossed over when power relations are not considered in an analysis of barriers to access.[56] For PEI women, obtaining an abortion outside of their home province was not simply a matter of choice. The dearth of information, harassment, and lack of options eroded personal autonomy in the PEI context.[57]

Women seeking an abortion in PEI at the time of this research project were not medical tourists who freely chose to travel to obtain a service that was not available at home. Multiple barriers coupled with experiences of persecution and alienation created a category of abortion refugees who had to travel for abortion services, often at a high cost financially, psychologically, and emotionally. Like many refugees, the focus of the participants in this project was on enduring these trials to the best of their ability and moving on with their lives.[58] As we reflect on the PEI government's evolving policies on abortion, we acknowledge the strength, resistance to oppression, and self-determination of the abortion refugees we studied.

Notes

1. For the purposes of this chapter, access to abortion service refers primarily to surgical abortions. In Canada, access to medical abortions is inconsistent and unreliable, and depends on the province and the individual physician. To date, medical abortions in PEI have occurred in a primarily clandestine manner. Only recently, in 2017, did the provinces of New Brunswick, Alberta, and Ontario announce that medical abortions would be offered and covered by the provincial medical plan at no cost. While this is a step in the right direction, adequate infrastructure, physician education, and universal availability at pharmacies remain a concern. In PEI, medical abortions have sometimes been offered by physicians; however, when women have needed follow-up medical care, they have been turned away from the hospital. See Kate McKenna, "Harrowing Experiences of Medical Abortions on Canada's Prince Edward Island Renews Criticism," *Vice News*, May 26, 2015, https://news.vice.com/article/harrowing -experiences-of-medical-abortions-on-canadas-prince-edward-island-renews -criticism for a detailed account of two PEI women's experiences trying to obtain a medical abortion.

2. Gretchen E. Ely et al., "Where Are They From and How Far Must They Go? Examining Location and Travel Distance in US Abortion Fund Patients," *International Journal of Sexual Health* 29, no. 4 (May 2017): 1–12. See also Rachel K. Jones and Jenna Jerman, "How Far Did US Women Travel for Abortion Services in 2008?," *Journal of Women's Health* 22, no. 8 (2013): 706–13.

3. Mary Gilmartin and Allen White, "Interrogating Medical Tourism: Ireland, Abortion and Mobility Rights," *Signs* 36, no. 2 (2011): 275–80. See also Christabelle Sethna and Marion Doull, "Spatial Disparities and Travel to Freestanding Abortion Clinics in Canada," *Women's Studies International Forum* 38 (May/June 2013): 52–62.

4. Joseph S. Alpert, "Medical Refugees in America," *Archives of Internal Medicine* 160, no. 4 (2000): 417–18. See also Arnold Milstein and Mark Smith, "America's New Refugees—Seeking Affordable Surgery Offshore," *New England Journal of Medicine* 355, no. 16 (2006): 1637–40.

5. Bennett Pafford, "The Third Wave—Medical Tourism in the 21st Century," *Southern Medical Journal* 102, no. 8 (2009): 810–13.

6. For a discussion on the evolution of persecution as a key defining factor in determining refugeehood, see José H. Fischel DeAndrade, "On the Development of the Concept of 'Persecution' in International Refugee Law," *Brazilian Yearbook of International Law*, no. 2 (2008): 114–36. DeAndrade notes that prior to World War II, it was lack of protection by the state, and not persecution, that was referenced when determining who constituted a refugee. Although the notion of persecution was implicit, it was not explicitly included in notions of refugeehood until after World War II. It was at this point that fear of future persecution, even in the absence of current persecution, was included in formal international legal documents. At the same time, persecution was not specifically defined in international law, and thus its meaning has evolved over time through academic, administrative, and judicial interpretations. Human rights norms are now typically used when determining which types of discrimination and harm constitute persecution. The UNHCR has further developed the interpretation of what constitutes persecution, and thus refugeehood, including "serious physical harm, loss of freedom, and other serious violations of human rights; discriminatory treatment which leads to consequences of a substantially prejudicial nature; and a combination of numerous harms, none of which alone constitutes persecution, but which, when considered in the context of a general atmosphere in a particular country, produces a cumulative effect which creates a well-founded fear of persecution." See the United Nations High Commissioner for Refugees, *Handbook on Procedures and Criteria for Determining Refugee Status* (Geneva: UNHCR, 1979, 1992). Furthermore, DeAndrade notes that recent case law has contributed to the notion that persecution can happen not only by the state but also by nonstate actors, and that there need not be any intent to harm for specific actions to be considered persecutory. Harm may be physical, but it can also be psychological as well, for example, if an individual suffers mental anguish as a result of their experiences. Persecution, or fear thereof, can also result from holding political opinions that are contrary to societal norms, and if a person is inhibited from expressing their political opinions for fear of harm or retribution.

7. This research was conducted between 2011 and 2014 by Dr. Colleen MacQuarrie, Dr. Jo-Ann MacDonald, and Cathrine Chambers. The research was partially funded through a CAD$7,000 research grant from the University of Prince Edward Island.

8. Katrina R. Ackerman, "In Defence of Reason: Religion, Science, and the Prince Edward Island Anti-Abortion Movement, 1969–1988," *Canadian Bulletin of Medical History* 31, no. 2 (2014): 117–38. See also Katrina R. Ackerman, "Not in the Atlantic Provinces: The Abortion Debate in New Brunswick, 1980–1987," *Acadiensis* 41, no. 1 (2012): 75–101.

9. Interministerial Women's Secretariat, *Women in PEI: A Statistical Review* (Charlottetown, PEI: Prince Edward Island Provincial Government, 2010); Prince Edward Island Advisory Council on the Status of Women, *Response to the Discussion Paper—Preventing and Reducing Poverty in Prince Edward Island: A Strategy for Engagement* (Charlottetown, PEI: Prince Edward Island Provincial Government, 2012); Prince Edward Island Provincial Government, *Preventing and Reducing Poverty in Prince Edward Island: A Strategy for Engagement—Discussion Paper* (Charlottetown, PEI: Prince Edward Island Provincial Government, 2011).

10. Brenda O'Neill and Lynda Erickson, "Evaluating Traditionalism in the Atlantic Provinces: Voting, Public Opinion and the Electoral Project," *Atlantis* 27, no. 2 (2003): 113–22.

11. Ackerman, "Not in the Atlantic Provinces."

12. Christina Clorey, "Votes and Vetoes: A Discursive History of Abortion Politics in Prince Edward Island from 1980–1996" (master's thesis, McMaster University, 2007). See also Chris Kaposy, "Improving Abortion Access in Canada," *Health Care Analysis* 18, no. 1 (2010): 17–34.

13. Godfrey Baldacchino, "Fixed Links and the Engagement of Islandness: Reviewing the Impact of the Confederation Bridge," *Canadian Geographer* 51, no. 3 (2007): 323–36.

14. For a discussion on the moral significance of the Confederation Bridge and its connection to abortion travel in PEI, see Joanna N. Erdman, "The Law of Stigma, Travel, and the Abortion-Free Island," *Columbia Journal of Gender and Law* 33, no. 1 (2016): 29–37.

15. Erdman, "The Law of Stigma, Travel, and the Abortion-Free Island."

16. Ackerman, "Not in the Atlantic Provinces"; and Ackerman, "In Defence of Reason."

17. Here the antichoice movement refers to individuals, groups, and community organizations who seek to block women's access to safe and legal abortions, for example, religious organizations, right-to-life organizations, and religiously funded "crisis pregnancy centers." Antichoice forces can also include individuals who seek to intimidate or influence women not to have an abortion, for example, those who protest or picket outside abortion clinics and hospitals, as well as antichoice doctors, medical professionals, government departments, and other community-based organizations whose aim is to block women from obtaining safe and legal abortions.

18. Heidi McDonald, "Maintaining an Influence: The Sisters of Saint Martha, Charlottetown, Respond to Social and Religious Change, 1965–85," *Atlantis* 32, no. 1 (2007): 91–101.

19. Nancy Bowes, Varda Burstyn, and Andrea Knight, *Access Granted—Too Often Denied: A Special Report to Celebrate the 10th Anniversary of the Decriminalization of Abortion* (Ottawa: Canadian Abortion Rights League, 1998). See also Howard A. Palley, "Canadian Abortion Policy: National Policy and the Impact of Federalism and Political Implementation on Access to Services," *Publius* 36, no. 4 (2006): 565–86.

20. Ackerman, "In Defence of Reason."

21. Lori Brown, J. Shoshana Erlich, and Colleen MacQuarrie, "Subverting the Constitution: Anti-Abortion Policies and Activism in the United States and Canada," in *Abortion: History, Politics, and Reproductive Justice after Morgentaler*, ed. Shannon Stettner, Kristin Burnett, and Travis Hay (Vancouver: University of British Columbia Press, 2017), 239–64.

22. Ackerman, "In Defence of Reason."

23. Katrina Ackerman, "A Region at Odds: Abortion Politics in the Maritime Provinces, 1969–1988" (PhD diss., University of Waterloo, 2015).

24. Ackerman, "In Defence of Reason."

25. Ackerman, "In Defence of Reason."

26. Brown, Erlich, and MacQuarrie, "Subverting the Constitution."

27. Catherine Dunphy, *Morgentaler: A Difficult Hero* (Toronto: Random House, 1996).

28. Katrina Ackerman, "Canada's Pro-Life Province: 30 Years without Abortion Access in PEI," ActiveHistory.ca, January 8, 2016, http://activehistory.ca/2016/01/canadas-pro-life-province-30-years-without-abortion-access-in-pei/.

29. See Clorey, "Votes and Vetoes"; Kaposy, "Improving Abortion Access"; and Ackerman, "In Defence of Reason."

30. Brown, Erlich, and MacQuarrie, "Subverting the Constitution."

31. Colleen MacQuarrie, Jo-Ann MacDonald, and Cathrine Chambers, "Trials and Trails of Accessing Abortion in PEI: Reporting on the Impact of PEI's Abortion Policies on Women" (Charlottetown: University of Prince Edward Island, 2014).

32. MacQuarrie, MacDonald, and Chambers, "Trials and Trails of Accessing Abortion in PEI."

33. Brown, Erlich, and MacQuarrie, "Subverting the Constitution."

34. PEI Reproductive Rights Organization, "Press Release: PRRO Calls on Elected Officials to Stand Up for the Rights of Women," PRRO, November 7, 2011, http://prro.lostwarren.com/2011/11/07/prro-calls-on-elected-officials-to-stand-up-for-the-rights-of-women-by-offering-equal-access-to-pregnancy-termination-services/ (website is under construction). See also PEI Reproductive Rights Organization, "Press Release: Ghiz Reverses Stance on Upholding Charter," PRRO, January 20, 2012, http://prro.lostwarren.com/2012/01/20/press-release-ghiz-reverses-stance-on-upholding-charter/ (website is under construction), and PEI Reproductive Rights Organization, "Press Release: PEI Reproductive Justice Groups Launch National Day of Action," October 15, 2012, http://prro.lostwarren.com/2012/10/16/release-pei/ (website is under construction).

35. "Women's Wellness Program and Sexual Health Services," Government of Prince Edward Island, accessed on February 12, 2018, https://www.princeedwardisland.ca/en/information/health-pei/womens-wellness-program.

36. Kevin Bissett, "New Brunswick Hospital to Offer Abortion Services for PEI Women," *Globe and Mail*, June 2, 2015, https://www.theglobeandmail.com /news/national/new-brunswick-hospital-to-offer-abortion-services-for-pei -women/article24746452/.

37. During our research, participants talked about needing the help of family and friends to travel off island to obtain an abortion. Whether it was financial support, needing someone to accompany them to the procedure and drive them home, asking for time off work, and/or getting a babysitter, women felt they needed to disclose that they were traveling to obtain an abortion in order to justify their requests. Some women also discussed their preference for obtaining an abortion at a private clinic, such as the Morgentaler clinic, as they felt their privacy and confidentiality would be better preserved there as opposed to in the public health system.

38. "Abortion Activists Keep Pressure on PEI Government," *CBC News*, June 17, 2015, http://www.cbc.ca/news/canada/prince-edward-island/abortion -activists-keep-pressure-on-p-e-i-government-1.3116643.

39. Women's Legal Education and Action Fund, "LEAF Proudly Supports Abortion Access Now PEI's Legal Challenge to Prince Edward Island's Discriminatory Abortion Policy," LEAF, January 5, 2016, http://www.leaf.ca/leaf-proudly -supports-abortion-access-now-peis-legal-challenge-to-prince-edward-islands -discriminatory-abortion-policy/. For an in-depth discussion of the significance of this action, see Joanna Erdman, "A Constitutional Future for Abortion Rights in Canada," *Alberta Law Review* 54, no. 3 (2017): 727–52.

40. Abortion Rights Network Prince Edward Island, "Abortion Access Now PEI Challenges PEI's Abortion Policy," Abortion Rights PEI, January 5, 2016, http://www.abortionrightspei.com/content/page/front_news/article/43. For an in-depth discussion of the significance of this action, see Erdman, "A Constitutional Future for Abortion Rights in Canada."

41. Sean Fine, "PEI Drops Opposition to Abortion, Plans to Provide Access by Year's End," *Globe and Mail*, March 31, 2016, https://www.theglobeandmail .com/news/national/pei-to-allow-abortions/article29474278/. See also Abortion Rights Network Prince Edward Island, "ARN Celebrates PEI Government Response to AAN-PEI Legal Challenge," *Abortion Rights PEI*, April 2, 2016, http://www.abortionrightspei.com/content/page/front_news/article/46.

42. Government of Prince Edward Island, "Women's Wellness Program."

43. Abortion Rights Network Prince Edward Island, "Medical Abortion Now Available Free in PEI," *Abortion Rights PEI*, November 17, 2017, http://www.abortionrightspei.com/content/page/front_news/article/51.

44. Canadian Broadcasting Corporation, "New Brunswick Women Will Be Able to Get Abortion Pill Free of Charge," *CBC News*, April 4, 2017, http://www .cbc.ca/news/canada/new-brunswick/abortion-pill-new-brunswick-1.4054517.

45. Andrea Woo, "BC Joins the Ranks of Provinces Offering Abortion Drug Mifegymiso," *Globe and Mail*, January 2, 2018, https://www.theglobeandmail .com/news/british-columbia/bc-becomes-latest-province-to-provide-free-access -to-abortion-pill-mifegymiso/article37475033/.

46. Government of Prince Edward Island, "Women's Wellness Program." See also Patty Skuster, "How Laws Fail the Promise of Medical Abortion: A Global Look," *Georgetown Journal of Gender and the Law* 18, no. 379 (2017): 379–90.

47. This participant was referring to violence against abortion providers in other provinces in Canada (British Columbia in 1994, Ontario in 1995, and Manitoba in 1997) and in the USA. To date, there have not been any abortion-related shootings, bombings, or property damage in the province of PEI. For a discussion on abortion-related violence in Canada and the USA as well as a chronology of events, see Richard B. Parent and James O. Ellis, *Right-Wing Extremism in Canada* (Waterloo: Network for Research on Terrorism, Security, and Society, 2014), https://www.publicsafety.gc.ca/lbrr/archives/cnmcs-plcng/cn31894-eng.pdf.

48. Office of the United Nations High Commissioner for Human Rights, *Information Series on Sexual and Reproductive Health and Rights: Abortion* (Geneva: OHCHR, n.d.), http://www.ohchr.org/Documents/Issues/Women/WRGS/SexualHealth/INFO_Abortion_WEB.pdf.

49. United Nations High Commission on the Status of Refugees, *Convention and Protocol Relating to the Status of Refugees* (Geneva: UNHCR, 2010), http://www.unhcr.org/3b66c2aa10.

50. Atle Grahl-Madsen, *The Status of Refugees in International Law: Volume II: Asylum, Entry and Sojourn* (Amsterdam: AW Sijthoff, 1972).

51. Andrew E. Shacknove, "Who Is a Refugee?" *Ethics* 95, no. 2 (1985): 274–84.

52. Jennifer Rinaldi, "The Public Pregnancy: How the Fetal Debut and the Public Health Paradigm Affect Pregnancy Practice," in *Without Apology: Writings on Abortion in Canada*, ed. Shannon Stettner (Edmonton: Athabasca University Press, 2016), 305–16.

53. Mary Hutchinson and Pat Dorsett, "What Does the Literature Say about Resilience in Refugee People? Implications for Practice," *Journal of Social Inclusion* 3, no. 2 (2012): 55–78. See also Robert Schweitzer, Jaimi Greenslade, and Ashraf Kagee, "Coping and Resilience in Refugees from the Sudan: A Narrative Account," *Australian and New Zealand Journal of Psychiatry* 41, no. 3 (2007): 282–88.

54. Organizations like Abortion Access Now PEI and the PEI Abortion Rights Network were founded during and following the research project. For example, PRRO was founded by the research participants themselves.

55. Erdman, "The Law of Stigma."

56. Abby Lippman, "Choice as a Risk to Women's Health," *Health, Risk and Society* 1, no. 3 (1999): 281–91; and chapters in Stettner, *Without Apology.*

57. Christabelle Sethna and Marion Doull, "Accidental Tourists: Canadian Women, Abortion Tourism, and Travel," *Women's Studies* 41, no. 4 (2012): 457–75.

58. Jessica R. Goodkind, "Promoting Hmong Refugees' Well-Being through Mutual Learning: Valuing Knowledge, Culture, and Experience," *American Journal of Community Psychology* 37, nos. 1–2 (2006): 129–40.

PART III DEMOCRATIC TRANSITIONS

[9]

Abortion Travel and the Cost of Reproductive Choice in Spain

AGATA IGNACIUK

I N 1970s and 1980s Spain, charter flights to London became synony-mous with Spanish women attempting to obtain an overseas abortion, a safer alternative to seeking a local abortion provider in the context of the total abortion ban that lasted in Spain until 1985. This association resurfaced in the Spanish public's imagination when the Law on Sexual and Reproductive Health (Ley Orgánica 2/2010, de 3 de marzo, de salud sexual y reproductiva y de la interrupción voluntaria del embarazo, LSRH), which in 2010 consolidated women's right to abortion on de-mand, came under threat. Just a year after the LSRH was approved, following elections won by the conservative Partido Popular, the then minister of justice, Alberto Ruiz-Gallardón, took on a political and per-sonal crusade to revoke the legislation and return Spain to the doctrine of partial decriminalization of pregnancy termination that had been in force for the previous two and a half decades. Legalization of abortion in a restricted set of medically justified circumstances was first proposed by the socialist government in 1983 but ultimately came into force in 1985. Gallardón's plea, more restrictive than the 1985 Abortion Law (Ley Orgánica 9/1985, de 5 de julio, de reforma del artículo 417 bis del Código Penal), as it removed fetal impairment as a possible medical jus-tification, attracted only limited political and social support and led to the minister's resignation in September 2014. It did, however, fuel spec-ulation about what would have happened if the ban went through, which refreshed in the public memory the experience of heading to the British capital in search of an affordable termination or accompanying a loved one on her potentially traumatic journey.

The aim of this chapter is to examine the options that were available to Spanish women who sought an abortion during the final years of General Francisco Franco's dictatorship and the democratic transition that followed his death in 1975. The period analyzed stretches from 1967, when the British Abortion Act made terminations available to nonresident women, including those coming from Spain, to 1985, when the Spanish Abortion Law was enacted. By focusing on the "supply" side of the phenomenon and comparing the offers from (illegal) abortion providers within Spain to that of overseas abortion clinics that specifically targeted Spanish women, I explore the realities of a time and place where "abortion was a crime"[1] that carried high financial and emotional costs for women at the same time as it constituted an attractive business opportunity for a variety of abortion suppliers, at home and abroad. I begin by examining Spanish reproductive policies before and during Franco's dictatorship and considering how these were progressively dismantled during the democratic transition. This discussion provides a useful context for the chapter to then analyze the opportunities available to women who sought an illegal abortion in Spain prior to 1985, including the option of travel to Britain, a geographical region explored in greater depth in this volume by Gayle Davis et al. and by Christabelle Sethna.

By contributing to the social and cultural history of abortion during the 1960s, 1970s, and 1980s, this chapter attempts to bridge the gap within the existing historiography, which has to date tended to focus heavily on the culture of abortion provision during the Second Spanish Republic (1931–1939)[2] and the early years of Franco's dictatorship.[3] Most of the existing scholarship on the period this chapter analyzes focuses on changing social and political attitudes to abortion, and attempts to quantify the scale of illegal terminations at this time while neglecting the personal and professional experiences of abortion.[4] Equally scarce is scholarship that focuses on Spanish women's abortion travel before the partial decriminalization of abortion in 1985, a phenomenon that has been studied much more from epidemiological and public health perspectives.[5] Interesting, yet tangential, contributions to the topic of abortion cultures and abortion travel in 1970s and early 1980s Spain can be found in the historiography of the Spanish feminist movement, which explores its role in promoting the decriminalization of contraception, achieved in 1978,[6] and in the recent historiography of Spanish family planning activism during the 1970s.[7]

This research is based on a range of print and oral sources. A systematic survey has been conducted of the daily press and women's magazines. These include *El País*, a very popular liberal daily newspaper; the progressive popular magazines *Cambio 16*, *Cuadernos para el Diálogo*, and *Triunfo*; and the women's magazines *Ama*, *Telva*, *Dunia*, and *Vindicación Feminista*. The titles *Ama* and *Telva* circulated during the 1960s and 1970s, and had a conservative profile, while the latter were born during the democratic transition and sought a more progressive (*Dunia*) or directly feminist (*Vindicación Feminista*) readership. I have also analyzed materials collected by the research team of two projects on the history of contraception and sexuality in post-1960 Spain, including oral history interviews with doctors, feminist and health activists involved in the Spanish family planning movement during the 1970s and 1980s, and documents obtained from the interviewees' personal archives.[8] Finally, I have conducted my own oral history interviews with women who traveled abroad for abortions during the 1970s and 1980s as well as with others who facilitated this travel.[9]

Legal Regulation of Abortion and Contraception in Franco's Spain

During the 1930s, Spanish territory saw the introduction of one of the world's earliest pieces of legislation relating to abortion on demand. At the dawn of the Spanish Second Republic, on December 25, 1936, the Cataluña regional government dictated a law that legalized abortion for therapeutic, neo-Malthusian, and ethical or "sentimental" reasons (Decreto de interrupción artificial del embarazo).[10] This meant that women who were anxious about their pregnancy could apply for a termination, though such operations were to be restricted to the first three months of pregnancy and to one abortion per year per woman. The law's contents were clearly emancipating as they equipped women with the right to reject the concept of undesired motherhood. According to the physician and psychologist Felix Martí Ibáñez, one of the main promoters of the reform, the Decreto freed women's sexuality from "egoistic masculine tyranny" and made motherhood a real choice.[11]

However, in practice, the Catalan abortion law was never really implemented after it came into force in early 1937.[12] Historian Mary Nash suggests several reasons for this. First, the doctors resisted performing abortions in cases that lacked therapeutic indications. While, according to Nash, most of the medical profession at that time accepted an abortion to save the pregnant woman's life, many perceived the Decreto as an anarchist imposition and entirely rejected abortion on demand. Second, only a limited number of women were aware of the fact that they could apply to terminate their pregnancy on "sentimental" grounds. Additionally, abortion on demand would publicly identify a woman as being sexually active but rejecting motherhood, which would be perceived as a heavy transgression of contemporary gender norms. Finally, the law was enacted a few months after the outbreak of the Spanish Civil War in the summer of 1936, which meant that the authorities prioritized health problems derived from the military conflict, including the care of the wounded and the fight against sexually transmitted diseases, over investing in an infrastructure for the provision of legal abortion.[13]

The Civil War ended after General Francisco Franco's victory over the Republican state in April 1939. Shortly thereafter, in January 1941, the newly constituted military regime under Franco's leadership enacted a law "for the protection of natality, against abortion and contraceptive propaganda."[14] In the text of this law, abortion was associated with the defeated Republican State and represented as a crime against "race" that impeded "many Spaniards from being born each year."[15] It criminalized not only "all abortion that is not spontaneous" but also the dissemination of contraceptive information and devices, although penalties for abortion-related crimes were substantially higher than those related to contraception.[16] This volume features several chapters that demonstrate the influence of the Catholic Church on the state and also examine the conflation of womanhood with marriage and motherhood. The Spanish case was no different. The law reflected the alliance between the dictatorship and the Catholic Church, whose moral teachings were translated into law by the regime. Other examples of laws that imposed conservative Catholic morals were the prohibition of divorce and the legal placement of women under the tutorship of their fathers and husbands.[17] Through these laws, the regime promoted a model of femininity that was based on the values of submission, selflessness, domesticity, and fertile motherhood, a model that was particularly strong during the early postwar years but that began to decline slowly in the 1960s as the regime aged along with the dictator.[18]

Fertility Limitation from the Dictatorship to the Democratic Transition

From 1959, when national economic policy moved away from autarchy and toward internationalization, Spain slowly but progressively transformed under the influence of the flow of goods (through participation in the international economy),[19] people (through the systematic influx of Western European tourism into the country and the massive emigration of Spaniards to Germany, France, and Switzerland),[20] and ideas (through an increase in the circulation of publications relating to feminism and "the woman question").[21] After Franco's death in 1975, which triggered the beginning of the Spanish democratic transition, the reversal of the legal ban on the sale and dissemination of contraceptives became a burning social issue and was finally enacted in 1978 as one of the first initiatives of the newly elected democratic parliament. The ban was removed smoothly and quickly as consensus grew that it was obsolete. Since at least the late 1960s, it had been the object of increasing public criticism by members of the medical profession and the progressive clergy, who favored married women's use of the contraceptive pill.[22]

The pill was officially in circulation on the Spanish market from the beginning of the 1960s. Initially, it was not commercialized as a contraceptive but as a drug to be used to treat a number of female ailments, including irregular and painful menstruation or functional sterility. Yet, the spectacular growth in its sales from the late 1960s onward suggests that it was prescribed and used for birth control purposes shortly after it was introduced.[23] While in Spanish medical journals many conservative doctors positioned themselves against the pill, for others the "therapeutic" value of oral contraceptives made it a useful product for women with ill health or those who already had large families or were facing economic hardship. Indeed, by the early 1970s, some doctors publicly argued that contraception was a human right.

Concurrently, oral contraceptives became a subject of lively debate in the Spanish media. These discussions contributed to the dissemination of information about birth control methods and stimulated social acceptance of contraception.[24] The feminist movement was another important agent responsible for stirring up discussion about improving women's access to birth control and abortion. Feminist efforts in this vein link together several contributions to this volume, notably those by Hayley Brown; Mary Gilmartin and Sinéad Kennedy; Cathrine Chambers, Colleen MacQuarrie, and Jo-Ann MacDonald; Anna Bogic; and Ewelina Ciaputa. Spanish feminists deployed slogans such as "Contraception to avoid abortion, (legal) abortion to avoid death" and "We want the right to abortion, but we don't want to have abortions," which became landmarks of feminist pro-choice activism during the late 1970s.[25] After contraception was legalized, access to legal abortion became one of the Spanish feminist movement's key goals.[26] As the aforementioned slogans demonstrate, abortion was discursively framed as the last resort, something the movement did not want per se. Rather, its illegality was linked to lethal danger for women who underwent clandestine procedures.

Paradoxically, the milestone for early mass feminist mobilizations around abortion in Spain was related to the defense of an illegal abortion provider. Similar legal struggles concerning Dr. Henry Morgentaler ended up in the Supreme Court of Canada, as Cathrine Chambers, Colleen MacQuarrie, and Jo-Ann MacDonald note briefly in their chapter. The Spanish "Bilbao trial" concerned eleven women and one man from Basauri, a working-class suburb of Bilbao, a large industrial city in the north of the country, all of whom were arrested in October 1976. One of the accused was a skilled lay abortion provider who had been offering cheap abortions to her neighbors, with no known harm to their health. Her mentally disabled daughter was accused of assisting in the operations, and the remaining nine women were clients or intended clients. The only man involved in the trial was accused of forcing his spouse to have a termination.[27] The trial, which started in May 1979, was covered extensively in the press and triggered support for the accused. These transformed into a variety of actions promoted by local and national feminist organizations, including public demonstrations, sit-ins, and mail campaigns. The latter consisted of flooding the courts with letters of self-inculpation by women who confessed to having had an illegal abortion and men who admitted to having helped women to obtain one. Through all these actions, the feminist movement claimed amnesty for the accused at the same time as it attempted to mainstream its plea for the liberalization of Spanish abortion law. In March 1982, the clients who had had the abortions were acquitted, and the abortion practitioner was granted amnesty.[28]

Meanwhile, public support for abortion law reform had grown. While in 1979, only 27 percent of Spaniards were found to be in favor of decriminalization, by 1981, according to one poll, 39 percent supported partial decriminalization,[29] and by 1983 that figure had climbed to 57 percent of the public.[30] A proposal to modify the penal code so that abortion would not be penalized in cases where pregnancy resulted from rape, where there was a diagnosis of fetal impairment, or where continuing with the pregnancy could be harmful to the woman's health was supported by the vast majority of the members of the Spanish Parliament. The conservative Alianza Popular appealed for the bill to be considered unconstitutional, but the Constitutional Tribunal authorized it to become law in the summer of 1985. No time limit was established for therapeutic abortion; those performed in cases of rape were limited to the first 12 weeks of pregnancy; and where fetal malformations were apparent, the time limit was 22 weeks.

Like the British Abortion Act of 1967,[31] the focus of the chapter by Gayle Davis et al. in this volume, a broad definition of "health"—conceptualized as a state of well-being rather than merely the absence of disease—made it possible for Spanish doctors to provide voluntary abortions locally and to use the mental health clause to authorize terminations.[32] In practice, after private clinics started to be authorized to become providers of "low-risk" abortions in November 1986,[33] most surgical terminations in Spain have been carried out in private abortion facilities licensed by regional authorities. In regions where no or few such clinics were established, women's access to abortion continued to depend on their ability to travel.

Home or Away? Women's Abortion Options

The phenomenon of illegal terminations, despite the fact that it is difficult if not impossible to accurately quantify, was central to Spanish studies of abortion during the late 1970s and early 1980s, as well as to media discussions of abortion. The most frequently quoted figure was that proposed by the Spanish Supreme Court in 1974, which estimated that 300,000 illegal abortions were being performed in Spain every year. While the Supreme Court's reasoning behind this figure lacked methodological grounding (perhaps due to its political utility),[34] this number was widely circulated in the press throughout the 1970s, to the point of becoming almost a standard reference for the number of illegal abortions in the country, and was also adopted by the feminist pro-choice movement. The high number of illegal abortions performed yearly in Spain was quoted frequently to characterize the existing law as inadequate and harmful to women, who were being placed into the hands of "back alley butchers."[35] As mentioned earlier, and similarly to other countries such as Canada and the United States of America (USA),[36] the health consequences of illegal abortions were used to promote the legalization of the procedure and appear as a common refrain in several chapters in this volume.

In 1985, the year abortion was decriminalized, the sociologist and demographer Josune Aguinaga Roustan prepared a report titled *Abortion in Spain: Data for the Planning of Social Policy*. Commissioned by the Women's Institute (Instituto de la Mujer), a public equality organization, the report proclaimed the total number of Spanish women's abortions to be 105,000 per year during the early 1980s, one-third of the widely circulated number of 300,000 published a decade earlier by the Supreme Court. According to Aguinaga Roustan, of these 105,000, approximately 60 percent were illegal abortions performed within the Spanish borders, and the remaining 40 percent resulted from abortion travel.[37]

Spanish women's abortion travel has been more adequately quantified only in the case of travel to Britain, where, under the 1967 Abortion Act, clinics were obliged to register nonresident women who underwent a termination and to communicate these figures to the British Office of Population Censuses and Surveys. According to this data, between 1974 and 1988, almost 200,000 Spanish women traveled to have an abortion in English and Welsh clinics, a figure that represents 2.7 percent of Spanish women born between 1935 and 1974.[38] It is also worth noting that throughout the 1970s, and especially during the second half of the decade, and in the early 1980s, Spanish women's abortions constituted an important proportion of all nonresident abortions performed in Britain. Indeed, according to Christopher Tietze and Stanley K. Henshaw, between 1978 and 1980, Spanish women's abortions, remarkably, constituted about half of all nonresident abortions.[39] Regardless, it was and is difficult to determine with great accuracy just how many nonresident women undergo abortions; both Christabelle Sethna and Niklas Barke, in their contributions to this volume, assume that the numbers are higher than presented.

As for other Spanish women's abortion travel itineraries, Aguinaga Roustan's report positioned France as the second most popular destination, with approximately 10,000 women seeking to have their pregnancy terminated there each year. Under the French Loi Veil, the abortion bill that in 1975 legalized early abortions on demand, residence for a period of three months was a precondition for women who wanted to have an abortion in France.[40] This, together with a compulsory one-week reflection period, would make France potentially less attractive for Spanish women. Nevertheless, the fact that the Spanish-French border could be crossed by car or train was an important incentive. Furthermore, French abortion clinics broke the law and offered their services to their southern neighbors and were favored by women from the north of Spain in particular, who could reach them and get back home the same day.[41] One such clinic in Biarritz, France, was reported by the Spanish newspaper El País to have closed in 1979 due to not having complied with the legal ban on abortion for nonresidents.[42]

Aguinaga Roustan also mentioned the significance of the Netherlands, with an estimate that some 6,000 Spanish women traveled to clinics in The Hague, Amsterdam, and Leiden every year after abortion was decriminalized there in 1981, and Portugal, which allegedly received some 3,000 Spanish women seeking abortions every year. The flow of Spanish women to its neighboring country of Portugal intensified after partial decriminalization of abortion was enacted in the country in May 1984 and private clinics opened their doors to Spanish clients. As in the case of France, the fact that cities such as Porto could be reached by car made travel more accessible. For women from the northeastern region of Galicia, whose local language is similar to Portuguese, the lack of a language barrier at Portuguese clinics was another asset. Another popular destination, although it was not mentioned in Aguinaga Roustan's report, was Morocco. Despite restrictive local laws, clinics that catered specifically to nonresident women operated in cities such as Tangier, sometimes called the "London of the South,"[43] a term that emphasizes the centrality of London as a destination hub for abortion services, as Christabelle Sethna does in this volume. Separated from Spain only by the Strait of Gibraltar, Tangier could be reached by car and ferry, and thus offered a potentially appealing alternative to Britain or the Netherlands for women from the southern Spanish region of Andalusia, highlighting the key role geographical proximity plays in obtaining an abortion, discussed in several chapters in this volume.

The aforementioned data suggests that having to arrange a clandestine abortion in Spain or a legal or illegal abortion abroad[44] was a relatively common experience for Spanish women during the last years of

Francoism and the democratic transition. The existing scholarship on abortion as well as many authors in this volume, such as Hayley Brown, and Mary Gilmartin and Sinéad Kennedy, demonstrate that each of these options requires the mobilization of a range of economic, social, and emotional resources, including collecting the money and activating a network of contacts in order to find an abortion practitioner and, where travel was concerned, organizing the trip.[45]

Analysis of the press and archival materials as well as oral history interviews with doctors and family planning activists situates medical abortion in Spain as the most expensive option available to women. The contemporary feminist and progressive press quoted 30,000–50,000 pesetas for a local medical abortion in 1977,[46] an amount similar to an average monthly salary and exceeding by 2.5 times the monthly minimum wage at the time.[47] In Madrid, a medical abortion in the late 1970s could cost 100,000 pesetas,[48] although some sources mention doctors who charged triple this sum.[49]

These high prices were a reflection of the ongoing controversy that abortion continued to create, contrary to contraception, which, even before decriminalization, enjoyed widespread social and medical support. They also suggest that most doctors were not willing to take risks and perform illegal terminations. Abortion was (at least officially) shunned by most early public and private family planning centers, established by doctors interested in offering women access to contraception when its advertisement and sale were still illegal. Doctors who in 1978 staffed the first semi-clandestine public family planning clinic funded as an outpatient surgery unit in a major teaching hospital in Seville, the capital city of the southern Spanish region of Andalusia, were reluctant, if not hostile, toward the concept of abortion.[50] They considered abortion "not their fight"[51] and something they "just didn't want to do."[52]

Abortion referral was nonetheless practiced on a large scale by at least three private family planning centers in Madrid: the Federico Rubio feminist family planning center, which operated between 1976 and 1978; the Instituto de Medicina Social, established in 1978 by the Communist Party; and the Pablo Iglesias family planning center, established in the same year and funded by the socialist party PSOE.[53] Federico Rubio and the Instituto de Medicina Social both had an unwritten agreement with one London clinic, according to which, due to the large volume of patients they were referring, they were able to send some women to have their abortions performed free of charge. Instituto de Medicina

Social and Pablo Iglesias also cooperated with a high-end travel agency, with whom they also negotiated a deal to obtain free flights and accommodation in London for women with financial difficulties.[54]

Indeed, traveling for an abortion, particularly to Britain, meant being able to obtain a "white-coat abortion" performed in a safer clinical setting, which was frequently cheaper than an illegal medical abortion at home. Yet, crossing borders added challenges to the process, especially while the dictatorship lasted. Before Franco's death, married women were legally treated as minors and, as such, needed the permission of their husband to apply for a passport. For single women, such an application was subjected to the completion of "social services," training in household management organized by Sección Femenina, the female branch of La Falange, the ruling fascist party.[55] Apart from the formalities necessary for crossing the border, the journey meant navigating strange roads and cities, and operating in a foreign language. Many of these journeys were carried out in solitude to avoid increasing the already-significant cost of the venture.

As I have explored elsewhere, abortion referral in Spain was commonplace not only in many socialist-inspired family planning clinics but in progressive circles more broadly. Left-wing political parties and progressive individuals frequently raised the money to fund abortion travel for their comrades, friends, and even anonymous women in need; distributed the addresses of foreign clinics; or accompanied women on their journeys.[56] London emerged as the leading destination, for reasons made clear in Christabelle Sethna's chapter, its popularity boosted by competitive "package holiday" prices that included the surgery, accommodation, and flights. After Franco's death in 1975, information about British and French abortion clinics started to circulate in Spain through several channels. One such channel was the press. As early as October 1976, the progressive daily newspaper *El País* dedicated several pages of their first Sunday magazine to abortion travel to London. In the years that followed, the information on abortion providers, including detailed descriptions of the clinics and their owners' names and addresses, circulated in the daily press.[57] These were also disseminated by Spanish feminist activists, both in writing and through word of mouth. In 1978, Leonor Taboada published *Cuaderno Feminista*, a self-help manual inspired by *Our Bodies, Ourselves*, a popular American feminist text that Anna Bogic analyzes in this volume.[58] *Cuaderno Feminista* included the contact details for three French and seven London clinics, annotating two of them as "cheap" and one as "they speak Spanish and pick you up at the airport."[59] Feminist groups in Barcelona, Madrid, and other cities also disseminated the clinics' contact information.[60]

Another source of information about London abortion clinics was Spanish doctors. While performing abortions was something most doctors rejected, abortion referral to British and other foreign clinics was likely a rather widespread practice for those physicians who, not willing to perform abortions themselves, nevertheless wished to offer abortion services in some way, a feature also discussed by Gayle Davis et al. in this volume. Moreover, the pre- and postabortion checkups, and perhaps also the referral itself, was a source of possible income without their having to take excessive risks. Indeed, evidence suggests that during the 1970s Spanish doctors were approached by commercial referral agencies who offered them kickbacks for every patient referred to them.[61] One doctor, the owner of a Harley Street surgery clinic who was fluent in Spanish, traveled to Spain in the mid-1970s to establish a network with Spanish gynecologists who would be willing to refer their abortion-seeking patients to his clinic. The clinic was staffed by Spanish-speaking nurses, and after surgery women were handed a letter in Spanish that provided information for their doctor back home who would be performing the postabortion checkup.[62] According to the clinic's own data, it served about one-quarter of all Spanish women who had their pregnancies terminated in the UK during the early 1980s.[63]

The price of the surgery in a private London clinic during the second half of the 1970s ranged from 5,000 to 14,000 pesetas, and the total cost of the trip totaled between 20,000 and 60,000 pesetas,[64] perhaps closer to 20,000 if purchased as a "package." Traveling to Holland, where such package trips were less common and the termination itself cost at least 20,000 pesetas, was a more expensive option. The whole trip in the early 1980s could cost as much as 75,000 pesetas.[65] Alternatively, France, Portugal, and Morocco, where it was possible to reach and return from on the same day, were probably much more cost-effective options. Private clinics in Porto after 1984 charged between 25,000 and 40,000 pesetas for the surgery.[66] A clinic in the aforementioned town of Biarritz, in France, close to the Spanish border, charged 15,000 pesetas in 1988,[67] which appears to have been a fairly standard charge by French clinics for an abortion without a general anesthetic or overnight stay.

The cost of an early abortion offered by the lay abortion groups the Valencia group (late 1970s–early 1980s) and the Health Collective, better known under the name "Los Naranjos" after the family planning and abortion clinic it established in Seville in 1980, was lower even than these "short-distance" abortion trips abroad. The Valencia group pioneered the use of vacuum aspiration in Spain, currently considered the safest procedure for an early surgical abortion. Established in Valencia, a city on the east coast of Spain with a population of 750,000, the group was comprised of local feminists and left-wing political activists (some of whom had nursing and medical training) as well as an experienced nonmedical abortion provider who traveled down to Valencia from Marseille several times a week in order to provide vacuum aspiration.[68] She later established herself in Valencia and trained a number of doctors and lay practitioners to perform abortions using homemade transportable aspiration devices, in which a bicycle pump was combined with a jar of Nescafé coffee, tubes, and a manometer.

The gynecologist Pere Enguix, a vocal defender of the legalization of abortion and one of the few doctors who openly broke the law by providing illegal terminations, for which he was imprisoned several times during the early 1980s,[69] was also involved with the group. Abortions were performed collectively in the flat of one of the pregnant women or, if this option was unavailable, in the houses of the collective's members or their friends. The constant change of location was intended to help avoid a possible police raid. The total price of a termination amounted to between 10,000 and 15,000 pesetas.[70] According to one of its members, the group was performing some 70 abortions per month throughout the two years it was most active.[71]

In late 1979, some members of the Valencia group, all of them lay providers who lacked formal medical training but had mastered the technique of early uterine vacuum aspiration, moved to Seville, where they funded the family planning center Los Naranjos. In this center, opened in January 1980, women seeking terminations first received a preabortion checkup to determine whether their stage of pregnancy was early enough to make them eligible for vacuum aspiration. A gynecologist was also available for pre- and postabortion checkups. Before the operation, women participated in a collective session during which self-exploration of the genitals and cervix were promoted. They also received a talk on contraception and sexuality, as well as detailed information about the abortion procedure itself. As in Valencia, abortions were not actually performed at the center but collectively in private flats. The procedure, as one of the members later recalled in his memoir, never exceeded 15 minutes, and none of the 416 women who used the center's services suffered from complications.[72] Having existed for ten months, in October 1980 the center was raided and its members were arrested. They were only acquitted in 1996, after a trial that lasted 16 long years.[73]

The pricing of the services was a controversial issue for the Los Naranjos group, as was the case in other abortion collectives such as Jane's underground feminist abortion services, which operated in Chicago between 1969 and 1973.[74] The Los Naranjos group, composed of four members—two women and two men—initially agreed on 30,000 pesetas as the monthly salary for each member, an amount established in relation to the official average monthly salary in Spain in 1980. Only after three months of activity did three of the members opt for the group to raise this salary by 50 percent, a decision voted for by the majority but not unanimously. According to different sources, the group charged women between 8,000 and 14,000 pesetas for the procedure.[75]

Both the Valencia and Los Naranjos groups treated women from different parts of Spain. Women traveled to Valencia not only from the Comunidad Valenciana region but from adjacent regions of Murcia, Castilla-La Mancha, and Andalusia.[76] Most clients of Los Naranjos came to Seville from its region, Andalusia; however, some crossed the country from the northern regions of Galicia and Basque Country. Some women even flew in from the Canary Islands.[77] Knowledge about their services circulated through word of mouth in progressive and feminist circles, despite the group's uneasy relationship with the organized feminist movement.[78]

Finally, for those women who did not know about the existence of abortion clinics abroad, or "revolutionary" lay abortion providers in Valencia and Seville, or who knew about them but could not reach them, using the services of lay practitioners with or without medical training was perhaps their only option, an option that Christabelle Sethna; Cathrine Chambers, Colleen MacQuarrie, and Jo-Ann MacDonald; Anna Bogic; and Ewelina Ciaputa likewise address in this volume. The price of such services started from as little as 2,000 pesetas. This amount was charged throughout the 1970s by the Bilbao lay abortion provider discussed earlier in the chapter, who also had an excellent safety record, an example of what historian Rickie Solinger has called "highly skilled and experienced practitioners, who compiled an astonishing record of successful procedures under extremely difficult conditions."[79] Similarly to what Solinger's work has emphasized for the pre–*Roe v. Wade* American context, it must be noted that in Spain those terminations that ended in the pregnant woman's serious injury or death were far more likely to be brought to trial, while the majority of those in which no complications occurred went unnoticed by the authorities.[80] Although the criminal investigations and trials for abortion-related crimes were conducted regularly while the dictatorship lasted (and beyond), during the last decades of Franco's rule there were as few as a maximum of 200 abortion-related trials per year.[81]

Conclusion

Despite the fact that abortion was criminalized in Spain until 1985, having an illegal abortion in the country or traveling abroad for the procedure was a fairly common experience for Spanish women. The high figures for illegal abortion and the juxtaposition of local backstreet abortions with abortion travel, the latter of which allegedly made a safe medical abortion available only to economically privileged women, were key themes of discussion in the progressive media during the late 1970s and early 1980s, and became pivotal arguments of the feminist movement's pro-choice campaigns.

Moving beyond the rhetoric of estimated illegal abortion figures, "package holidays" to London, and "back alley butchers," however, helps to uncover the complexities of the abortion trade in pre-1985 Spain. As I have shown in this chapter, for women who could afford and were determined to have a medical abortion, organizing a trip to Britain could be cheaper than seeking a medical abortion at home, especially if a woman was able to purchase a package deal or received support from a progressive family planning clinic, whose staff arranged to bridge the gap between well-off and less well-off women's access to overseas abortion services. Many women were directed toward these clinics by their private gynecologists or by comrades from feminist and/or left-wing activist groups. Women who belonged to left-wing political parties or the feminist movement could also have reached abortion providers, who operated in Valencia from the late 1970s through the early 1980s and in Seville in 1980. Women without such contacts would rely on lay providers, probably for the most part safer than their back-alley butcher reputation in the public imaginary, or resort to scarce and extremely expensive services of local gynecologists.

Acknowledgments

This research was developed within the research project "London Calling: Embodied Mobility, Abortion Tourism and the Global City" (Social Sciences and Humanities Research Council of Canada, SSHRC ref. no. 435-2016-1397. PI: Christabelle Sethna).

Notes

1. Leslie J. Reagan, *When Abortion Was a Crime: Women, Medicine, and Law in the United States, 1867–1973* (Berkeley: University of California Press, 1998).

2. Mary Nash, "Género, Cambio Social y la Problemática del Aborto," *Historia Social*, no. 2 (1988): 19–36.

3. Clive Beadman, "Abortion in 1940s Spain: The Social Context," *Journal of Gender Studies* 11, no. 1 (2002): 55–66; Inmaculada Blasco Herranz, "Actitudes de las Mujeres Bajo el Primer Franquismo: La Práctica del Aborto en Zaragoza durante los Años 40," *Arenal: Revista de Historia de las Mujeres* 6, no. 1 (1999): 165–80.

4. Gerardo Hernández Rodríguez, "Actitudes y Criterios Sobre el Aborto y la Planificación Familiar," *Revista Española de Investigaciones Sociológicas*, no. 1 (January 1978): 205–49; Gerardo Hernández Rodríguez, "Aborto y Planificación Familiar: Aspectos Sociológicos," *Revista Española de Investigaciones Sociológicas*, no. 5 (1979): 137–63; Gerardo Hernández Rodríguez, "El Aborto en España: Análisis de un Proceso Socio-Político" (PhD diss., Universidad Complutense de Madrid, 1992); José Luis Ibáñez y García Velasco, *La Despenalización del Aborto Voluntario en el Ocaso del Siglo XX* (Madrid: Siglo Veintiuno, 1992); Magda Teresa Ruiz Salguero, Teresa Castro Martín, and Montse Solsona Pairó, *Anticoncepción y Salud Reproductiva en España: Crónica de una (R)Evolución* (Madrid: Consejo Superior de Investigaciones Científicas, Instituto de Economía y Geografía, 2005).

5. Rosana Peiró et al., "Does the Liberalisation of Abortion Laws Increase the Number of Abortions? The Case Study of Spain," *European Journal of Public Health* 11, no. 2 (2001): 190–94; Rosana Peiró et al., "Abortos Inducidos en Mujeres Españolas en Inglaterra y Gales (1974–1988)," *Gaceta Sanitaria* 8, no. 41 (1994): 57–62.

6. Mercedes Agustín Puerta, *Feminismo, Identidad Personal y Lucha Colectiva: Análisis del Movimiento Feminista Español en los Años 1975 a 1985* (Granada: Universidad de Granada, 2003); Carmen Martínez Ten, Purificación Gutiérrez, and Pilar González, eds., *El Movimiento Feminista en España en los Años 70* (Madrid: Cátedra, 2009).

7. Teresa Ortiz-Gómez and Agata Ignaciuk, "The Fight for Family Planning in Spain during Late Francoism and the Transition to Democracy, 1965–1979," *Journal of Women's History* 32, no. 2 (2018): 38–62; Agata Ignaciuk and Teresa

Ortiz-Gómez, *Anticoncepción, Mujeres y Género: La "Píldora" en España y Polonia (1960–1980)* (Madrid: Catarata, 2016); Teresa Ortiz-Gómez et al., "Activismo Feminista y Movimiento Asociativo por la Planificación Familiar en España," in *Transmisión del Conocimiento Médico e Internacionalización de las Prácticas Sanitarias: Una Reflexión Histórica*, ed. María Isabel Porras Gallo et al. (Ciudad Real: Sociedad Española de Historia de la Medicina, 2011); Eugenia Gil García, Teresa Ortiz-Gómez, and Agata Ignaciuk, "El Movimiento de Planificación Familiar en Sevilla durante la Transición Democrática," in *Investigación y Género. Logros y Retos*, ed. Isabel Vázquez Bermúdez (Seville: University of Seville, 2011), 726–36.

8. These research projects were conducted between 2010 and 2017: "PF" (La constitución de la planificación familiar en España durante los últimos años del franquismo y la transición democrática, 1975–1985, Ministerio de Ciencia e Innovación, HAR2008-05809-HIST) and "ASYS" (Anticoncepción, sexualidad y salud: memorias de vida y prácticas sanitarias en España durante el franquismo y la Transición Democrática, Ministerio de Economía y Competitividad, HAR2012-39644-C02-01). The principal investigator of both projects was Teresa Ortiz-Gómez, and the recordings, transcripts, and personal documents collected during this research are currently deposited in the archives of the Department of the History of Science at the University of Granada.

9. In 2017, within the aforementioned "London Calling" project, I carried out a number of in-person, telephone, and Skype interviews with women who traveled for abortions abroad, people who accompanied them on their journeys, and those who helped organize these trips.

10. Mariacristina Sogos, "L'Impatto Sociale dell'Aborto. L'Analisi del Discorso sull'Interruzione Volontaria di Gravidanza nella Stampa Spagnola" (master's thesis, University of Granada/University of Bologna, 2013).

11. Nash, "Género, Cambio Social."

12. Salguero, Martín, and Pairó, *Anticoncepción y Salud*.

13. Nash, "Género, Cambio Social."

14. Ignaciuk and Ortiz-Gómez, *Anticoncepción, Mujeres*.

15. "Ley de 21 de Enero para la Protección de la Natalidad, contra el Aborto y la Propaganda Anticoncepcionista," *Boletín Oficial del Estado* 33 (1941): 768–69.

16. Ignaciuk and Ortiz-Gómez, *Anticoncepción, Mujeres*.

17. María del Rosario Ruiz Franco and Gloria Nielfa Cristóbal, *"Eternas Menores": Las Mujeres en el Franquismo* (Madrid: Biblioteca Nueva, 2007); Aurora G. Morcillo, *The Seduction of Modern Spain: The Female Body and the Francoist Body Politic* (Lewisburg, PA: Bucknell University Press, 2010).

18. Jordi Roca i Girona, "Esposa y Madre a la Vez: Construcción y Negociación del Modelo Ideal de Mujer Bajo El (Primer) Franquismo," in *Mujeres y Hombres en la España Franquista: Sociedad, Economía, Política, Cultura*, ed. Gloria Nielfa Cristóbal (Madrid: Editorial Complutense, 2004), 45–65.

19. Pablo Martín Aceña and Elena Martínez Ruiz, "The Golden Age of Spanish Capitalism: Economic Growth without Political Freedom," in *Spain Transformed: The Late Franco Dictatorship, 1959–75*, ed. Nigel Townson (Basingstoke: Palgrave Macmillan, 2007), 30–85.

20. Sasha D. Peck, "Tourism and Political Change in Franco's Spain," in Townson, *Spain Transformed*, 47–66.

21. Ortiz-Gómez and Ignaciuk, "The Fight for Family Planning."

22. Ignaciuk and Ortiz-Gómez, *Anticoncepción, Mujeres*.

23. Ignaciuk and Ortiz-Gómez, *Anticoncepción, Mujeres*.

24. Teresa Ortiz-Gómez and Agata Ignaciuk, "'Pregnancy and Labour Cause More Deaths than Oral Contraceptives': The Debate on the Pill in the Spanish Press in the 1970s," *Public Understanding of Science* 24, no. 6 (2015): 658–71.

25. *Vindicacción Feminista*, January 1, 1978, 27.

26. Augustín Puerta, *Feminismo*.

27. Joaquina Prades, "Yo Las Ayudé a Abortar porque me Daban Mucha Lástima, Llenas de Problemas y sin un Duro," *El País*, October 18, 1979, http://elpais.com/diario/1979/10/18/espana/309049234_850215.html; Joaquina Prades, "Abortaron por Problemas de Salud y Falta de Medios Económicos," *El País*, October 17, 1979, http://elpais.com/diario/1979/10/17/espana/308962811_850215.html; Joaquina Prades, "Juicio Contra 11 Mujeres Acusadas de Practicar o Someterse a Abortos," *El País*, October 3, 1979, http://elpais.com/diario/1979/10/03/espana/307753230_850215.html. See also Oihane López Grande, "Juicios por Aborto a 11 Mujeres de Basauri: Nueve Años del Largo y Duro Proceso," in *La Defensa del Derecho al Propio Cuerpo y la Construcción del Movimiento Feminista: Juicio por Aborto a 11 Mujeres de Basauri, 1976–1985* (master's thesis, University of the Basque Country, 2011), 37–50.

28. The sentence was appealed to the Supreme Court, which in 1983 acquitted only four women and condemned the rest to fines and imprisonment. In the final instance, the Constitutional Court rectified the Supreme Court's ruling, but the lay abortion provider's amnesty was upheld. See López Grande, "Juicios por Aborto," 45–49.

29. Merike Blofield, *The Politics of Moral Sin: Abortion and Divorce in Spain, Chile and Argentina* (New York: Routledge, 2006), 63–95.

30. Blofield, *The Politics of Moral Sin*, 63–95.

31. Melanie Latham, *Regulating Reproduction: A Century of Conflict in Britain and France* (Manchester: Manchester University Press, 2002), 262.

32. Sogos, *L'Impatto Sociale Dell'Aboro*; Augustín Puerta, *Feminismo*.

33. Real Decreto 2.409/1986, de 21 de Noviembre, sobre Centros Sanitarios Acreditados Dictámenes Perceptivos para la Práctica Legal de la Interrupción Voluntaria del Embarazo, reproduced in V. A. Arrufat Gallén and J. Ll. Carbonell i Esteve, *Análisis de la Demanda de Interrupción Voluntaria de Embarazo: Informe Técnico* (Valencia: Edicions Vicent Llorens, 1988).

34. Josune Aguinaga Roustan, *El Aborto en España: Datos para la Planificación de una Política Social* (Madrid: Instituto de la Mujer, 1985).

35. Rickie Solinger, ed., *Abortion Wars: A Half Century of Struggle* (Berkley: University of California Press, 1998), 49.

36. Solinger, ed., *Abortion Wars*; Reagan, *When Abortion Was a Crime*; Christabelle Sethna, "All Aboard: Canadian Women's Abortion Tourism, 1960–1980," in *Gender, Health, and Popular Culture: Historical Perspectives*, ed. Cheryl Lynn Krasnick Warsh (Waterloo, ON: Wilfrid Laurier University Press, 2011), 89–108.

37. Aguinaga Roustan, *El Aborto en España.*

38. Peiró et al., "Abortos Inducidos."

39. Christopher Tietze and Stanley K. Henshaw, *Induced Abortion: A World Review* (New York: Guttmacher Institute, 1986), 51–52.

40. Jean C. Robinson, "Gendering the Abortion Debate: The French Case," in *Abortion Politics, Women's Movements and the Democratic State*, ed. Dorothy McBride Stetson (Oxford: Oxford University Press), 87–110.

41. Mary Nash, *Dones en Transició: De la Resistència Política a la Legitimitat Feminista: les Dones en la Barcelona a la Transició* (Barcelona: Ayuntamiento de Barcelona, 2007), 203–23.

42. Feliciano Fidalgo, "Cerrada en Biarritz una Clínica donde las Españolas Iban a Abortar," *El País*, June 17, 1979, http://elpais.com/diario/1979/12/09 /ultima/313542005_850215.html.

43. José Ángel Lozoya Gómez, *Aborto: Historias de Combate y Resistencia* (Seville: Fundación Iniciativa Social, 2014), 216.

44. While in Britain and the Netherlands it was legal for nonresident women to obtain terminations, this was not the case for countries where residency requirements were in place (France) or restrictive abortion laws ruled out abortion on demand (Portugal and Morocco). This is why the abortions that Spanish women obtained in the latter three countries were still formally considered to be illegal abortions.

45. Leslie J. Reagan, "Crossing the Border for Abortions: California Activists, Mexican Clinics, and the Creation of a Feminist Health Agency in the 1960s," *Feminist Studies* 26, no. 2 (2000): 323–48; Christabelle Sethna and Marion Doull, "Accidental Tourists: Canadian Women, Abortion Tourism, and Travel," *Women's Studies* 41, no. 4 (2012): 457–75; Beth Palmer, "Lonely, Tragic but Legally Necessary Pilgrimages: Cross Border Travel for Abortions," in *Choices and Compromises: The Abortion Movement in Canada 1969–1988* (PhD diss., University of York, 2012), 143–94; Katrina Ackerman, "The 'Dark' and 'Well-Kept Secret': Abortion Experiences and Feminist Activism," in *A Region at Odds: Abortion Politics in the Maritime Provinces, 1969–1988* (PhD diss., University of Waterloo, 2015), 135–75; and Jennifer Nelson, "Thank You for Your Help . . . Six Children Are Enough: The Abortion Birth Control Referral Service," in *More Than Medicine: A History of the Feminist Women's Health Movement* (New York: New York University Press, 2015), 57–89.

46. Ismael Fuente Lafuente, "La Situación en España," *El País*, February 18, 1977, http://elpais.com/diario/1977/02/18/sociedad/225068423_850215.html.

47. Ana Ortas and Victor Peña, "Ganar la lotería de navidad en los 70," December 9, 2014, http://www.rtve.es/noticias/20081217/ganar-loteria-navidad -70/208330.shtml.

48. CMP, gynecologist, interview by Teresa Ortiz-Gómez, Madrid, July 14, 2010. See also Trini de León Sotelo, "España. El Aborto: Batalla en las Próximas Cortes," *Blanco y Negro*, May 18, 1977, 24–27; "Doscientos Mil Abortos en España Cada Año?," *Blanco y Negro*, September 21, 1974, 82–83.

49. Lozoya Gómez, *Aborto.*

50. Gil García, Ortiz-Gómez, and Ignaciuk, "El Movimiento de Planificación Familiar."

51. JC, gynecologist, interview by Eugenia Gil-García, Seville, January 15, 2010.

52. SR, gynecologist, interview by Eugenia Gil-García, Seville, December 15, 2009.

53. Ortiz-Gómez and Ignaciuk, "The Fight for Family Planning."

54. CMT, gynecologist, interview by Teresa Ortiz-Gómez, Madrid, April 13, 2010; CMP, interview.

55. Concepción Cifrián, Pilar Martínez Ten, and Isabel Serrano, *La Cuestión del Aborto* (Barcelona: Icaria, 1986).

56. Agata Ignaciuk, "An Underground Public Health Service? Abortion Travel Networks in Spain before 1985" (Paper presented at the European Association for the History of Medicine and Health conference, "The Body Politic: States in the History of Medicine and Health," Bucharest, September 1, 2017).

57. Ignaciuk, "An Underground Public Health Service?"

58. Teresa Ortiz-Gómez, "Conocer el Propio Cuerpo para Acabar con el Patriarcado: Publicaciones Feministas sobre Salud en España durante la Transición Democrática," in *Medicina y Poder Político: Actas del XVI Congreso de la Sociedad Española de Historia de la Medicina*, ed. Ricardo Campos Marín et al. (Madrid: Sociedad Española de Historia de la Medicina, 2014), 259–63.

59. Leonor Taboada, *Cuaderno Feminista, Introducción al Self-Help* (Barcelona: Fontanella, 1978).

60. Augustín Puerta, *Feminismo*.

61. De León Sotelo, "España."

62. GC, psychologist, interview by Agata Ignaciuk, July 24, 2017; Joaquín Abad, "A través del Centro Pablo Iglesias, se Aborta en Londres," *El Alcázar*, November 4, 1979, 21.

63. Handwritten statistics of abortions performed in the clinic, 1981–1983, personal archive of the doctor (identity preserved upon request).

64. "Costumbres: Las Extranjeras a Londres, donde el Aborto es Legal," *Blanco y Negro*, April 16, 1975, 65; Neliana Tresigni, "Abortar en Londres," *El País*, October 3, 1976, http://elpais.com/elpais/2011/11/24/actualidad /1322120268_850215.html; De León Sotelo, "España"; Abad, "A través del Centro"; Hernández Rodríguez, "El Aborto en España"; "Yo he Abortado Voluntariamente, Decían Mil Trescientas Mujeres," *El País*, October 10, 1979, https://elpais.com/diario/1979/10/20/espana/309222005_850215.html; Marisa, "Aquel Fin de Semana en Londres," *Dossier Dones en Lluita*, no. 21 (1983): 21; and Josefina Jiménez, nurse and feminist activist, interview by Agata Ignaciuk, Granada, July 13, 2017.

65. Luisa Fortes, "Algunos Consejos Útiles," *Dossier Dones en Lluita*, no. 21 (1983): 33–34; and CN, scholar, interview by Agata Ignaciuk, Granada, August 13, 2017.

66. Amaia Pérez, physician, interview by Agata Ignaciuk, July 20, 2017; and "Abortar—Más fácil fuera de la Ley," *El Globo*, July 25, 1988. Reproduced in *Dossier de Prensa*, ed. Instituto de la Mujer (Madrid: Instituto de la Mujer, 1989).

67. "Abortar."

68. Consuelo Catalá, "Penalización y Despenalización Parcial del Aborto: Situación Actual de la I.V.E en el Estado Español y el Caso de Nicaragua: El

Derecho al Aborto en la Comunidad Valenciana y 30 Años del Feminismo," in *30 Anys de Feminisme al País Valenciá*, ed. Assemblea Jornades Feministes País Valenciá (Valencia: Gauda Impresores, 2007), 165–68.

69. Manuel Muñoz, "El Médico Valenciano Pedro Enguix Presentó los Nombres de Más de 2.700 Mujeres que Declaran Haber Abortado," *El País*, September 27, 1983, http://elpais.com/diario/1983/09/27/sociedad/433465204 _850215.html; Manuel Muñoz, "Tribunales: El Ginecólogo Pedro Enguix, Encarcelado por Practicar Abortos, Sale en Libertad Provisional," *El País*, November 18, 1983, http://elpais.com/diario/1983/11/18/sociedad/437958002 _850215.html; Manuel Muñoz, "El Doctor Enguix Dirigirá unas Jornadas para Promover la Erradicación del Aborto," *El País*, April 29, 1985, http://elpais.com /diario/1985/04/29/sociedad/483573604_850215.html; Fluvia Nicolás, "Pedro Enguix Afirma que el Colectivo Médico que Dirige Ha Seguido Practicando Abortos," *El País*, March 2, 1985, http://elpais.com/diario/1985/03/02/sociedad /478566004_850215.html.

70. Lozoya Gómez, *El Aborto: Historias de Combate*; Francoise, abortion practitioner, interview by Agata Ignaciuk and Teresa Ortiz-Gómez, Alicante, July 5, 2017.

71. Lozoya Gómez, *El Aborto*.

72. Lozoya Gómez, *El Aborto*.

73. Lozoya Gómez, *El Aborto*.

74. Laura Kaplan, *The Story of Jane: The Legendary Underground Feminist Abortion Service* (Chicago: University of Chicago Press, 1997).

75. José Ángel Lozoya Gómez, educator and activist, cofounder of Los Naranjos, interview by Eugenia Gil García, Seville, January 11, 2010; FH, activist who worked for Los Naranjos, interview by Eugenia Gil García, Seville, January 17, 2010.

76. Consuelo Catalá, nurse, politician, and feminist activist, interview by Agata Ignaciuk and Teresa Ortiz-Gómez, Alicante, July 5, 2017; SCA, administrative worker, interview by Agata Ignaciuk, August 18, 2017.

77. "Los Naranjos—Instrucción," handwritten statistics from the clinic, personal archive of José Ángel Lozoya Gómez.

78. Lozoya Gómez, *El Aborto*.

79. Rickie Solinger, "Pregnancy and Power before *Roe v. Wade*, 1950–1970," in *Abortion Wars*, 15–32.

80. Rickie Solinger, *The Abortionist: A Woman against the Law* (Berkeley: University of California Press, 1994).

81. Ibáñez y García Velasco, *La Despenalización*.

[10]

"The Import Problem"

The Travels of *Our Bodies, Ourselves* to Eastern Europe

ANNA BOGIC

CROSSING BORDERS in search of abortion services is sometimes re-ferred to as "abortion tourism."[1] However, the notion that women "travel" and that their experiences can be described as "tourism" can be interpreted as unfortunate euphemisms, since their search for abortion services is often fraught with anxiety, shame, financial burdens, and even danger.[2] While women from the United States of America (USA) have in the past crossed state and international borders, including traveling to communist Eastern Europe during the Cold War in the hope of finding safe and legal abortion services,[3] they have also organized widely in the name of abortion legalization. During the late 1960s and early 1970s, American women wrote countless books and pamphlets that contributed to the formulation of a decidedly pro-choice position. One of the best-known examples of an American feminist pro-choice text is *Our Bodies, Ourselves* (*OBOS*) (1971), written by the Boston Women's Health Book Collective (hereafter the Boston collective) when abortion was still illegal in many regions of the USA.[4] *OBOS* is often featured in studies of the American women's health movement and the landmark struggle for abortion legalization in 1973.[5] *OBOS* has also traveled to other parts of the world as an important source of pro-choice discourse and women's empowerment within the context of women's reproductive rights.

This chapter examines one case of the travel of *OBOS*: the Serbian translation of *OBOS*, *Naša tela, mi* (*NTM*), published in the former Yugoslav republic of Serbia in 2001, some 30 years after the first publication of the American version in 1971.[6] Women in socialist Yugoslavia enjoyed liberal abortion laws during the Cold War period (1945–1989), and American women at times traveled there in the hope of terminating unwanted pregnancies and escaping restrictive abortion laws in the USA. This legal situation took an abrupt turn in the 1990s, during the violent disintegration of Yugoslavia. For the first time, Yugoslav women had to organize in opposition to the governments' attempts to restrict abortion laws.[7] During the period of socialism, women's position was unique as they did not need to struggle for those basic rights for which women in Western Europe had to fight for years, such as the right to abortion, divorce, maternity leave, property rights, and employment. The "only" issue that remained for women in socialist countries to tackle was to ensure the actual realization of these rights.[8] But in the turbulent 1990s, after the fall of several communist regimes, women in Serbia (one of Yugoslavia's successor states), and elsewhere in Eastern Europe, began to organize against the anti-feminist policies of newly established democratic governments. This time, instead of traveling to Yugoslavia for abortion services, women from the USA traveled to the fractured region, copies of *OBOS* in their hands, in order to support Yugoslav feminists in their fight for reproductive rights. Simultaneously, in the USA, women witnessed a renewed series of attacks against their own reproductive rights, including hundreds of state laws restricting abortion access, as well as violence directed against abortion doctors and clinics.[9] The 1992 edition of *OBOS* that American women brought with them contained a pro-choice discourse shaped by these battles on the home front.

In what follows, I briefly describe the origins of the Boston collective and its *OBOS* project, followed by a discussion of the American abortion laws and their impact on women's travel for abortion services. I draw a comparison of liberal abortion laws in Eastern Europe during the Cold War, focusing specifically on socialist Yugoslavia (and, later, Serbia), a country with a communist regime but with an open cross-border travel policy, unlike the rest of Eastern Europe under socialism.[10] The role of the American feminists' travel to the disintegrating Yugoslavia in the 1990s and the women's influence in spreading a pro-choice discourse by bringing copies of *OBOS* to local feminist groups for translation and further distribution is examined in the last section. The chapter concludes with a look at the intertwined travels of women and *OBOS* to the Yugoslav region in their efforts to strengthen the resistance to the clamping down on one of the most controversial areas of women's reproductive rights.

OBOS and the Boston Collective

The beginnings of the Boston collective can be traced back to the late 1960s and specifically to a conference held in May 1969 at Emmanuel College in Boston.[11] The gathering, titled "Female Liberation Conference," attracted hundreds of women who were willing to question power structures in an American society already shaken by civil rights battles, anti-war protests, and new social protest movements emerging out of the New Left.[12] The conference workshop on reproductive health brought together a group of women, many of whom would eventually become founding members of the Boston collective and embark on a decades-long collaboration. Workshop papers from the conference were further researched and developed, and subsequently turned into a women's health course text that became the feminist classic *OBOS*.[13] The first edition came out one year after the conference and was a product of intense feminist activism, research, and consciousness-raising meetings.

It is from such consciousness-raising meetings that the now-famous second-wave feminist slogan "The personal is political" arose.[14] No longer isolated from one another or thinking that their seemingly unique experiences were just individual matters, many women came to the realization that their often troubling experiences were shared by many other women across the USA. By identifying their commonalities, women in such discussion groups were able to identify the link between individual experiences and the wider structures of oppression. This was that aha moment experienced in the 1970s, "the bread and butter of consciousness-raising."[15] One of the Boston collective's founders, Wendy Sanford, explains how her activism sprang from her experiences of postpartum depression and paternalistic treatment from her doctor, who admonished her not to "want too much" and continued: "This is what I like to tell my new mothers: get out to a library once in a while to keep your mind going and your spirits up, but be satisfied. You are raising a new generation. You are taking care of your husband when he comes home from a busy day."[16] Wondering how soon before sexual intercourse she should insert a diaphragm, Sanford's doctor advised further: "Dinner, dishes, diaphragm,"[17] a phrase that encapsulates the era's gender relations, as alluded to by Christabelle Sethna in her contribution to this volume. Women's personal accounts of their encounters with doctors suggest that such treatment was common at the time, but they also inadvertently provided a growing impetus for women to search for answers elsewhere, notably, from other women in consciousness-raising groups. The power of the slogan "The personal is political" came from the ability to name effectively the systems that shaped women's everyday lives.

OBOS provided information on women's anatomy, as well as on sexuality, lesbian relationships, masturbation, healthy relationships, violence against women, self-care and self-defense, contraception (including the controversial birth control pill), abortion, pregnancy, birth, and aging. Most importantly, OBOS adapted medical information and combined it with intimate first-person accounts. It also included photographs and drawings of real women's bodies, which gave women readers an essential and empowering knowledge base about topics that were usually treated as taboo, rarely discussed, and if discussed articulated in shameful terms. The text's message was highly political, and it addressed its readers with a voice that called upon women to join the feminist movement.

Importantly, OBOS provided an entire chapter dedicated to the abortion procedure together with its political, medical, and legal implications. In the section on illegal abortion, quite common before 1973 in most of the USA,[18] the Boston collective provided invaluable information for its female readers, illustrating just what was at stake for women seeking abortions at the time: "It is important for a woman to know the whole range of abortion methods, so that she will know what she is talking about with her doctor, and more important, so she can judge the methods of an illegal abortionist and find the courage to walk out if her life is in danger (Don't pay in advance if you can help it.)."[19] OBOS's strong pro-choice message reflected the political ambiance of the time and contributed to the consciousness-raising of thousands of women, many of whom were engaged in the battle for the legalization of abortion. Significantly, Sarah Weddington, the lawyer for Jane Roe, credits OBOS for having shaped her own awareness of women's reproductive health issues. Weddington's efforts on behalf of her client resulted in the landmark 1973 Roe v. Wade decision, in which the United States Supreme Court legalized abortion. Weddington would later acknowledge that when she was a young law student, she and her boyfriend left their home in Austin, Texas, and crossed the border for an abortion in a nearby Mexican town.[20] Such journeys, notes Lori A. Brown in this volume, were made by many American women, although abortion was technically illegal in both the USA and Mexico at the time. She holds that the Texas state legislature's multipronged attacks on abortion services have resulted in pre–*Roe v. Wade* conditions for women.

The impact of *OBOS* was immediate, and soon it became highly influential, given the treatment of American women's bodies and their sexual and reproductive needs. Before its appearance, there was "virtually no open discussion of sex and reproduction in schools or the popular media, and physicians condescended to women and regularly withheld medical information from their female patients."[21] Growing interest in the women's health course developed by the Boston collective led to large sales of *OBOS*. It became a great "underground success" and sold more than 200,000 copies in the first few months, mostly through newly established women's centers and by word of mouth.[22] When the demand for *OBOS* became too overwhelming for the publisher (the New England Free Press) to manage, the Boston collective's members struck a contract with a commercial publisher, Simon and Schuster, in 1972. This somewhat controversial transfer from a leftist movement publisher to a capitalist, commercial publishing house was debated among the collective members, but in the end, the need to reach as many women across the USA as possible prevailed.[23]

Despite attempts to censor *OBOS*,[24] it remained widely available and became what Byllye Avery calls "the bible for women's health."[25] As a powerful feminist manifesto, *OBOS* contributed to the transformation of doctor-patient relationships as increasing numbers of women educated themselves by participating in a growing women's health movement. Women not only demanded better treatment from doctors, but some doctors also started to use *OBOS* in their practice.[26] Referring to the importance of *OBOS*, Sheryl Ruzek suggests: "Historians often ponder how books change history. *Our Bodies, Ourselves*, the enormously popular and influential work, will long be studied for igniting and sustaining a worldwide women's health movement."[27] In her work on the women's health movement in the USA, Sandra Morgen argues: "It would be difficult to exaggerate the impact of *Our Bodies, Ourselves*. . . . Erupting into the void (there were few popular books about women's health before it), *Our Bodies, Ourselves* created its own niche."[28]

Nine editions of *OBOS* have been published since its debut (1971, 1973, 1976, 1979, 1984, 1992, 1998, 2005, and 2011). The content has evolved in step with various feminist communities and feminist ideas. New concepts and perspectives have been added over time, such as reproductive justice principles and experiences of transgender individuals. The tone of the text has also been transformed, following changes to terminology and the retreat of the radical feminism so emblematic of the late 1960s and 1970s in the USA. Since 1971, *OBOS* has sold more than 4.5 million copies and has entered American popular culture through television, films, and books. Throughout its nine editions, the Boston collective remained committed to feminist activism and the women's health movement but also to a highly collaborative process of knowledge production. Each edition is a product of research and collaboration between dozens and even hundreds of contributors; for example, the 2011 edition includes contributions by more than 500 people.

As soon as *OBOS* reached mass domestic readership, translations and adaptations began to appear. Today, there are more than 30, in addition to about a dozen new translation and adaptation projects currently in preparation.[29] Ranging from direct translations to cultural adaptations and "inspired adaptations," *OBOS* was taken up by publishers, feminist activist groups, and women's health organizations,[30] a point reinforced in this volume by Agata Ignaciuk's assessment of the influence of *OBOS* on the Spanish scene in the 1970s. In this way, American feminist, pro-choice messages and women's personal narratives, as Kathy Davis has argued, traveled around the world, including to Eastern European countries, where they were adapted within a postcommunist context of the retraditionalization of women's roles.[31] In order to understand fully the pro-choice discourse in *OBOS* and its capacity to travel internationally, it is important to trace its roots within the history of American abortion laws and, specifically, to situate it within the context of the *Roe v. Wade* decision.

Abortion Laws in the USA before and after *Roe v. Wade*

The first statutes regulating abortion appeared in the 1820s and 1830s in the form of poison-control laws, banning the sale of commercial abortifacients.[32] By the end of the nineteenth century, abortion was criminalized state by state across the USA, following a vigorous physician-led campaign to criminalize it. As Leslie J. Reagan explains, the campaign of the American Medical Association (AMA) to criminalize abortion had much to do with power struggles between physicians, midwives, and homeopaths for the control over medical practices including abortion. Reagan raises an important point: while doctors were behind the criminalization of abortion in the late nineteenth century, they were also the main providers of abortion. Many of them continued to operate while charging considerable fees.[33] While the AMA had been behind the anti-abortion campaigns, it fought not only women who sought out abortions but also physicians who continued to provide them either out of sympathy for the women or because of financial motives. The law, however, allowed for the shaming and humiliating of women caught in police raids on abortion clinics: "Public exposure of a woman's abortion—through the press or gossip—served to punish women who had abortions, as well as their family members."[34] In the politically repressive decade of the 1950s, even these underground abortions became difficult to obtain, and the rate of botched operations from illegal practitioners and unsuccessful attempts at self-abortion increased, building and leading in the end to the feminist campaigns for abortion legalization of the late 1960s and early 1970s.[35] At the same time, women of color brought much-needed attention to sterilization abuses that saw thousands of them sterilized against their will in the 1940s and 1950s, and advocated for the "need to combine their opposition to sterilization abuse with solid support for safe, legal abortion and birth control.[36]

The movement for abortion law reform gathered strength in this period thanks to a growing number of women's groups, civil liberties, and population groups, as well as some church groups. As a result of these pressures, the first states (Alaska, Hawaii, and Washington) reformed their abortion laws in 1970, allowing for abortion on request, with residency requirements, for women whose pregnancy was less than 24 weeks. In the same year, the state of New York also repealed its abortion law, removing the residency requirement. The newly reformed abortion laws were modeled after the proposal made by the liberal American Law Institute, whose guidelines allowed abortion in the following cases: in the case of rape or incest, if the woman had rubella (German measles), if she were younger than 15 years of age, or if her health were seriously endangered by the pregnancy.[37] Feminists, however, insisted that even these reformed abortion laws continued to humiliate women by forcing them to provide a reason for requesting an abortion; it was a degrading procedure that also suggested that only certain women "deserved" an abortion.[38] In the present volume, Cathrine Chambers, Colleen MacQuarrie, and Jo-Ann MacDonald observe that Canadian feminist groups raised similar objections to the establishment of hospital-based Therapeutic Abortion Committees. These committees had the power to approve or deny women's requests for legal abortions and were considered demeaning to women seeking abortion services.

Roe v. Wade legalized abortion for American women during the first trimester, allowing for the possibility of increasing restrictions in the following two trimesters. The Supreme Court "invalidated all state laws limiting women's access to abortions during the first trimester of pregnancy . . . and associated the right to abortion with the privacy right named in *Griswold v. Connecticut*."[39] Although a series of subsequent judicial rulings and legislation altered negatively the rights created by *Roe v. Wade*, the court case remains a judicial landmark.[40]

Abortion Travel before *Roe v. Wade*

Before *Roe v. Wade*, the state of New York was the overwhelming destination for women wishing to terminate their pregnancies, indicating, as do several chapters in this volume, the significance of domestic travel for abortion services, particularly when countries or regions are geographically vast. As mentioned previously, in 1970, this state had struck down its anti-abortion statute, together with the states of Alaska, Hawaii, Washington, and the District of Columbia.[41] However, New York was the only state that did not require women to reside there at least 30 days before the operation. Consequently, in 1972, the year before abortion legalization in the USA, some 100,000 women had traveled from states such as Michigan, Pennsylvania, and Illinois to New York for abortion services.[42] In fact, some 50,000 women were willing to travel more than 500 miles (or 800 kilometers), or even 1,000 or 2,000 miles from across the USA, to obtain a legal abortion in New York City.[43] The lack of residency requirements in the 1967 British Abortion Act spurred travel for abortion services to Britain and is explored in more detail in this volume by Christabelle Sethna and also by Agata Ignaciuk. Before the legalization in New York in 1970, American women, but also Canadian women, who had the financial means traveled to

Britain for abortion services following the passage of the 1967 Abortion Act.[44] The Guttmacher Institute reported that in the last three months of 1969 alone, more than 600 American women had made the trip to Britain for the services,[45] and by 1970, "package deals (including round-trip airfare, passports, vaccination, transportation to and from the airport and lodging and meals for four days, in addition to the procedure itself) were advertised in the popular media."[46] From the 1970s onward, thousands of Canadian women from the province of Ontario made the trip to New York for abortion services every year,[47] signaling once more in this volume the important role neighboring regions play in terms of abortion provision.

The 1973 edition of *OBOS* reported to its American readers that abortion was legal and available on demand "in communist Russia and the Eastern Bloc countries" since the 1950s, in a tone that suggested that in these countries women's reproductive rights were more progressive than in the USA.[48] Likewise, another very popular source on reproductive health, the *Birth Control Handbook*, published in 1968 by a group of McGill University students in Montreal, Quebec, informed its readers that communist countries such as "Poland, Cuba, and China appeared more enlightened because they were the only regimes to permit abortion on demand."[49] In this way, these texts pitted the "backward" USA against its ideological enemies by showing the latter as more advanced in regard to the status of women. Moreover, in 1972, an in-depth report on Eastern Europe's so-called abortion culture was published in a widely read newspaper, the *Washington Post*.[50] The American journalist Dan Morgan investigated the effects of communist countries' liberal abortion laws on abortion rates, state population policies, family formation, and local attitudes toward abortion, family, and work. Importantly, Morgan discovered that by and large abortion was not viewed as a moral issue ("The moral discussion ended in the 1950s," he writes) but also that communist Eastern European countries, and in particular Yugoslavia, had become destinations or "potential havens" for American and Western European women seeking abortions. In one section of the article titled "The Import Problem," Morgan observed with a sense of irony that while Eastern Europeans may be migrating to the West in search of jobs, "the flow is the other way around for abortions."[51]

Ewelina Ciaputa in this volume shows that at certain points in time Poland was, like Yugoslavia, an appealing destination for women from abroad who sought abortion services. Although the Yugoslav government forbade foreign nationals from accessing abortion on demand, the country had a policy of unrestricted travel and open borders. Legal hurdles were overcome "through connections." Some family doctors in Yugoslavia were willing to issue the necessary certifications of pregnancy for local hospitals.[52] A number of Yugoslav feminist activists and scholars engaged in feminist debates at the time remember visiting American women in search of abortion services for unintended pregnancies.[53] While such evidence is anecdotal and scarcely recorded because of the gray areas of Yugoslav bureaucratic procedures, Morgan's article and the recollections of these Yugoslav feminists suggest that a certain kind of abortion tourism flowed in the direction of Eastern Europe, especially in the 1970s.

In particular, Belgrade, then the capital city of Yugoslavia, offered a wide range of gynecological clinics where every day, dozens of women of all ages and marital status gathered for the purpose of obtaining a legal abortion. Morgan writes, "for most city women living under communism, an abortion carries about as much social stigma as a visit to the hairdresser."[54] Writing for the *Washington Post* and, therefore, for the American audience during the Cold War and in the months leading to the *Roe v. Wade* decision, Morgan was certain to arouse interest. Undoubtedly, his reportage also contributed to the popular Western image of communists as godless people for whom abortion did not warrant any moral discussion. However, comparing abortion to a mere haircut is not supported by research, which shows that even though abortion, together with coitus interruptus, were the most preferred methods of birth control among Yugoslav women, a certain amount of stigma was always associated with abortion.[55] Despite the availability of contraceptives, rates of abortion remained high. The birth control pill, or, more accurately, the oral contraceptive pill, was made available in Yugoslavia in 1964 and the intrauterine device (IUD) in 1967; both were available in pharmacies, particularly in the cities.[56] Nevertheless, women did not use them widely because these medical methods were seen as disruptive to sexual relationships between men and women. Only 20 percent of women in Belgrade used contraceptives in the late 1960s and early 1970s.[57] Abortion was, and continues to be, treated as a taboo topic even among women, and is rarely spoken of publicly and openly; this silence suggests that there remains something shameful about the procedure.[58] Although abortion was largely accessible and had "become a part of a woman's life and accepted as such," it nevertheless carried its own stigma, even in countries such as Yugoslavia, with its liberal abortion policies.[59]

Abortion Laws in Socialist Yugoslavia

According to Lena Lennerhed in this volume, Sherri Finkbine's 1962 flight from the USA to Sweden for a legal abortion spotlighted Sweden's abortion laws and clinical practices, and generated enormous national and global publicity. Yet it was communist and socialist countries that were among the first in the world to liberalize abortion. In fact, data about abortion techniques and abortion safety in Eastern European countries bolstered the Abortion Law Reform Association's campaign for abortion law reform in Britain, as is argued by Christabelle Sethna in this volume. The Soviet Union, which was a leader "in the liberalization of abortion legislation in 1920, restricted abortion in 1936, and then re-liberalized it in 1955, an action eventually followed by all the socialist countries of Central and Eastern Europe except Albania."[60] In the 1960s, declining fertility rates became a major concern in Eastern Europe. Due to these demographic concerns, socialist countries introduced a series of pronatalist programs starting in the mid-1960s and 1970s.[61] Hoping to increase fertility rates, many governments resorted to "positive incentives" for couples, such as paid maternity leave, unpaid leave with job guarantees, increased family allowances, birth payments, and housing, among others.[62] This pronatalist discourse was rooted in demographic concerns and did not go unnoticed at the time. During her tour of some of the communist countries in the late 1970s, American feminist scholar Sheila Tobias warned presciently of future struggles for women's reproductive rights in the countries she visited (Yugoslavia, Hungary, and Czechoslovakia): "I found motherhood considered everywhere as essential for every female. There is concern for underpopulation that bodes ill for abortion rights."[63]

Under the leadership of Josip Broz Tito, the Yugoslav government liberalized its abortion policy as early as 1952. The liberalization occurred within the context of rapid economic growth and a pressing need for women's labor in the workforce. After the end of World War II, the Yugoslav government enshrined women's equality in legislation, including policies such as voting rights, equal pay, access to education, maternity leave, childcare, abortion access, and political representation.[64]

However, the gap between Yugoslav laws and women's lived experiences was never completely removed. Gendered labor divisions persisted, and women continued to experience discrimination in all areas of life. In particular, women continued to shoulder the largest portion of responsibility for housework, reproductive labor, and domestic duties.[65] Reproduction, sexuality, and domestic violence were rarely discussed publicly and were generally treated as taboo topics.[66] Nevertheless, medical doctors urged the government to legalize abortion, given the detrimental health consequences of unsafe illegal abortions, which included infertility.[67] The progressive abortion law adopted in the 1950s had roots in the earlier efforts dating to the 1920s and 1930s, when the medical association of gynecologists called for the decriminalization of abortion and advocated for the removal of prison sentences for women who had undergone an abortion, in place since 1929.[68]

Following the widespread criminalization of abortion in the middle of the nineteenth century (when the Yugoslav regions were still scattered under the Austro-Hungarian and Ottoman Empires), the procedure became legally possible only for medical reasons—to save the woman's life—in 1929.[69] Under this law, both the woman and the individual performing the abortion could be prosecuted and imprisoned. However, in 1952, the socialist government adopted a new, elaborate law in which it specified more clearly the conditions under which an abortion committee comprising three doctors would approve the abortion request under medical, legal-ethical (rape, incest), and sociomedical conditions within the first three months of gestation.[70] This last condition essentially opened wide the door to abortion services: "owing to the broad and rather vague definition of the provision which also allowed the possibility of termination of pregnancy when childbirth could lead to deterioration of the woman's health due to her difficult financial, personal or family circumstances, the possibility was created, in practice, to perform abortions also in situations when the child was simply unwanted."[71]

Although the 1952 law introduced the sociomedical conditions and specified that the procedure must be performed only in hospitals, it did not prevent women whose abortion requests were rejected by the abortion committee from seeking illegal abortions elsewhere. Resolutions adopted by the government in 1960 and 1969 further liberalized the abortion law by clarifying the somewhat vague "sociomedical conditions" clause and by developing a position on the concept of "family planning."[72] In 1974, the Yugoslav constitution established family planning, including contraception, as a human right, and in accordance, in 1977 the local Serbian government (still part of the socialist Yugoslav federation) adopted a new abortion law containing a provision that guaranteed "the right of a woman to freely decide on childbearing."[73] There were no limitations on abortions and no abortion committees necessary in the first trimester, while the procedure was limited to 20 weeks of gestation except in cases of a threat to the woman's life or severe damage to her health.

The extent of abortion access in Yugoslavia in the 1970s can also be measured by the willingness of Yugoslav women living in Western European countries to return home for the procedure. In her survey of 258 Yugoslav female migrant workers living in France, West Germany, and Sweden in the late 1970s, Mirjana Morokvašić found that coitus interruptus and abortion were their most preferred methods of birth control.[74] The migrants she studied often traveled back home to Yugoslavia for abortion services. Morokvašić explains, "Coming from a country in which it is relatively easy to have an abortion and where it has become a part of a woman's life and accepted as such, Yugoslav migrants probably experience difficulty in getting an abortion in the new and very different social context. In Sweden for example, abortion is not viewed as an acceptable means of fertility control. It is only 'designed as a humanitarian measure to protect women's life and health.' . . . In France and Germany abortion was only legalized in 1975 and 1976 respectively."[75] Her study shows that rather than having an abortion in their country of residence, most of the women traveled back to Yugoslavia, even though this decision incurred financial cost and the risk of job loss. Moreover, the Yugoslav women's decision to return home reveals that despite the local feminist movements and their pressure for abortion legalization in France, Germany, and Sweden, these three Western European countries remained socially conservative in this regard, and abortion was still heavily interpreted through a moral lens.

However, the progressive trend in abortion legislation in Yugoslavia, and after its disintegration, its successor state, Serbia, was interrupted by the adoption of a more restrictive law on the termination of pregnancy in 1995.[76] This new law, which excluded the sociomedical conditions for women seeking abortion after the first trimester, followed in the footsteps of a series of increasingly restrictive abortion laws that were adopted by Eastern European democratic governments elected after the fall of communism in 1989.[77] This trend is mirrored by Poland's experience, as Ewelina Ciaputa shows convincingly in her contribution to this volume.

OBOS Travels to Serbia in the 1990s

The transition away from communism that gradually began in the 1980s and took an abrupt turn in 1989 with the first democratic elections in decades had a dramatic impact on the standard of living in Eastern European countries. Although this supposed transition to democracy and a market economy was expected to expand human rights, it also significantly eroded women's rights in all areas of women's lives, including reproductive rights.[78] Abortion was targeted early on. Writing in 2000, Susan Gal and Gail Kligman were compelled to ask: "Why was abortion among the first issues raised, after 1989, by virtually all the newly constituted governments of East Central Europe?"[79] Romania, after Nicolae Ceauşescu's draconian dictatorship, and Bulgaria initially liberalized their abortion laws after decades of a total ban (Romania) and serious restrictions (Bulgaria). However, as Adriana Băban reports: "Nationalists and demographers blame the declining birthrate on unrestricted access to abortion," resulting in the resurgence of public debates on limiting women's abortion access.[80]

The breakup of Yugoslavia, and its division into five independent republics—Slovenia, Croatia, Bosnia and Herzegovina, Macedonia, and the "new" Yugoslavia consisting of Serbia and Montenegro—was accompanied by a series of wars and brutal violence in the 1990s.[81] Amid the chaos of the armed conflicts and displacement of more than two million people, the governments of the succession republics still found it necessary to threaten women's access to abortion services.[82] Attempts to restrict women's reproductive rights were closely linked to pronatalist discourses sparked by the fears of a "dying nation" and to low fertility rates prevalent in the former Yugoslav republics, which declined further during the war. They were also tied to governments' unwillingness to deal with the growing numbers of women refugees who had become pregnant as a result of wartime rape.[83]

Examples of pro-choice feminist activism in national and international arenas are a prominent feature of many chapters in this volume. In the Serbian example, as a response to the wars, the attack on women's reproductive rights, and, particularly, to the sexual violence targeting women, a transnational feminist network developed, offering all forms of assistance in the name of feminist solidarity.[84] American feminist activists and scholars traveled to the Yugoslav region, in addition to many other groups and individuals coming from Germany, Sweden, Austria, the UK, France, and Switzerland, among others. In Serbia and the rest of the Yugoslav region, autonomous feminist groups flourished, thanks to two simultaneous but contradictory conditions: increasing opportunities for women's autonomous organizing (but also rollbacks of women's rights under new governments democratically elected after 1989) and increasing privatization.[85] Although American women's abortion access in the 1990s was also under threat in the USA through a series of legal challenges and right-wing fundamentalist assaults on abortion clinics,[86] American feminists traveled to the Yugoslav region, including to the city of Belgrade, Serbia, bringing with them material and financial support in a strong show of solidarity.

American feminists also brought heaps of books, most notably English-language feminist classics on the topics of women's human rights, violence against women, and feminist theory, which helped local feminists build their own libraries and documentation centers. In Belgrade, American feminists brought copies of the 1992 *OBOS* in the belief that such a text could contribute to women's consciousness-raising, especially in the area of women's reproductive rights.[87] In the introduction to their politically framed chapter on abortion, the Boston collective wrote: "Women have always used abortion as a means of fertility control. Unless we ourselves can decide whether and when to have children, it is difficult for us to control our lives or participate fully in society. Legal, safe and affordable abortions help to give us that control."[88] But in addition to this introduction to the abortion chapter, which dates back to the early 1970s, the 1992 edition informed its readers of the growing backlash against the legalization of abortion in the USA: "[In] the current political situation our right to legal abortions is in serious danger."[89] In the chilling political climate of the 1990s, American feminists faced backlash against abortion by the state as well as by anti-abortion groups that engaged increasingly in violence against abortion providers. Although separated by different political contexts, the Belgrade feminists also encountered a clamping down on women's reproductive rights. A feminist organization, the Autonomous Women's Center (AWC), located in Belgrade, eventually adapted the 1992 English-language version of *OBOS* for local women, publishing it in Serbian as

Naša tela, mi (NTM) in 2001. But first, a short, translated excerpt from *OBOS* appeared in 1994 in their yearly publication *Feminističke sveske* (*Feminist Notebooks*). In that same year, the Belgrade feminists fought against the new Serbian government's attempt to limit women's access to abortion.

The Belgrade feminists' interest in *OBOS* needs to be understood within the context of sexual violence against women in the 1990s as Yugoslavia split apart. It also reflected a larger shift in translation trends that occurred in that decade. While the Yugoslav feminism of the 1980s inspired translations into Serbo-Croatian[90] and other languages spoken in Yugoslavia of feminist theory on Marxism, psychoanalysis, and lesbianism written in English, French, and Italian, this trend was interrupted in the 1990s when translations of texts on violence against women became more urgent. Feminist activists working at the AWC were motivated to translate *OBOS* into Serbian as they hoped to contribute to women's sense of empowerment. In the specific Serbian context, this meant resisting dominant wartime patriarchal discourses of nation building and those discourses justifying and legitimating violence against women. A group of about 16 women from Belgrade was formed around the topic of women's health with the objective of raising women's awareness about their bodies and their reproductive rights. This gathering of women echoed in many ways the beginnings of *OBOS* in Boston in the late 1960s and early 1970s, when American women formed their consciousness-raising groups and organized for the purpose of improving their rights and health.

NTM was the first textual project that addressed taboo topics such as women's sexuality, reproduction, and violence against women through an avowedly feminist lens pertinent to women in Serbia. It did so in defiance of the traditional patriarchal customs according to which women are discouraged from knowing about their bodies and from sharing this knowledge with other women and girls, and at the same time as the state continued to regulate such vital issues as abortion access and population policies in the 1990s. *NTM* offered women a tool with which they could learn about their reproductive rights and break the silence around taboo topics such as abortion. The resulting 23-page chapter on abortion in *NTM* was by far the most elaborate source of information on pregnancy termination then available to Serbian women. The chapter provided very detailed information about the abortion procedure and the different medical techniques used. It also framed abortion as a reproductive right and as an important choice for women. Women's feelings of guilt after having an abortion were acknowledged but so too were social pressures, such as compulsory motherhood and the devaluation of women's lives over that of the fetus. These were analyzed with an eye to opponents of abortion.

Given the context of increasing intolerance toward women's rights, the publication of the translation was timely. In the late 1980s and throughout the 1990s, women's reproductive behavior and their liberal access to abortion were criticized and frequently described as "immoral" and "unnatural."[91] In literature and newspapers, a number of male intellectuals in Serbia laid the blame on the socialist government's promotion of women's emancipation, and particularly on women who were understood to reject their prescribed gender role.[92] Ewelina Ciaputa, in her contribution to this volume, argues that Polish women who insist on reproductive rights are understood as influenced by Western values that betray the Polish nation. Similarly, in refusing to have many children by resorting to birth control and abortion, Serbian women have been seen as morally corrupt, paradoxically by socialist feminism *and* capitalist consumerism, the latter a reference to Western values that were said to pose a threat to the stability of the Serbian nation.[93]

The Serbian government's adoption of the 1995 law sent the message to women that the state was growing less tolerant of women's autonomous reproductive decision making and that their bodies were to be subjected to greater state scrutiny. A detailed analysis of this abortion law and the debate leading up to it illustrates how ideological shifts produce material consequences for women and their reproductive rights.[94] The debate on abortion began with a 1993 draft bill to ban abortion completely in the neighboring Republika Srpska, a newly formed, mainly Serb-populated entity in Bosnia, politically very close to Serbia, and then continued with a discussion about a separate, less draconian but also restrictive, abortion draft bill in Serbia in 1994. In May 1994, the government under president Slobodan Milošević scrapped the 1994 draft bill, deemed too restrictive, but then introduced a new abortion bill. This new bill maintained women's access to abortion services until the tenth week of gestation, available upon request, but restricted access past this time period, allowing for only a few medical reasons. It effectively removed the sociomedical conditions under which abortions could be accessed in the past.[95] Additionally, this draft of the bill did not recognize pregnancy as a result of rape as a legitimate reason for abortion past the tenth week of gestation.[96] The debate that ensued in the parliament revealed that abortion, together with its wide availability, was seen as the primary cause of Serbian women's low fertility rates, thereby endangering national survival.

The contributions of Mary Gilmartin and Sinéad Kennedy; Ewelina Ciaputa; and Cathrine Chambers, Colleen MacQuarrie and Jo-Ann MacDonald to this volume demonstrate how Irish, Polish, and Canadian feminists, respectively, have resisted government's attempts to curtail access to legal abortion. Similarly, Serbian feminist groups organized protests, demanded amendments, circulated a petition, and wrote in newspaper editorials.[97] A group of activists demonstrated on March 18, 1993, in Belgrade with overtly political slogans that accused the Serbian Orthodox Church and the "fascist" state of curtailing women's fundamental rights. Their banners read: "Less church, more condoms," "Free abortion: A condition of democracy," and "We will not be birth machines for the church, state, and the nation."[98] The activists' point of view was largely ignored, including their demand for amendments. However, one amendment that was eventually successful allowed for rape as a legitimate reason for access to abortion. Despite the opposition expressed by feminist groups, opposition parties, and some medical experts, a new version of the abortion draft bill was passed in parliament in December 1994 and officially became law in May 1995.[99]

This new abortion law was restrictive when compared to the previous socialist abortion law, but it mainly targeted abortion requests past the tenth week of gestation. Since most abortions were performed before the tenth week of gestation (98 percent), only a small number would be affected by the new law (2 percent). However, given that 95 percent of requests for abortion after the tenth week were based on sociomedical conditions, the new law did represent a significant abridgement of women's reproductive rights.[100] After a close study of the legal changes to the abortion law, Slobodanka Konstantinović-Vilić and Nevena Petrušić concluded that the new law imposed great limitations on women's ability to decide freely about childbirth. In their final analysis, they state: "It is obvious that by denying the right to abortion, which means denying the woman the right to control her own body, women are being sent the message that their bodies do not belong to them, but to some collective entity, which is usually identified with the nation.[101] As documented by Konstantinović-Vilić and Petrušić, the percentage of women denied access to abortion may be small, but the consequences of this denial of abortion services and forced carrying to term of unwanted pregnancies are of tremendous significance and devastating for women's lives.[102]

Conclusion

Given the rollback of women's reproductive rights in Serbia in the 1990s, the Belgrade feminists' translation of *OBOS* was seen as an important "feminist alphabet."[103] However, in this travel of the *OBOS* pro-choice discourse, a certain contradiction developed. Women in Yugoslavia had had access to legal abortion for decades, placing them somewhat ahead of American women in this respect. The pro-choice discourse in the 1992 version of *OBOS* was closely intertwined with the feminist battles for abortion in the USA. Since Yugoslav women did not have to fight for the legalization of abortion, they did not necessarily connect to this pro-choice discourse. However, with the changes in the politics of reproduction, the 1990s brought a clamping down on women's reproductive rights in Serbia with the new, restrictive 1995 abortion law, ironically making the *OBOS* pro-choice discourse in the translation highly relevant to women in Serbia. Indeed, the *OBOS* philosophy and consciousness-raising principles became essential tools for the activists.

American women were among those many activists who traveled to the Yugoslav region, including Belgrade, and who held the belief that the sharing of knowledge and expertise was key to strengthening the local feminist movement in its activism and opposition to the government.[104] Rather than traveling to Yugoslavia for abortion access, this time around American women were traveling because of their desire to show solidarity with women who were fighting for their reproductive rights, all the while socially conservative groups and politicians in the USA threatened American women's access to abortion.

Both the American and Yugoslav, and later Serbian, histories of abortion law testify to the ephemeral state of women's reproductive rights. The waxing and waning of state repression in the arena of women's health has over the decades forced women to seek solutions to unintended pregnancies elsewhere, that is, to travel across state and international borders, leading to the phenomenon of abortion tourism. Ironically, American women traveled to communist countries such as Yugoslavia during the Cold War, when communist regimes were depicted as dark enemies of the so-called free world, where women were supposedly to lead lives of liberty. Yugoslav migrant workers also chose to return to Yugoslavia for the abortion procedure even when they lived and worked in France, Germany, and Sweden—Western European countries with robust autonomous feminist movements. In contrast to these countries, in the communist countries of Eastern Europe, the state was the agent behind liberal abortion access.

In their fight for abortion legalization, American women produced an empowering pro-choice discourse that became the driving force behind the women's health movement in the USA. *OBOS*, as a direct result of this feminist activism, figured as a textual legacy, and as such it has traveled to more than 30 countries in the form of translations and cultural adaptations. In the case of the Serbian translation, *OBOS* served as a key feminist source on women's health at an extremely uncertain moment in Serbia's history, which produced both an ideological and physical assault on women's bodies, rights, and health. Lastly, women's travels, either in search of abortion or in support of other women's battle for reproductive rights, continue to build a transnational feminist network of solidarity as the future of women's reproductive rights remains uncertain.

Notes

1. Dan Morgan, "East Europe's Abortion Culture," *Washington Post*, July 9, 1972, B1, B4, refers to the "import problem." For more information about "abortion tourism," see Christabelle Sethna and Marion Doull, "Accidental Tourists: Canadian Women, Abortion Tourism, and Travel," *Women's Studies* 41, no. 4 (2012): 457–75.

2. Christabelle Sethna, "All Aboard? Canadian Women's Abortion Tourism, 1960–1980," in *Gender, Health, and Popular Culture: Historical Perspectives*, ed. Cheryl Krasnick Warsh (Waterloo, ON: Wilfrid Laurier University Press, 2011), 89–108.

3. Ted Joyce, Ruoding Tan, and Yuxiu Zhang, "Abortion Before and After *Roe*," *Journal of Health Economics* 32, no. 5 (2013): 804–15.

4. Abortion was legalized at the federal level in the USA in 1973, after the legal challenge of *Roe v. Wade*. A number of states (California, Colorado, Maryland, and New York, among others) had, however, already in 1969 and early 1970 reformed their laws to include more indications allowing for a "therapeutic abortion," making the procedure somewhat more accessible. The early editions of *OBOS* explain the abortion laws in detail. See Boston Women's Health Book Collective (BWHBC), *Our Bodies, Ourselves* (New York: Simon and Schuster, 1970, 1971, 1973, 1976); see also Leslie J. Reagan, *When Abortion Was a Crime: Women, Medicine, and the Law in the United States, 1867–1973* (Berkeley: University of California Press, 1997).

5. Sandra Morgen, *Into Our Own Hands: The Women's Health Movement in the United States, 1969–1990* (New Brunswick, NJ: Rutgers University Press,

2002); Sheryl Ruzek, "Transforming Doctor-Patient Relationships," *Journal of Health Services Research and Policy* 12 (2007): 181–82; Wendy Kline, *Bodies of Knowledge: Sexuality, Reproduction, and Women's Health in the Second Wave* (Chicago: University of Chicago Press, 2010).

6. Autonomni ženski centar, *Naša tela, mi* [*Our Bodies, Ourselves*] (Belgrade: Autonomni ženski centar, 2001).

7. See Vlasta Jalušič, "Women in Post-Socialist Slovenia: Socially Adapted, Politically Marginalized," in *Gender Politics in the Western Balkans: Women and Society in Yugoslavia and the Yugoslav Successor States*, ed. Sabrina Ramet (University Park, PA: Pennsylvania State University Press, 1999), 109–29, and Žarana Papić, "Women in Serbia: Post-Communism, War and Nationalist Mutations," in Ramet, *Gender Politics in the Western Balkans*, 153–69.

8. Rada Iveković, "Studije o ženi i ženski pokret" ["Women's Studies and Women's Movement"], *Marksizam u svetu* [*Marxism in the World*], nos. 8–9 (1981): 46–47.

9. Gloria Feldt, *The War on Choice: The Right-Wing Attack on Women's Rights and How to Fight Back* (New York: Bantam Books, 2004); Susan Faludi, *Backlash: The Undeclared War on American Women* (New York: Anchor Books, 1992).

10. Ana Dević, "Anti-War Initiatives and the Un-Making of Civic Identities in the Former Yugoslav Republics," *Journal of Historical Sociology* 10, no. 2 (1997): 143.

11. Kathy Davis, *The Making of "Our Bodies, Ourselves": How Feminism Travels across Borders* (Durham, NC: Duke University Press, 2007), 89; BWHBC, *Our Bodies, Ourselves* (1971), 3.

12. Todd Gitlin, *The Sixties: Years of Hope, Days of Rage* (Toronto: Bantam Books, 1987).

13. Between 1970 and 1971, the title changed from *Women and Their Bodies* to *Our Bodies, Ourselves*.

14. Davis, *The Making of "Our Bodies, Ourselves,"* 22.

15. Davis, *The Making of "Our Bodies, Ourselves,"* 91.

16. Joan Ditzion, Nancy Miriam Hawley, Paula Doress-Worters, and Wendy Sanford, "Formative Years: The Birth of *Our Bodies, Ourselves*" (Conference paper presented at "A Revolutionary Moment: Women's Liberation in the Late 1960s and Early 1970s," Boston University, March 27–29, 2014), https://www.bu.edu/wgs/files/2013/10/Ditzion-Formative-Years-The-Birth-of-Our-Bodies-Ourselves.pdf.

17. Ditzion et al., "Formative Years," 7.

18. For a detailed study of the prevalence of illegal abortion before 1974, see Reagan, *When Abortion Was a Crime*.

19. BWHBC, *Our Bodies, Ourselves* (1973), 148.

20. Sarah Weddington, *A Question of Choice* (New York: Feminist Press, 2013), 15–19. See also Rachel Cooke, "Sarah Weddington, Roe v. Wade Attorney, on Trump's Threat to Abortion Rights," *Guardian*, March 12, 2017, https://www.theguardian.com/world/2017/mar/12/sarah-weddington-roe-v-wade-lawyer-legalise-abortion-america-donald-trump.

21. Linda Gordon and Berrie Thorne, "Feminist Subversions: *Our Bodies, Ourselves*," in *Required Reading: Sociology's Most Influential Books*, ed. Dan Clawson (Amherst: University of Massachusetts Press, 1998), 182.

22. Wendy Coppedge Sanford, "Working Together, Growing Together: A Brief History of the Boston Women's Health Book Collective," *Heresies* 2, no. 3 (1979): 85.

23. Davis, *The Making of "Our Bodies, Ourselves."*

24. The Boston collective's archived documents housed at the Schlesinger Library at Harvard University contain dozens of news articles and letters documenting the attempts by conservative and religious groups to censor the book by removing it from public libraries and schools. Collections: BWHBC. MC503 and BWHBC. MC667.

25. Byllye Avery, "Preface to the 25th Anniversary Edition," in *Our Bodies, Ourselves,* ed. Boston Women's Health Book Collective (New York: Simon and Schuster, 1996), 8.

26. Morgen, *Into Our Own Hands,* 19.

27. Ruzek, "Transforming," 181.

28. Morgen, *Into Our Own Hands,* 19.

29. See the "OBOS Global Initiative," Our Bodies Ourselves, accessed October 18, 2017, http://www.ourbodiesourselves.org/global-projects/global-initiative/.

30. Davis, *The Making of "Our Bodies, Ourselves,"* 50–58.

31. Anna Bogic, "Translating into Democracy: The Politics of Translation, *Our Bodies, Ourselves,* and the 'Other Europe,'" in *Translating Women: Different Voices and New Horizons,* ed. Luise von Flotow and Farzanah Farahzad (New York: Routledge, 2016), 56–75. *OBOS* translations appeared in Serbia (2001), Bulgaria (2001), Moldova (2002), Poland (2004), Albania (2006), and Russia (2007). These translations are a product of converging factors, such as a volatile political climate, burgeoning feminist activism, and availability of foreign funding, among others.

32. Reagan, *When Abortion Was a Crime.*

33. Reagan, *When Abortion Was a Crime,* 72.

34. Reagan, *When Abortion Was a Crime,* 125.

35. Rosalyn Baxandall and Linda Gordon, eds., *Dear Sisters: Dispatches from the Women's Liberation Movement* (New York: Basic Books, 2000); Linda Gordon, *The Moral Property of Women: A History of Birth Control Politics in America* (Urbana: University of Illinois Press, 2002), 299.

36. Jennifer Nelson, *Women of Color and the Reproductive Rights Movement* (New York: New York University Press, 2003), 76.

37. BWHBC, *Our Bodies, Ourselves* (1973), 141.

38. BWHBC, *Our Bodies, Ourselves* (1973), 142.

39. Rickie Solinger, *Reproductive Politics: What Everyone Needs to Know* (New York: Oxford University Press, 2013), 28–29.

40. Solinger, *Reproductive Politics,* 31–33.

41. BWHBC, *Our Bodies, Ourselves* (1973), 144.

42. Rachel Benson Gold, "Lessons from before Roe: Will Past Be Prologue?," *Guttmacher Report* 6, no. 1 (March 2003), https://www.guttmacher.org/gpr/2003/03/lessons-roe-will-past-be-prologue; Joyce et al., "Abortion Before and After Roe."

43. Benson Gold, "Lessons from before Roe."

44. Christabelle Sethna, Beth Palmer, Katrina Ackerman, and Nancy Janovicek, "Choice, Interrupted: Travel and Inequality of Access to Abortion Services since the 1960s," *Labour/Le Travail* 71 (Spring 2013): 29–48.

45. Benson Gold, "Lessons from before Roe."

46. Benson Gold, "Lessons from before Roe."

47. Sethna, "All Aboard?," 96–97.

48. BWHBC, *Our Bodies, Ourselves* (1973), 141. Although there are some overlaps, Eastern Europe is not to be confused with the Eastern Bloc, which was an officially defined group of countries under direct Soviet influence: East Germany, Poland, Hungary, Czechoslovakia, Bulgaria, and Romania. Yugoslavia was considered to be part of Eastern Europe but not an Eastern Bloc member country. Under the leadership of Josip Broz Tito, Yugoslavia was a founding member of the Non-Aligned Movement and was not under direct Soviet influence. Socialist Yugoslavia followed its own model of communism particularly after the Tito-Stalin split in 1948. See P. H. Liotta, "Paradigm Lost: Yugoslav Self-Management and the Economics of Disaster," *Balkanologie* 5, nos. 1–2 (2001), https://balkanologie.revues.org/681. Yugoslavia, the Eastern Bloc, and the Soviet Union were all governed by a communist party and enjoyed the so-called state socialism—an encompassing political, ideological, and economic system of governance and wealth distribution. Hence, academic literature on these countries tends to describe them as both "socialist" and "communist."

49. Christabelle Sethna, "The Evolution of the *Birth Control Handbook*: From Student Peer Education Manual to Feminist Self-Empowerment Text, 1968–1975," *Canadian Bulletin of Medical History* 23, no. 1 (2006): 97.

50. Morgan, "East Europe's Abortion Culture."

51. Morgan, "East Europe's Abortion Culture," B4.

52. Morgan, "East Europe's Abortion Culture," B4.

53. Anna Bogic, "Our Bodies, Our Location: The Politics of Feminist Translation and Reproduction in Post-socialist Serbia" (unpublished PhD diss., University of Ottawa, 2017), 136.

54. Morgan, "East Europe's Abortion Culture," B1.

55. Mirjana Morokvašić, "Sexuality and the Control of Procreation," in *Of Marriage and the Market: Women's Subordination in International Perspective*, ed. Kate Young, Carol Wolkowitz, and Roslyn McCullagh (London: CSE Books, 1981), 132; Rada Drezgić, *"Bela kuga" medju Srbima: O naciji, rodu i radjanju na prelazu vekova ["White Plague" among the Serbs: On the Nation, Gender and Birth at the Turn of the Century]*, Fronesis ed. (Belgrade: Albatros Plus, 2010); Bogic, "Our Bodies, Our Location."

56. Rada Drezgić, "(Re)producing the Nation: The Politics of Reproduction in Serbia in the 1980s and 1990s" (PhD diss., University of Pittsburgh, 2004), 197.

57. Vera Gudac-Dodić, *Žena u socijalizmu: Položaj žene u Srbiji u drugoj polovini 20. veka [Woman in Socialism: Women's Status in Serbia in the Second Half of the 20th Century]* (Belgrade: Institut za noviju istoriju Srbije, 2006), 145.

58. Drezgić, *"Bela kuga,"* 45–48.

59. Morokvašić, "Sexuality," 132. On the ways in which criminal abortion laws create stigma, see also Rebecca J. Cook, "Stigmatized Meanings of Criminal Abortion Laws," in *Abortion Law in Transnational Perspective: Cases and Controversies*, ed. Rebecca J. Cook, Johanna N. Erdman, and Bernard M. Dickens (Philadelphia: University of Pennsylvania Press, 2014), 347–70.

60. Henry P. David and Robert J. McIntyre, *Reproductive Behavior: Central and Eastern European Experience* (New York: Springer, 1981), 91.

61. David and McIntyre, *Reproductive Behavior*, 16–17.

62. David and McIntyre, *Reproductive Behavior*; John F. Besemeres, *Socialist Population Politics: The Political Implications of Demographic Trends in the USSR and Eastern Europe* (White Plains, NY: M. E. Sharpe, 1980).

63. Sheila Tobias, "International Notes," *Signs* 2, no. 3 (1977): 705. It is important to note that Tobias's tour was arranged by the United States Information Agency, a government body in charge of promoting American policies and culture abroad in direct competition with the Soviet influence. This fact sheds a different light on this way of channeling information on feminism.

64. Vera Gudac-Dodić, "Domestic Violence against Women in Serbia," *Tokovi istorije*, no. 3 (2014): 143–58; Gudac-Dodić, *Žena u socijalizmu*; Barbara Jancar, "Neofeminism in Yugoslavia," *Women and Politics* 8, no. 1 (1988): 1–30.

65. Susan Woodward, "The Rights of Women: Ideology, Policy, and Social Change in Yugoslavia," in *Women, State, and Party in Eastern Europe*, ed. Sharon L. Wolchik and Alfred G. Meyer (Durham, NC: Duke University Press, 1985), 234–54.

66. Gudac-Dodić, "Domestic Violence."

67. Mirjana Rašević, *Ka razumevanju abortusa u Srbiji* [*Toward an Understanding of Abortion in Serbia*] (Belgrade: Institut društvenih nauka, Centar za demografska istraživanja [Institute for Social Sciences, Centre for Demographic Research], 1993), 47–48.

68. Rašević, *Ka razumevanju abortusa*, 48; Jasmina Stevanović, "Reproduktivna prava u Srbiji" ["Reproductive Rights in Serbia"], in *Neko je rekao feminizam? Kako je feminizam uticao na žene u XXI veku* [*Somebody Said Feminism? How Feminism Has Influenced Women in the 21st Century*], ed. Adriana Zaharijević (Belgrade: Heinrich Boll Stiftung, 2008), 86.

69. Rašević, *Ka razumevanju abortusa*, 48. Yugoslav regions were consolidated into the Kingdom of Serbs, Croats, and Slovenes in 1918. In 1929, the kingdom was renamed the Kingdom of Yugoslavia.

70. Rašević, *Ka razumevanju abortusa*, 48–49.

71. Slobodanka Konstantinović-Vilić and Nevena Petrušić, "Abortion Rights—Legislation and Practice," in *Women's Rights and Social Transition in FR Yugoslavia*, ed. Vesna Nikolić-Ristanović (Belgrade: Center for Women's Studies, Research and Communication, 1997), 23–24.

72. Rašević, *Ka razumevanju abortusa*, 49–50.

73. Konstantinović-Vilić and Petrušić, "Abortion Rights," 24–25.

74. Morokvašić, "Sexuality."

75. Morokvašić, "Sexuality," 132.

76. Konstantinović-Vilić and Petrušić, "Abortion Rights," 26.

77. See Susan Gal and Gail Kligman, eds., *Reproducing Gender: Politics, Publics, and Everyday Life after Socialism* (Princeton, NJ: Princeton University Press, 2000).

78. Gal and Kligman, eds., *Reproducing Gender*. See also Susan Gal and Gail Kligman, *The Politics of Gender after Socialism* (Princeton, NJ: Princeton University Press, 2000); Barbara Einhorn, *Cinderella Goes to Market: Citizenship,*

Gender, and Women's Movements in East Central Europe (London: Verso, 1993); Nanette Funk and Magda Mueller, eds., *Gender Politics and Post-Communism: Reflections from Eastern Europe and the Former Soviet Union* (New York: Routledge, 1993).

79. Gal and Kligman, *Reproducing Gender*, 3.

80. Adriana Băban, "Women's Sexuality and Reproductive Behavior in Post-Ceauşescu Romania: A Psychological Approach," in Gal and Kligman, eds., *Reproducing Gender*, 239.

81. Susan Woodward, *Balkan Tragedy: Chaos and Dissolution after the Cold War* (Washington, DC: Brookings Institution, 1995).

82. Jeremy Shiffman, Marina Skrabalo, and Jelena Subotic, "Reproductive Rights and the State in Serbia and Croatia," *Social Science and Medicine* 54, no. 4 (2002): 625–42.

83. Laura Pitter and Alexandra Stiglmayer, "Will the World Remember: Can the Women Forget?" *Ms.* (March/April 1993): 19–22; Inger Skjelsbaek, "Victim and Survivor: Narrated Social Identities of Women Who Experienced Rape during the War in Bosnia-Herzegovina," *Feminism and Psychology* 16, no. 4 (2006): 373–403; Drezgić, *"Bela kuga"*; Elissa Helms, *Innocence and Victimhood: Gender, Nation, and Women's Activism in Postwar Bosnia-Herzegovina* (Madison: University of Wisconsin Press, 2013).

84. Bogic, "Our Bodies, Our Location"; Cynthia Cockburn, *From Where We Stand: War, Women's Activism and Feminist Analysis* (London: Zed Books, 2007).

85. Jill Benderly, "Feminist Movements in Yugoslavia, 1978–1992," in *State-Society Relations in Yugoslavia, 1945–1992*, ed. Melissa K. Bokovoy, Jill A. Irvine, and Carol S. Lilly (London: Macmillan, 1997), 196. Many of the new autonomous women's groups had roots in the previous Yugoslav feminist movement that sprang up in the 1970s and was active in the 1980s across Yugoslavia. However, it was a small, urban feminist movement that remained outside the mainstream political discourse. See Marijana Stojčić, "Proleteri svih zemalja—ko vam pere čarape? Feministički pokret u Jugoslaviji 1978–1989" ["Proleterians of the World—Who's Washing Your Socks? Feminist Movement in Yugoslavia 1978–1989"], in *Društvo u pokretu: Novi društveni pokreti u Jugoslaviji od 1968 do danas* [*Society on the Move: New Social Movements in Yugoslavia from 1968 to Today*], ed. Djordje Tomić and Petar Atanacković (Novi Sad, Serbia: Cenzura Publishing, 2009), 108–21. The Yugoslav feminism of this period refuted the socialist Yugoslav government's assertion that the "woman question" had been resolved by the Yugoslav revolution and that the "solving of the class issues solves the 'Woman Question'" (Jancar, "Neo-feminism in Yugoslavia," 21).

86. Solinger, *Reproductive Politics*; Feldt, *The War on Choice*; Faludi, *Backlash*.

87. Bogic, "Our Bodies, Our Location."

88. BWHBC, *Our Bodies, Ourselves* (1992), 353.

89. BWHBC, *Our Bodies, Ourselves* (1992), 361.

90. In socialist Yugoslavia (1945–91), the official language was Serbo-Croatian, spoken by a large majority of Yugoslav citizens living in the six Yugoslav republics. Following the breakup of the Yugoslav federation in the early 1990s, the term "Serbo-Croatian" became highly politicized and contro-

versial, and subsequently "Croatian" became the official language of Croatia and "Serbian" of Serbia.

91. Marina Blagojević, "Mizoginija: Nevidljivi uzroci, bolne posledice" ["Misogyny: Invisible Causes, Painful Consequences"], in *Mapiranje mizoginije u Srbiji. Diskursi i prakse, Vol. I* [*Mapping Misogyny in Serbia: Discourses and Practices, Vol. I*], ed. Marina Blagojević (Belgrade: Asocijacija za žensku inicijativu, 2000), 44.

92. Drezgić, *"Bela kuga,"* 99. Drezgić specifically analyzes texts by two male professors, Milan Vojnović and Marko Mladenović.

93. Drezgić, *"Bela kuga,"* 103F.

94. Rada Drezgić, "Religion, Politics and Gender in Serbia: The Re-traditionalization of Gender Roles in the Context of Nation-State Formation." Final Report. United Nations Research Institute for Social Development (2009). http://www.unrisd.org/80256B3C005BCCF9/(httpPublications)/3C57C157BE2D09D18025790D004F8E82.

95. Drezgić, "Religion, Politics and Gender in Serbia," 16.

96. Drezgić, "Religion, Politics and Gender in Serbia," 16; Žarana Papić, "Women in Serbia," 163.

97. Nadežda Ćetković, "Beogradski ženski lobi" ["Belgrade Women's Lobby"], in *Ka vidljivoj ženskoj istoriji: Ženski pokret u Beogradu 90-ih* [*Toward a Visible Women's History: The Women's Movement in Belgrade in the 1990s*], ed. Marina Blagojević (Belgrade: Centar za ženske studije, istraživanja i komunikaciju, 1998), 65.

98. Beogradski ženski lobi [Belgrade Women's Lobby], "Protest ženskog parlamenta protiv odluke skupštine Republike Srbije o učešću osiguranika u troškovima zdravstvene zaštite" ["Protest of the Women's Parliament against the Decision of the Parliament of the Republic of Serbia on the Insurer's Contribution to Health Expenses"], *Feminističke sveske*, nos. 3–4 (1995): 31.

99. Drezgić, "Religion, Politics and Gender in Serbia," 18.

100. Drezgić, "Religion, Politics and Gender in Serbia," 18; Konstantinović-Vilić and Petrušić, "Abortion Rights," 26; Rašević, *Ka razumevanju abortusa.*

101. Konstantinović-Vilić and Petrušić, "Abortion Rights," 38.

102. Konstantinović-Vilić and Petrušić, "Abortion Rights," 34–38.

103. Bogic, *Our Bodies, Our Location*, 142.

104. See Ann Snitow, "Feminist Future in the Former East Bloc," in *Eastern European Feminist Conference: What Can We Do for Ourselves?*, ed. Marina Blagojević, Daša Duhaček, and Jasmina Lukić (Belgrade: Centar za ženske studije, istraživanja i komunikaciju, 1995), 141–55.

[11]

Abortion and the Catholic Church in Poland

EWELINA CIAPUTA

I am 34 years old, have two daughters, a husband, higher education, a job, an apartment, a car and no debts. Two weeks ago, I found out that I was pregnant for the third time!!! Terrified, my husband and I started seeking help. I went through a nightmare!!! From visits to gynecologists looking at me like I was a murderer, to opinions on the internet, [telling me] what a monster I am going to be and how it [the abortion] will change my life. . . . For a week, alternating with my husband, we cried, yelled, [and] for a while accepted the facts. Finally, under the pressure of time we decided to go to Slovakia to an abortion clinic. I felt like I was in another world, like a normal person, like a woman who has the right to decide not only about herself but also about the fate of her family. Everything went without pain, including the care of my mental and physical health. On the second day, when we got back home, I felt great relief; everything was back to normal. Why did I do it??? BECAUSE WE CANNOT AFFORD A THIRD CHILD!!! Because I think about the future of my daughters, whom I love more than life itself. The situation in which I found myself opened my eyes to what kind of country I live in, and that scares me the most. I've never been for abortion or against it . . . until it happened to me. Today, taking full responsibility for my words, I can say that I am for early, legal abortion to the ninth week—period. And one more thing: no one has the right to judge us; that kind of decision is not taken quickly and easily.[1]

This quotation is from a reader's letter published in 2012 in one of the most influential and progressive newspapers in Poland, *Gazeta Wyborcza*. Although it was not the first time that a woman's personal struggle with abortion legislation was publicized,[2] this story makes two important points. First, it confirms that the phenomenon of "abortion tourism" in Poland exists; women did, do, and will continue to travel to have their reproductive needs met when mental, physical, or socioeconomic circumstances constitute an obstacle to bearing and raising a child. Second, it demonstrates that many years of neglect and ignorance concerning women's reproductive health and rights on behalf of a state deeply influenced by the Catholic Church has strengthened social stigma against abortion and has contributed to ongoing problems with access to abortion services.

The Federation for Women and Family Planning, one of the most important feminist pro-choice organizations in Poland advocating for women's reproductive rights, estimates that every year thousands of Polish women travel outside the country for abortion services. Women who are better situated socially and economically can afford to travel to Belgium, the Netherlands, Germany, Austria, and Britain, while those lower on the socioeconomic ladder choose less expensive clinics in Lithuania, Ukraine, the Czech Republic, or Slovakia, on the other side of the Tatra Mountains. While most of the clinics in these countries translate their webpages into Polish and/or have Polish-speaking personnel and consultants, such as the GynMed Clinic for Abortion and Family Planning in Austria,[3] some of the latter even organize transportation to and from Poland, as does MediKlinik in Slovakia.[4] However, there are also Polish women we must not forget: those women from rural areas and smaller cities who cannot afford to go abroad and therefore must seek help inside Poland instead. These women are forced to use financial credit, or borrow money from relatives and friends to pay for the abortion and the attendant costs, and if that is not possible, they are forced to use health- and life-threatening solutions such as swallowing pills of unknown origin, taking a mixture of drugs, or inserting sharp objects into the uterus to induce a miscarriage.[5] In this volume, Cathrine Chambers, Colleen MacQuarrie, and Jo-Ann MacDonald see the same connection between a lack of resources and self-induced abortions emerge out of their study on Prince Edward Island.

In this chapter, I argue that the restrictiveness of Polish abortion laws has its effects in the number of women seeking help both from the illegal abortion underground inside Poland and through abortion tourism outside the country. Although these two phenomena are not new, politicians in the postcommunist era have been especially reluctant to recognize the illegal abortion underground and abortion tourism abroad as serious predicaments in need of a rapid response from the state, mainly because of pressure exercised by the Catholic Church. The Church does not function only as a religious institution but as a major political actor as well, a contention strongly supported in this volume by Mary Gilmartin and Sinéad Kennedy's research on the Republic of Ireland (hereafter Ireland), and by Agata Ignaciuk's analysis of Spain, among others. Most Polish politicians take into account the Church's opinions when making policy decisions concerning antidiscrimination and gender equality issues, and Church leaders often serve as experts on parliamentary committees on education, social, and health policy.[6] As demonstrated by Mirosław Chałubiński, since the collapse of communism in 1989, the Catholic Church in Poland has affected, among other matters, election results and judicial decisions. It frequently functions as a lobby group, impacting directly and indirectly the declarations made by some political parties. It has also had a major impact on the push to restrict access to abortion services.[7]

There is no official data on the illegal abortion underground or on abortion tourism from Poland, which is a major challenge when estimating their scale. Drawing upon available statistics, ministerial reports, articles published on the internet and in the press (in *Gazeta Wyborcza* and *Polityka* but also *Wysokie Obcasy* and *Duży Format*), readers' letters published in *Bluszcz* (a feminist magazine),[8] and nongovernmental organization reports as well as women's testimonies published in secondary sources,[9] this chapter provides an account of the interplay between the beliefs of the Polish Catholic Church, the Polish government's opposition to abortion, and Polish national identity.

Poland's Abortion Legislation, the Catholic Church, and Women's Reproductive Rights

Poland now has, after Ireland and Malta, the most restrictive abortion policy in Europe. As observed by many feminist scholars and activists, women's right to decide freely and independently how to manage their reproductive lives has been gradually eroded over the past 25 years.[10] Polish women's hopes for safeguarding their reproductive rights after the country's political transition from a regime ruled by a Communist government to a parliamentary democracy initiated in 1989 had to be set aside due to the political struggles over the new direction for the Polish economy and the construction of a "new neoliberal citizen."[11] Anna Bogic's contribution to this volume ascertains that in regard to Serbia, the postcommunist transition to democracy did not safeguard women's reproductive rights, because of the state's pronatalist agenda for women. In a related manner, Anne-Marie Kramer's observations about postcommunist states such as Poland and their relationship to women's reproductive rights are particularly relevant here. Kramer comments, "Contestations around reproductive policy are arguments about the proper shape of post communist states, political arrangements and civil society. . . . Debate around reproduction serves as a substitute issue where wider concerns and anxieties around the proper ordering of the re/constructed postcommunist polity, (gendered) citizens and nation/state are played out, and where the legitimacy of political authority is articulated and contested. Despite having real and material effects on women's lives, postcommunist abortion debates are thus explained as being more properly about the nature of democracy and the character of the nation-state, than simply about reproduction."[12] Public discussions concerning women's decision making about reproduction are not only part of a political game, as argued in the previous quotation, but should also be seen as a highly ideological contest.[13]

As has been indicated by Polish antidiscrimination legal experts, the current legislation on abortion excludes women from making decisions regarding their own fertility.[14] Recent studies have shown that access to reproductive services in Poland depends on gender, legal age of consent, socioeconomic circumstances, and (dis)ability, in addition to place of residence, public funding for effective contraception, and availability to access safe, affordable, and legal abortion services.[15] While the social roles of women are defined through an obligation to be mothers, wives, and guardians of the Polish nation,[16] a woman striving for reproductive rights is seen as an example of the ideological blindness or false consciousness stemming from Western values.[17] Anna Bogic addresses similar accusations that are made against Serbian women in her chapter in this volume. The notion that reproductive rights are contrary to the Polish national identity is undoubtedly connected with the power exercised by the Catholic Church.[18] This identity is founded on an ethno-religious basis that emphasizes homogeneity and prioritizes community over the rights of individuals.[19] Women's reproductive rights are subordinated to the nation, and a woman herself is considered the property of the community. Discussions about abortion can be understood as resulting primarily from the influence of the Catholic Church on politicians' views of women and the status attributed to an embryo—increasingly understood in postcommunist Poland as an unborn human being and citizen entitled to civil rights. This contention is well illustrated by events that occurred two years before Poland's accession to the European Union (EU). Although Polish politicians said they would liberalize the country's abortion laws due to EU pressure, the Church hierarchy resisted, demanding that Poland maintain its strict antichoice stance in exchange for the Church's support for Poland's membership in the EU.[20] Nowadays, attempts to liberalize abortion laws are presented as pro-Communist, anti-Catholic, and anti-nationalist.[21]

Abortion in Poland before World War II and during the Second Republic

In the Middle Ages, Polish common law considered abortion as equal to manslaughter.[22] The 1818 Penal Code of the Kingdom of Poland recognized abortion as a criminal act, demanding punishment or incarceration for the first time in Polish history.[23] Late eighteenth- and nineteenth-century concerns about overpopulation as a main reason for poverty, common to authors such as Thomas Malthus, Jeremy Bentham, James Mill, and John Stuart Mill, as well as Robert Dale Owen, brought into sharp focus the link between economy and fertility. During the interwar period in Poland, the idea of downsizing the Polish population in order to improve the economic standing of individuals was adopted by Polish intellectuals who made the poor the main target of a birth control movement.[24] Polish laws in regard to abortion reflected the complex influence of the penal codes of three powers—Austria-Hungary, Prussia, and Russia—that occupied Poland at various points in its history.[25] In 1918, when Poland gained its independence after 123 years under partition, state leaders decided to create a Codification Commission that was responsible for harmonizing civil and criminal legislation in the Second Polish Republic.[26] In 1929, the commission proposed the first draft of an abortion law that endowed the fetus with the right to live. The pregnant woman and any other person responsible for pregnancy termination could be sentenced to prison for up to five years. In debates about the law that were broadcast in the popular press, physicians such as Justyna Budzińska-Tylicka, Henryk Kłuszyński, Leonard Lorentowicz, Tadeusz Boy-Żeleński, and Irena Krzywicka, in addition to authors such as Maria Pawlikowska-Jasnosrzewska and Wanda Melcer, continued to raise the issue of uncontrolled fertility among the nation's poorest. A Polish abortion law was eventually passed in 1932.[27]

During the interwar period, Poland was not as industrialized and modernized as were other states in Western Europe. As indicated by Andrzej Gawryszewski, at the beginning of the twentieth century, 59 percent of Poles were involved in agriculture as their main livelihood.[28] Although in other European countries industrialization went hand in hand with a decrease in the number of infants born, Poland noted an escalation of its birth rate. For instance, between 1926 and 1930, there were 1.4 births for every 1,000 inhabitants in France, while in Poland the birth rate was 15.5 per 1,000 Poles.[29] Magdalena Gawin explains that this discrepancy is the effect of a slower industrialization process in Poland, while Gawryszewski attributes it to the upheaval resulting from postwar repatriation and migration of Germans from Pomerania, Wielkopolska, and Upper Silesia.[30]

The interwar period in Poland could be characterized by upper-class trends to regulate the number of children born to families on the basis of their material conditions. This trend started to penetrate slowly into the middle classes and peasantry. However, it was not followed by an increased awareness of the use of contraception, which quickly led to the popularization of illegal (and risky) abortion as a method of birth control.[31] During this period, Poland experienced the growth of abortion tourism inside Poland. As described by Gawin,[32] in rural areas, middlemen took women willing to terminate their pregnancies to abortion providers who were quacks, midwives, or paramedical personnel in cities. Importantly, abortion was not solely a lower-class matter; it was also widely practiced by the Polish intelligentsia. When costs linked to travel were too high, women tried to bring on a menstrual period by using dangerous and harmful do-it-yourself methods.[33] Given the illegal status of abortion, it was difficult to estimate the number of pregnancy terminations. Some information on this matter could be derived from medical questionnaires distributed in the early 1930s and analyzed by Marcin Kacprzak. As indicated by Gawin, according to Kacprzak's findings, a majority of physicians admitted that very few of the women they treated had had only one abortion; nearly three times the number of their patients had had multiple abortions.[34]

The Lawyers' Congress rejected the Codification Commission's first draft of the abortion legislation in 1929. Subsequently, two more relatively lenient drafts were proposed. One permitted abortion due to economic, medical, or eugenic reasons, while the other allowed a woman to abort because of her difficult material conditions. The latter was rejected as a result of episcopal pressure.[35] The Catholic Church treated abortion as tantamount to homicide,[36] and during public discussions about the proposed abortion legislation it accused liberated women of causing the moral degradation of society and the decline of the birth rate: "Since modern woman began to turn away from the natural purpose [motherhood] that God intended for her, her soul started to become ill. . . . Instead of grasping her children by the hand and leading them to God . . . she grabbed the steering wheel, she stepped on the tennis court, drowned herself in fashion, sport and dance, and sold her love for profit and sensual pleasure."[37]

In contrast, birth control activists raised the issue of the uncontrolled fertility of the poor, who were said to be the most affected by abortion legislation. Progressive physician and activist Tadeusz Boy-Żeleński, one of the founders of a network of "conscious motherhood" clinics[38] and the author of one of the most important texts that contributed to public discussions about abortion at that time, *Piekło kobiet* (*The Women's Hell*), argued: "criminalization of pregnancy termination is the biggest crime committed by criminal law." As documented by Kazimiera Szczuka, Boy-Żeleński insisted that the criminalization of abortion did not limit the number of terminations. Rather, it led to the death of women due to botched abortions. He also concurred that poverty was the reason women sought abortions at home or traveled to obtain them.[39]

Abortion law reform was also widely debated in women's magazines. *Głos Kobiet* (*Women's Voice*), connected to the Polish socialist party, and *Kobieta Współczesna* (*Modern Woman*), a progressive independent weekly on women's issues, both positioned themselves in favor of decriminalizing abortion. A lively debate also took place in *Bluszcz*. Zofia Galicka, author of a letter published in this magazine, favored the decriminalization of abortion, writing: "A woman, unmarried or married, who due to personal, health or material reasons does not want to bear a child, cannot be forced to do so under threat of incarceration. It is unethical!"[40] Her opinion gave rise to several contrary responses. These were often underpinned by claims that the Second Polish Republic, restored after more than a century of partition, should be founded on Catholic morals that extended to a rejection of abortion. One letter writer even insisted that for Catholic women, state law was meaningless "if it is opposed to the law of Christ. We cannot forget that the

Church condemns every mother who commits a crime against her innocent baby by disregarding the commandments of God: 'do not kill.'"[41]

Although existing laws banned abortion, it was commonly undertaken illegally. As indicated by Aleksandra Czajkowska,[42] women's lack of differentiation between abortion and contraception meant that many women trying to control their fertility died because of the unhygienic conditions under which so many illegal abortions were performed. The deadly consequences of illegal abortions led some women, feminists, liberals, and socialists to promote the idea of conscious motherhood. They created a birth control clinic within the Robotnicze Towarzystwo Służby Społecznej (Workers' Social Service Society) as well as a conscious motherhood clinic. Both were established in Warsaw in 1931 but spread to other Polish cities as well. Their main aim was to create a space where Poles could gain knowledge of the use and effectiveness of contraception,[43] because contraceptive use was limited mostly to urban intelligentsia.[44] In her contribution to this volume, Anna Bogic expounds upon the curious relationship of contraception to abortion in the former Yugoslavia, noting that although abortion was somewhat stigmatized, only a minority of women turned to contraceptive devices, with a majority preferring coitus interruptus as a means of birth control. In Poland, clinics collected data on their clients, including information about abortion in cities such as Warsaw. The biggest problem that the clinics had to deal with, especially at the beginning of their existence, was that working-class women seeking abortion services did not distinguish between the termination of a pregnancy and the prevention of conception.[45]

The establishment of the birth control and conscious motherhood clinics combined with intense public discussions about proposed abortion laws to trigger a reaction within the Catholic community. Catholic leaders wrote a letter to the Codification Commission expressing their dissatisfaction and opposition to any draft legislation that liberalized abortion laws.[46] In 1931, a third draft legislation was announced, but the public was not kept well informed.[47] Finally, in 1932, a new penal code that included regulations concerning abortion was introduced. According to this code, termination of pregnancy was permitted only if the pregnancy was the result of a criminal act or if a woman's health or life was in danger. Penalties for performing an abortion under circumstances other than indicated in the penal code were as follows: a three-year period of imprisonment for the woman in question and a five-year

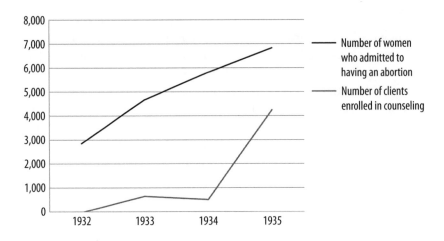

Figure 11.1. Abortion after introduction of the 1932 Penal Code in Poland.
Gawin, Magdalena. "Planowanie rodziny—hasła i rzeczywistość." In *Równe prawa i nierówne szanse: Kobiety w Polsce międzywojennej*, edited by Anna Żarnowska and Andrzej Szwarc, 221–39. Warsaw: Wydawnictwo DIG, 2000.

period of punishment for a physician who performed the surgery.[48] A few weeks after the 1932 Penal Code was introduced, national leaders introduced an executive act, the Ordinance of the President of the Republic of Poland. The ordinance specified that abortion could be performed legally by a physician only if two different doctors approved termination due to medical indications. In the case of pregnancy as a result of a criminal act (rape or incest), a public prosecutor's testimony was needed.[49]

Available data from Warsaw's conscious motherhood clinic[50] about abortions obtained from women during medical interviews indicates that the introduction of the 1932 Penal Code and the partial liberalization of abortion resulted in an increase in the terminations performed (see figure 11.1). In 1933, 15 percent of 4,624 clients admitted to having an abortion, but in 1935 it was more than 62 percent of 6,821 clients. These numbers are proof of a wider trend among Polish women to treat termination of pregnancy as a main method of birth control. The ineffectiveness of the 1932 legislation to regulate legal abortion, as well as its discriminatory consequences for working-class women, who often could not afford to provide for yet another child but could not abort legally because of a lack of financial or social indicators,[51] provided the main arguments for law reform. Unfortunately, attempts to revise the 1932 law were interrupted by the start of World War II.

Poland as an Abortion Tourism Destination in the Mid-Twentieth Century

Immediately after the end of the war, public discussions about abortion emerged yet again. As maintained by Barbara Klich-Kluczewska, "the concept of the numerical strength of the national community and (related directly to it) the need to replace the casualties from World War II had become an axiom of public discourse in post-war Poland, particularly during the reconstruction (1945–1948) and Stalinist (1949–1955) periods."[52] Between 1947 and 1948, opposition to the 1932 legislation prevailed among physicians, Catholic leaders, and conservative politicians due to the significant depopulation of the Polish nation, but no new legislation was introduced.[53] The government decided to apply policy measures to increase the role of the family and change women's attitudes toward motherhood.[54] Nevertheless, as contraceptive use throughout society was low, and there were no national campaigns to promote the importance of contraceptives, women continued to have illegal abortions in Poland.[55] As indicated by the Ministry of Justice, Polish hospitals in 1951 registered 70,919 miscarriages (a great percentage of which were possibly self-induced or actually were illegal abortions), and in 1955 this number increased to 101,597. Moreover, as Klich-Kluczewska indicates, between 1950 and 1955, it is estimated that 300,000 women had illegal abortions, 80,000 of whom were "hospitalized in a serious condition and there diagnosed to have had a miscarriage earlier."[56] Some other sources indicate that the number of illegal terminations at that time reached 500,000 per year.[57]

Growing numbers of clandestine terminations and a trend initiated by the Soviet Union toward the legalization of abortion on social grounds[58] accelerated the introduction in 1956 of new abortion legislation. The Law on the Admissibility of Abortion allowed pregnancy termination on socioeconomic grounds. The main argument for this new legislation was to protect women from the consequences of backstreet abortions, preserve women's reproductive and productive capacities, and promote the quality, rather than quantity, of socialist citizens.[59] However, in reality, women in postwar communist bloc countries were trapped by a "double burden." They were mothers and homemakers but also employees who worked inside and outside the home.[60]

A Six-Year Plan introduced by the Polish government and realized between 1950 and 1955 aimed at increasing the employment of women and raising their standard of living by improving perinatal care and childcare, and creating maternity wards and counseling clinics, as well as nurseries and kindergartens.[61] The establishment in 1957 of the Polish Society for Conscious Motherhood could be perceived as a sign of state leaders' willingness to ensure maximum effectiveness of the 1956 abortion legislation.[62] Yet, as indicated by Agata Ignaciuk, who in addition to her contribution to this volume has also analyzed the publications of this particular Polish organization between 1957 and 1980, abortion was generally represented as a harmful necessity potentially affecting women's fertility and the physical and psychological capabilities of any future offspring.[63]

The realization of the Six-Year Plan did not make all women's lives better or easier; women from rural areas and smaller cities experienced limited access to healthcare and had little information about contraception. The realities of the labor market did not encourage couples to reproduce, and women employed outside the home experienced several labor rights violations, including employers' reluctance to hire a woman because of the costs of maternity and sick child leave, as well as reduced earnings.[64]

The 1956 abortion legislation allowed termination of pregnancy on socioeconomic grounds, but the execution of this premise proved to be difficult at first.[65] The Polish healthcare system suffered from a lack of adequate equipment in hospitals, an insufficient number of gynecologists and properly qualified personnel, and a scarce supply of medications.[66] Even though the law did not include a conscience clause, some physicians still refused to perform the procedure because of their Catholic beliefs. Economic matters also played a significant role. Some physicians declined to perform abortions in public clinics and hospitals, hoping that the most desperate women would seek them out in private practices, where they would pay higher fees for the procedure.[67] The concern that abortion provision could line the pockets of doctors in the private sector is raised by Christabelle Sethna and by Gayle Davis et al. in their respective discussions of opposition to the 1967 British Abortion Act found in this volume.

Nevertheless, the main problem that arose due to the implementation of the 1956 legislation was related to the tortuous process women had to follow in order to have an abortion justified by their difficult economic and/or social situations. Doctors were obliged to authorize abortions based on documents submitted by a woman that provided proof of her difficult socioeconomic circumstances. However, doctors were unsure how to evaluate them.[68] Although physicians could refuse to carry out terminations, there were no mechanisms through which women could appeal the refusal. As a result, women continued to rely on the abortion underground.[69]

Difficulties with the interpretation and implementation of this legislation as well as changes to the state's policies toward reducing the birth rate[70] resulted in an executive order from the Ministry of Health in December 1959. It allowed women to appeal physicians' refusal to authorize an abortion. Furthermore, it removed physicians' obligation to evaluate the documents a woman produced and introduced only a written statement as a basis for a termination. Additionally, the same doctor who issued a referral for pregnancy termination could perform the abortion. In practice, the executive order allowed women to exercise their right to abortion on demand, which was provided free of charge in public hospitals.[71] Available statistics on abortions performed in public hospitals and their outpatient departments during the period from 1957 to 1966 show that after the introduction of the 1956 legislation, the number of terminations carried out in hospitals increased, possibly because the large number of abortions that were performed earlier in secret were now being carried out legally in hospitals (see figures 11.2 and 11.3).[72] More importantly, abortions performed on socioeconomic grounds far outnumbered therapeutic abortions, and these increased in number after 1960 as the consequence of the 1959 executive order from the Ministry of Health.[73]

While a variety of contraceptives were available for purchase, their quality was not always satisfactory, which may be a reason why there were another 50,000 to 60,000 abortions per year that were performed by unqualified individuals or physicians in private practice.[74] Data presented by Czajkowska also includes information on the number of abortions initiated outside the hospital and completed in outpatient clinics.[75] Although distinguishing between illegally performed terminations and spontaneous miscarriages seems impossible,[76] these figures allow us to

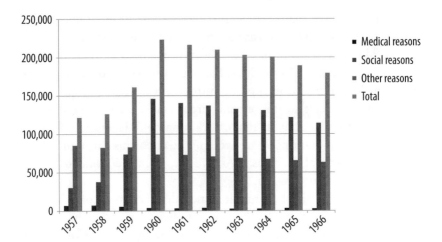

Figure 11.2. Abortions performed in public hospitals, 1957–1966. Author's own extrapolation based on Czajkowska, "O dopuszczalności przerywania ciąży," 180.

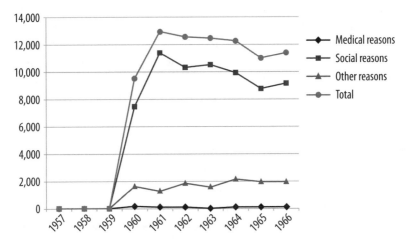

Figure 11.3. Abortions performed in other hospitals, 1957–1966. Author's own extrapolation based on Czajkowska, "O dopuszczalności przerywania ciąży," 180.

assume that the 1959 abortion legislation did not eliminate altogether the problem of the illegal abortion underground (see table 11.1).

The adoption of the more liberal abortion policies by the state was highly criticized by Catholic organizations.[77] For instance, members of an ad hoc Moral Regeneration Committee appealed to the government to protect unborn children on the grounds that they would be major

Table 11.1. Abortions performed in outpatient clinics in Poland, 1962–1966

Year	Total
1962	48,421
1963	43,925
1964	33,936
1965	33,849
1966	30,347

Czajkowska, Aleksandra. "O dopuszczalności przerywania ciąży: Ustawa z dnia 27 kwietnia 1956 r. i towarzyszące jej dyskusje." In *Kłopoty z seksem w PRL: Rodzenie nie całkiem po ludzku, aborcja, choroby, odmienności*, edited by Marcin Kula, 180. Warsaw: Wydawnictwa Uniwersytetu Warszawskiego, 2012.

assets to Poland in the future: "We all have an understanding and a sense of major responsibility to save the lives of unborn children. Among these innocent victims are ordinary people but also geniuses, great leaders of the nation, artists, thinkers, and scientists. Their sacrifice has been impoverishing our nation in a way that cannot be reversed."[78]

Similar arguments were brought forward by the Catholic Church, which was perceived as a defender of human rights, the icon of the struggle for freedom from communism, and the mediator between the government and its opposition.[79] From 1965 on, as Jacqueline Heinen and Anna Matuchniak-Krasuska illustrate, public attitudes toward abortion were increasingly influenced by Church leaders.[80] They designed and implemented actions aimed at ending the "mass killing of the unborn" and supported the mainstreaming of mandatory premarital courses for Catholic future spouses, family counseling in local congregations, religion courses for medical students, and seminars and congresses for physicians and theologians.[81]

Poland's liberal abortion policies proved to be tempting for women from Western countries where abortion services were still illegal. Official statistics on abortion tourism to Poland are unknown, but according to a number of scholars specializing in the history of abortion travel, in the 1960s Poland became somewhat of an abortion destination for a few Canadian women and for some Swedish women who were denied that right in their home countries.[82] At about the same time that Sherri Finkbine traveled to Sweden from the USA for an abortion in the early 1960s, a journey Lena Lennerhed examines in this volume, Swedish women traveled to Poland, where abortion on demand was legal. Information about Swedish women coming to Poland for abortions was made public in 1964 at a "Sex and Society" international conference held in Stockholm, during which one of the participants spoke about her Polish abortion experience. It should be noted that the conference organizer, as well as the woman whose testimony was made public, helped approximately 1,000 women contact Polish physicians.[83] Abortion tourism to Poland had its effect on Swedish abortion policies, because in 1974 a new Swedish law granted women the right to abortion on demand.[84]

In 1970s Poland, concerns about dropping birth rates led state authorities to design policies aimed at stimulating population growth.[85] They initiated pronatalist policies based on the long-standing assumption that a woman's main role was to bear and raise children.[86] Pronatalist policies included the extension of voluntary, unpaid maternity leave from one year to three years and paid maternity leave from three to four months after giving birth.[87] Paid leave for women caring for a sick child was also introduced.[88] However, women continued to try to limit their families, even though "the most popular birth control techniques . . . were non-medicalized and relatively insecure methods, such as *coitus interruptus* and different forms of the rhythm method."[89] There was marginal use of condoms. Catholic Church propaganda against oral contraception, its limited availability, and fears of its side effects were the main reasons for its unpopularity among Polish women. Moreover, as shown by Peter Mazur, contraceptive use was correlated with women's level of education; the higher the level, the more frequently the women used contraception. Surprisingly, urban women more often relied on natural family planning and condoms than rural women.[90] Abortion continued to be used as a method of birth control for women in general. Scholars estimate that the number of induced abortions in 1975 was between 250,000 and 1.4 million but officially registered only at 138,900.[91]

Abortion Tourism in the Third Polish Republic

In the early 1980s, public discussions about abortion shifted from a focus on demographic issues to an emphasis on the moral reconstruction of Polish society. The first Catholic pro-life organizations were established, among them Troska o Życie (Care for Life), Gaudium Vitae (Joy of Life), and Pro Familia (Pro-Family). They organized awareness campaigns on the moral consequences and health risks of abortion, and sought to help pregnant women and young mothers.[92] In this context, the Ministry of Health and Social Policy issued in late 1980 a regulation defining a specialty in gynecology and obstetrics as the legal qualification a physician needed to terminate a pregnancy.[93] The following year, an instruction issued by the Ministry of Health directed physicians to reduce the number of abortions performed in Poland by discouraging the woman from her intention to end her pregnancy.[94]

The rhetoric of Catholic Church leaders and pro-life organizations that prevailed in the public discussion contributed to stigmatization of abortion, which led to the growth of the illegal abortion underground and abortion tourism.[95] In 1988, the Klub Inteligencji Katolickiej (Club of Catholic Intelligentsia) from Szczecin submitted to the Polish Parliament a proposal to repeal the abortion legislation of 1956, but a parliamentary committee concluded that it would only worsen the situation by forcing women to use the illegal abortion underground. The Catholic Church disagreed with the committee's opinion and began preparing a draft of the Unborn Child Protection Bill.[96] Opposition to this bill gave rise to independent women's organizations such as Pro Femina (For Woman), Ruch Samoobrony Kobiet (Women's Self-Defense Movement), Godność kobiety (Woman's Dignity), and Polskie Stowarzyszenie Feministyczne (Polish Feminist Association), which, shortly after the collapse of communism, became active in advocating for women's reproductive rights.[97]

The transformation of the Polish state associated with the collapse of communism, the adoption of a democratic political system as the basis for reviving the state and the nation, and the development of a collective Polish Catholic identity shaped postcommunist discussions about abortion.[98] In fact, as Anne Kramer brilliantly argues, the social and political transformation of Poland was effected discursively *through* the abortion debate.[99] This debate is marked by a clash of human rights: the fetus's right to live and pregnant women's right to freedom.[100] Antichoice sentiments have penetrated deeply into post-Communist Polish society. For example, in 1992, 47 percent of public opinion held that a woman's socioeconomic circumstances could be grounds for an abortion, but in 2016 this number plummeted to just 11 percent.[101]

In 1993, the Polish Parliament yielded to the pressure exercised by the Catholic Church and introduced a law on "Family planning, protection of the human embryo and the conditions for the termination of pregnancy," popularly known as the "Anti-Abortion Law." This law authorizes abortion if: (1) the pregnancy threatens a pregnant woman's life or physical health, (2) fetal abnormalities are detected, and (3) the pregnancy occurs as the result of a criminal act. Furthermore, the 1993 law states that termination of pregnancy could be performed only when a public prosecutor issues a confirmation of rape or incest. In the case of a woman's health or life being in danger, legal grounds for abortion were met when a physician issued a written opinion. Significantly, the language used in this law reflects the pro-life rhetoric of the Catholic Church, for example, replacing the word "fetus" with "unborn child."[102]

The Anti-Abortion Law proved to be very restrictive and quickly reduced the number of legally performed terminations. In 1978, 223,000 abortions were registered in Poland, approximately half of them performed in public hospitals and the rest in private clinics. However, experts considered abortions in private clinics to be largely underreported and estimated that the total number of abortions performed in Poland throughout the state-socialist period oscillated between 300,000 and 500,000 terminations per year.[103] By contrast, in 1993, the number of legal abortions dropped to 1,240,[104] and this trend has continued into the new millennium. Only 1,040 legal abortions were recorded in Poland in 2015.[105] This number is extremely low given the current size of the Polish population at 38 million.[106] It is a common practice for entire hospitals to invoke conscientious objector status and refuse to provide abortion services altogether.[107] Those few hospitals that agree to perform abortions face regular harassment from anti-abortion protesters.[108] They are also scattered throughout the country, forcing women to travel to them even for legal terminations. "Agata," a 14-year-old girl who became pregnant as a result of rape, was denied access to a legal abortion in two hospitals and then forced to journey 400 kilometers away from her home to end her pregnancy.[109] There have also been other instances in which physicians have dissuaded women from accessing legal abortions, as in the case of Alicja Tysiąc, a woman pregnant for the third time and suffering from vision problems that pregnancy could worsen. Denied access to legal abortion on health grounds by several physicians, she gave birth but was compared in a Catholic newspaper, *Gość Niedzielny*, to a Nazi war criminal for wanting to murder her own child.[110]

The position of the Catholic Church in Poland was strengthened further by the signing of a concordat with the Holy See that was ratified in 1998. With this agreement, the Polish state made a commitment to provide every child with access to religious education, which resulted in the introduction of religious classes into schools and the promotion of Catholic values in the education system.[111] Even though the illegal abortion underground is a present-day reality in Poland, the state has chosen to ignore it. The Anti-Abortion Law is supplemented by provisions in the penal code, which state that certain behaviors resulting in the termination of a pregnancy shall be punished with imprisonment from six months to eight years. Even though these provisions are aimed at limiting abortions performed illegally by physicians, there are only a few cases of penal code violations, which means that the illegal abortion underground is not significantly persecuted.[112] In the early 2010s, nongovernmental organizations estimated the total number of clandestine abortions performed in Poland at around 85,000 to 90,000 per year, with an additional 10,000 to 15,000 women traveling abroad for abortions yearly.[113]

Shortly after the introduction of the Anti-Abortion Law, abortion referral agencies mushroomed in Poland, with demand peaking in the first three months after it was passed. One anonymous individual who helped Polish women access abortion services abroad stated: "We had contacts in two private surgeries, a private clinic, two public hospitals, six gynaecologists, three anaesthesiologists and a few nurses in one of the neighbouring countries. This way we were able to help about 220–250 women get terminations. Later, in 1993 we were referring 60–70 a month for abortions. In 1994, we sent between 40 and 50 women [abroad] each month for abortion. During this whole period, we managed to help organize approx. 1,200 terminations [outside Poland]."[114] Abortion referral agencies, as Christabelle Sethna, Hayley Brown, and Agata Ignaciuk discuss in their respective chapters on Britain, New Zealand, and Spain in this volume, have played a significant part in the history of travel for abortion services. Polish women were sent to Russia, Ukraine, Lithuania, Belarus, the Czech Republic, and Slovakia. Women with economic means traveled to the Netherlands, Germany, Belgium, and Austria, where the conditions under which abortion services operated were often better than their Eastern European counterparts. Poland's abortion referral agencies were located in 20 cities, among them Kraków, Lublin, Łódź, Gdańsk, and Olsztyn. The Federation for Women and Family Planning estimates that between 1993 and 1994, these agencies facilitated approximately 16,000 abortions abroad per year, but this figure excludes abortions practiced on women living in border areas who organized their own travel to access abortion services.[115]

Penal code provisions meant that individuals involved in abortion referral faced the risk of arrest and imprisonment.[116] After several trials that resulted in prison sentences for those organizing abortion travel abroad, the work of abortion referral agencies dwindled.[117] Moreover, the transitory liberalization of the Anti-Abortion Law in 1996, when abortion due to socioeconomic difficulties was briefly relegalized, also interrupted their efforts. Although access to legal termination during this short time was more difficult than during most of the state-socialist period, the number of legal abortions multiplied. In 1996, only 505 legal terminations were registered, but in 1997 this number reached 3,047, with 87 percent of these abortions performed after invoking the law's socioeconomic clause.[118]

In 1997, the Polish Constitutional Tribunal, a constitutional body that is independent from the president, parliament, and the Council of Ministers, ruled against the reliberalization of the abortion law.[119] The return to the more restrictive version of the Anti-Abortion Law once again forced Polish women to seek help in the abortion underground or to travel abroad to access abortion services. Many women who were denied access to legal abortion in Poland turned to the Federation for Women and Family Planning.[120]

In the late 1990s, abortion travel outside Poland received only limited coverage in the press. However, one article in *Gazeta Wyborcza* published in 1997 explored the ways in which EU membership could facilitate abortion tourism from countries with restrictive abortion laws to those with more liberal approaches to abortion services: "But why do we need national regulations, since in uniting Europe one can benefit from a hospital in any country? The French woman who settled in the south of the country, and to whom the gynecologist refused an abortion, gets in a car and after a few hours she is in a Spanish maternity ward. Italians and Irish women travel to Britain, German and Belgian women to the Netherlands. Ninety percent of abortions performed in late pregnancy in Dutch clinics are foreigners. The number of women using treatments abroad is estimated at 15 thousand."[121] This excerpt showcases the valuable role of the EU in terms of access to abortion services, and one with which Niklas Barke grapples in his contribution to this volume, as well as the importance of neighboring regions that provide abortion services, a recurring theme in several chapters.

Poland became an EU member in 2004, but a year earlier, it was a target of a pro-choice campaign by Women on Waves (WOW). Founded in 1999, WOW has brought to light a lack of abortion services in several countries by sailing a Dutch ship that provides sexual and reproductive health services and includes an abortion clinic on board. The organization now concentrates mainly on web-based abortion counseling and on supplying women internationally with abortion pills mifepristone and misoprostol by mail to procure a medical abortion.[122] Poland also joined the Schengen Agreement in 2007, which facilitates the free movement of people, goods, services, and capital across the borders of 26 European states, and is discussed in this context by Niklas Barke in his chapter in this volume. This agreement has contributed greatly to Polish women's access to abortion services abroad. Polish women now travel, preferably to Germany, Czech Republic, Austria, and Slovakia for abortion services. They also go to Britain, which is not a Schengen Area country but is, like Poland, a member of the EU. This kind of abortion tourism is an attractive alternative to the illegal abortion underground.[123]

Some Polish feminist organizations have used abortion tourism as a pretext to bring public attention to the inaccessibility of abortion services and the negative treatment of women using the illegal abortion underground, mirroring developments in many chapters in this volume. In 2010, an informal pro-choice women's group, Separatystyczne Rewolucyjne Oddziały Maciczne (Separatist Revolutionary Womb Brigades), from the city of Łódź organized a publicity campaign because access to medical abortions was still effectively limited. It distributed a poster featuring a young, white, slim, blond-haired woman wearing a white bra and panties and leaning against a brick wall. The slogan "MY CHOICE" appears in English in red paint across her exposed stomach. The poster's Polish-language text resembles a contemporary advertising campaign promoting the use of Mastercard to purchase a list of desirable items on credit. It encourages women to participate in abortion tourism to access safe and legal abortion services rather than resort to the illegal abortion underground, a choice also promoted among Spanish women, as Agata Ignaciuk investigates in this volume. The Polish-language text reads:

Return ticket to England: special offer—300 zloty
Accommodation—240 zloty
Medical abortion in a public clinic—0 zloty

Relief after termination performed under good
conditions—PRICELESS.
For everything you pay less than for an underground abortion in
Poland.

This campaign circulated widely in the media, but it soon attracted the interest of the public prosecutor, who wanted to determine whether it constituted a violation of the existing abortion law. However, nobody was arrested or convicted. Other Polish cities took up the campaign to draw attention to the problem of the illegal abortion underground.

Polish women's abortion tourism has intensified in the 2010s and so too has Polish women's pro-choice activism. As indicated by Wanda Nowicka, the president of the Federation for Women and Family Planning, due to the growing numbers of Polish clients, abortion clinics in Britain and Germany translated information on their websites into Polish. In the present volume, authors Anna Bogic and Agata Ignaciuk individually review in more depth the significance of translating information about abortion or access to abortion services from English into local languages. In August 2010, the federation, together with Marek Balicki, a Polish politician and former minister of health, organized public hearings on abortion tourism. Gynecologists Dr. Christian Fiala from Vienna, Austria, and Dr. Janusz Rudziński from Prenzlau, Germany, testified at the hearings and estimated that the number of Polish women seeking abortion at their clinics ranged from 200 to 400 annually.[124] Most clients of such clinics were well-off, educated women from large Polish cities such as Warsaw, Poznań, and Wrocław.[125]

In June 2015, the limited access to abortion services in Poland served as the basis for another WOW pro-choice campaign. An Abortion Drone campaign was organized in cooperation with activists from a women's group in Berlin called Ciocia Basia (Aunty Basia) that assists Polish women traveling to Berlin for abortion services. Founded by one German and one Polish woman, this group emerged because of the difficulties Polish women face when ordering abortion pills from WOW for delivery to Poland because Polish customs officers withhold their parcels. The group provides help with translation, counseling, and accommodation services, and sometimes even financial support. Some women needing late-term abortions are sent to the Netherlands, where termination remains legal until 22 weeks of pregnancy.[126] Other feminist organizations joined Aunty Basia, including the Polish Feminoteka

Foundation (Feminist Foundation) and Stowarzyszenie Porozumienie Kobiet 8 Marca (March 8th Women's Coalition Association), and a Berlin-based group supporting Irish women seeking abortion services called Berlin-Ireland Pro-Choice Solidarity.

Taking cues from Google and Amazon, globally successful businesses that have tested drones to deliver goods to customers, WOW launched for the first time on June 27, 2015, a drone carrying two packages of abortion pills from Frankfurt an der Oder to the Polish border town of Słubice.[127] Despite interventions by the German police, the drone landed in Słubice without incident, its flight captured by its camera. After the drone landed, one of the participating Polish activists immediately swallowed the first set of pills. The second package was destined for another Polish woman.[128] The abortion drone received widespread media coverage, with some detractors expressing concern that the campaign would lead to the extinction of the Polish nation. Dr. Antoni Zięba, president of the pro-life organization Polskie Stowarzyszenie Obrońców Życia Człowieka (Polish Association of Human Life Defenders), compared the delivery of abortion pills by drone from Germany to Poland to "the darkest elements of Polish-German relations during the Second World War, when Hitler planned to destroy Poland through the promotion of abortion and contraception."[129] Such opinions are quite prevalent, and they aim at presenting abortion as a destructive foreign influence on this Catholic nation. Consequently, pro-choice supporters are othered as pro-Communist, anti-Catholic, and antipatriotic; abortion is equated with genocide; and pregnant women are highly sentimentalized as blessed by God.

Since the Abortion Drone campaign, there have been several attempts to limit Polish women's reproductive rights by an aggressively pronatalist government led by the Law and Justice Party that is supported by the Catholic Church. In September 2015, members of parliament debated a draft of a "Stop Abortion Law" that proposes to ban abortion except to preserve the pregnant woman's life and criminalizes both doctors who perform abortions and women who end their pregnancies for any other reason.[130] Two months later, the Ministry of Health began to question the over-the-counter availability of emergency contraception, eventually classifying it as a prescription-only drug. The Polish government also decided to replace a state-subsidized IVF program with a national procreation program founded on naprotechnology (natural procreative technology). State sanction of this faith-based model of biomedical reproductive healthcare is considered proof of the stigmatization of many reproductive health services for women and the domination of these services by the Catholic Church and right-wing politicians after 1989.[131]

A major protest against the proposed Stop Abortion Law took place in September 2016, featuring large numbers of women (and some men) outside parliament. Acknowledging that approximately 150,000 illegal abortions were taking place in Poland every year, Krystyna Kacpura, the executive director of the Federation for Women and Family Planning, was moved enough by the rally to state: "It is as if Polish women have woken up from a long dream. We had grown accustomed to our [1993] abortion law (the wealthy merely paid for the plane tickets and medical procedures needed to work around it) and everyone seemed to accept it as a measure to keep the peace in our predominantly Catholic country. But even Catholic women are appalled at the move by the Law and Justice party to restrict our already limited reproductive rights [with the proposed Stop Abortion Law]. 'Not one step further,' goes the rallying cry."[132] When parliament refused to consider feminist draft legislation in the place of the proposed Stop Abortion Law, the aforementioned protest was followed by "Black Monday," a national women's strike held on November 3, 2016, to call attention to the threat of the further criminalization of abortion and its consequences for women. The strike was a great success in terms of women's solidarity. And because it managed to inject the language of reproductive rights into public debate, it may be a sign of positive change on the horizon.[133]

Conclusion

Polish women have waged a long and difficult battle for their reproductive rights since the end of the Communist era. It is significant that public discussions concerning women's reproductive rights are conjoined by wider concerns and anxieties about postcommunist Polish national identity. Women's reproductive rights are very problematic in Poland. On the one hand, over the past years, state authorities have been reluctant to introduce any changes to the 1993 Anti-Abortion Law. On the other hand, the influence of the Catholic Church impedes a comprehensive public debate on the matter of abortion. One main reason for state authorities' reluctance to secure abortion access lies in Catholic pro-life beliefs held by right-wing politicians, healthcare providers, pharmacists, and pro-life activists who do not recognize a woman's right to make choices freely and independently in regard to their reproductive lives. Moreover, they actively deny women this right by focusing far more on the right of the unborn to live. While some women are provided with high-standard reproductive healthcare, especially if they are socioeconomically privileged, most have to rely on limited, state-provided, and/or state-funded medical treatment. Polish authorities actually do very little to change the situation of Polish women. Even though the Polish government is obliged to issue annual reports about family planning counseling and legal abortion, it does not take into serious consideration the consequences of the 1993 law, turning its back on the illegal abortion underground and abortion tourism.

Acknowledgments

I would like to thank Christabelle Sethna and Agata Ignaciuk for comments and editing that greatly improved this chapter. All translations by author.

Notes

1. "Miałam aborcję na Słowacji," *Wysokie Obcasy*, October 9, 2012, http://www.wysokieobcasy.pl/wysokie-obcasy/1,96856,12548978,Mialam _aborcje_na_Slowacji.html. All translations in this chapter are by the author.

2. See Federation for Women and Family Planning, *Piekło kobiet trwa: Historie opowiedziane podczas II Trybunału na rzecz Prawa Kobiet do Samostanowienia O GODNOŚĆ KOBIETY* (Warsaw: Federation for Women and Family Planning, 2007); Federation for Women and Family Planning, *20 lat tzw. ustawy antyaborcyjnej w Polsce: Raport 2013* (Warsaw: Federation for Women and Family Planning, 2013), http://federa.org.pl/wp-content/uploads/2017/07 /raport_federacja_2013.pdf.

3. "Koszt aborcji," GynMed, accessed August 10, 2017, https://www.gynmed .at/pl/aborcja/koszt.

4. "Transport do kliniki," MediKlinik, accessed August 10, 2017, http://www .mediklinik.sk/pl/transport-do-kliniki; Agnieszka Hreczuk, "Ciocie Basie," *Polityka*, February 28, 2017, https://www.polityka.pl/tygodnikpolityka/swiat /1695412,1,kim-sa-kobiety-pomagajace-polkom-dokonujacym-w-niemczech -aborcji.read; Marta Syrwid, "Polki jadą po aborcję na Słowację," *Duży Format*, January 28, 2016, http://wyborcza.pl/duzyformat/1,127290,19540669,polki -jada-po-aborcje-na-slowacje.html; Federation for Women and Family Planning, *20 lat*, 7, 22.

5. Federation for Women and Family Planning, *20 lat*, 21–22; Federation for Women and Family Planning, "Skutki ustawy antyaborcyjnej—Raport Federacji 1996," unpublished report, 2–3; "Zabieg wykonałam wieszakiem," in *A jak hipokryzja: Antologia tekstów o aborcji, władzy, pieniądzach i sprawiedliwości*, ed. Claudia Snochowska-Gonzalez (Warsaw: O Matko!, 2011), 76.

6. Magdalena Środa, "Kobiety, Kościół, katolicyzm," in *Czarna księga kobiet,* ed. Christine Ockrent (Warsaw: Wydawnictwo W. A. B., 2007), 655.

7. Mirosław Chałubiński, "Polityka, kościół, aborcja," in *Polityka i aborcja,* ed. Mirosław Chałubiński (Warsaw: Scholar, 1994), 107, 135. See also Jacek Raciborski, "Kościół i wybory," in Chałubiński, *Polityka i aborcja,* 157, and Joanna Mishtal, "Quietly 'Beating the System': The Logics of Protest and Resistance under the Polish Abortion Ban," ed. Silvia De Zordo, Joanna Mishtal, and Lorena Anton, *A Fragmented Landscape: Abortion Governance and Protest Logics in Europe* (New York and Oxford: Berghahn Books, 2017), 226–44.

8. When searching for articles about the illegal abortion underground and abortion tourism, I used search engines available in newspapers and internet archives by entering these keywords/phrases: "abortion," "termination of pregnancy," "abortion tourism," and "abortion underground." Time frame: from 1993 to 2017. To access articles published in *Bluszcz* magazine, I used the archives of the Digital Library of Wielkopolska, available at: http://www.wbc .poznan.pl/dlibra?action=ChangeLanguageAction&language=en.

9. See Federation for Women and Family Planning, *Piekło kobiet. Historie współczesne* (Warsaw: Federation for Women and Family Planning, 2001); Federation for Women and Family Planning, *Piekło kobiet trwa* (Warsaw: Federation for Women and Family Planning, 2007); Claudia Snochowska-Gonzalez, ed., *A jak hipokryzja: Antologia tekstów o aborcji, władzy, pieniądzach i sprawiedliwości* (Warsaw: O Matko!, 2011), 11, 24, 37, 55, 76, 87, 124, 147.

10. Wanda Nowicka and Eleonora Zielińska, "Zdrowie kobiet w Polsce," in *Raport Kobiety dla Polski. Polska dla kobiet: 20 lat transformacji 1989–2009,* ed. Joanna Piotrowska and Agnieszka Grzybek (Warsaw: Fundacja Feminoteka, 2009), 288; Wanda Nowicka, "Prawa reprodukcyjne w Polsce," in *Czarna księga kobiet,* ed. Christine Ockrent (Warsaw: Wydawnictwo W. A. B., 2007); Kazimiera Szczuka, *Milczenie owieczek—rzecz o aborcji* (Warsaw: Wydawnictwo W. A. B., 2004). See also Eleonora Zielińska, "Between Ideology, Politics, and Common Sense: The Discourse of Reproductive Rights in Poland," in *Reproducing Gender: Politics, Publics, and Everyday Life after Socialism,* ed. Susan Gal and Gail Kligman (Princeton, NJ: Princeton University Press, 2000), 23–57.

11. Jacek Kochanowski, preface to Polish edition to *The Social Construction of Sexuality,* ed. Steven Seidman (Warsaw: Wydawnictwo Naukowe PWN, 2012), 15.

12. Anne-Marie Kramer, "The Polish Parliament and the Making of Politics through Abortion," *International Feminist Journal of Politics* 11, no. 1 (2009): 82, http://doi.org/10.1080/14616740802567824.

13. See also Anna Bogic, "Our Bodies, Our Location: The Politics of Feminist Translation and Reproduction in Post-socialist Serbia" (PhD diss., University of Ottawa, 2017).

14. Monika Płatek, "Rzecz o bezpieczeństwie kobiet w prawie karnym," in *Czarna Księga Kobiet,* ed. Christine Ockrent (Warsaw: Wydawnictwo W. A. B., 2011); Eleonora Zielińska, "Prawo wobec kobiet: Refleksja w dwudziestą

rocznicę kontraktu Okrągłego Stołu," in *Gender w społeczeństwie polskim*, ed. Krystyna Slany, Justyna Struzik, and Katarzyna Wojnicka (Kraków: Nomos, 2011); Katarzyna Szumlewicz, "Kobiety i transformacja ustrojowa w Polsce," *Lewą Nogą: Półrocznik Polityczno-Artystyczny* 16, no. 4 (2004): 225–31.

15. Ewelina Ciaputa et al., "Macierzyństwo kobiet z niepełnosprawnościami ruchu, wzroku i słuchu," *Studia Socjologiczne* 2, no. 213 (2014): 203–25; Agata Chełstowska, "Sprawiedliwość społeczna i sprawiedliwość reprodukcyjna," in Snochowska-Gonzalez, *A jak hipokryzja*; Izabela Desperak, "Ile to kosztuje? Edukacja, antykoncepcja, aborcja i rynek," in Snochowska-Gonzalez, *A jak hipokryzja*; Nowicka and Zielińska, "Zdrowie kobiet w Polsce."

16. Anna Titkow, *Tożsamość polskich kobiet: Ciągłość, zmiana, konteksty* (Warsaw: Wydawnictwo Instytutu Filozofii i Socjologii Polskiej Akademii Nauk, 2007), 71; Katarzyna Zielińska, "W poszukiwaniu nowej wspólnoty? Feministki o narodzie, obywatelstwie i demokracji," in *Ponad granicami: Kobiety, migracje, obywatelstwo*, ed. Marta Warat and Agnieszka Małek (Kraków: Wydawnictwo Uniwersytetu Jagiellońskiego, 2010), 68.

17. Agnieszka Graff, *Magma i inne próby zrozumienia, o co tu chodzi* (Warsaw: Wydawnictwo Krytyki Politycznej, 2010), 33.

18. See Agnieszka Graff, *Rykoszetem: Rzecz o płci, seksualności i narodzie* (Warsaw: Wydawnictwo W. A. B., 2008); and Joanna Mishtal, *The Politics of Morality: The Church, the State, and Reproductive Rights in Postsocialist Poland* (Athens: University of Ohio Press, 2015).

19. Zielińska, "W poszukiwaniu nowej wspólnoty," 63. See also Irena Borowik, *Procesy instytucjonalizacji i prywatyzacji religii* (Kraków: Wydawnictwo Uniwersytetu Jagiellońskiego, 1997); Zdzisław Mach, "The Roman Catholic Church and the Transformation of Social Identity in Eastern and Central Europe," in *New Religious Phenomena in Central and Eastern Europe*, ed. Irena Borowik and Grzegorz Babiński (Kraków: Nomos, 1997), 63–79; Graff, *Magma*, 64–65.

20. Alicia Czerwinski, "Sex, Politics, and Religion: The Clash between Poland and the European Union over Abortion," *Denver Journal of International Law Policy* 32, no. 4 (2004): 659.

21. Rachel Alsop and Jenny Hockey, "Women's Reproductive Lives as a Symbolic Resource in Central and Eastern Europe," *European Journal of Women's Studies* 8, no. 454 (2010): 461, https://doi.org/10.1177/1350506810080404.

22. Aleksandra Czajkowska, "O dopuszczalności przerywania ciąży: Ustawa z dnia 27 kwietnia 1956 r. i towarzyszące jej dyskusje," in *Kłopoty z seksem w PRL: Rodzenie nie całkiem po ludzku, aborcja, choroby, odmienności*, ed. Marcin Kula (Warsaw: Wydawnictwa Uniwersytetu Warszawskiego, 2012), 108.

23. Eleonora Zielińska, *Przerywanie ciąży: Warunki legalności w Polsce i na świecie* (Warsaw: Wydawnictwo Prawnicze, 1990), 33, 38.

24. Contacts between activists for "birth control" were initiated in the 1930s but continued after the second global military conflict, mainly via letters exchanged between Margaret Sanger and Polish physician Herman Rubinraut. See Sylwia Kuźma Markowska, "Transatlantyckie kontakty działaczy na rzecz kontroli urodzeń w Polsce i Stanach Zjednoczonych (1931–1960)," *Dzieje*

Najnowsze 39, no. 4 (2007): 199–214. See also Magdalena Gawin, "Planowanie rodziny—hasła i rzeczywistość," in *Równe prawa i nierówne szanse: Kobiety w Polsce międzywojennej*, ed. Anna Żarnowska and Andrzej Szwarc (Warsaw: Wydawnictwo DIG, 2000): 221–22.

25. Czajkowska, "O dopuszczalności przerywania ciąży," 108–9.

26. Michał Pietrzak, "Sytuacja prawna kobiet w Drugiej Rzeczypospolitej," in Żarnowska and Szwarc, *Równe prawa i nierówne szanse*, 83.

27. Jerzy Kolarzowski, "Polski spór o aborcję: Konsekwencje rozstrzygnięć legislacyjnych," in *Polityka i aborcja*, ed. Mirosław Chałubiński (Warsaw: Scholar, 1994), 173. See also Pietrzak, "Sytuacja prawna kobiet w Drugiej Rzeczypospolitej," 83; Zielińska, *Przerywanie ciąży*, 48; and Szczuka, *Milczenie owieczek*, 209.

28. Andrzej Gawryszewski, *Ludność Polski w XX wieku* (Warsaw: Instytut Geografii i Przestrzennego Zagospodarowania imienia Stanisława Leszczyckiego Polskiej Akademii Nauk, 2005), 337.

29. Gawin, "Planowanie rodziny—hasła i rzeczywistość," 223. See also Gawryszewski, *Ludność Polski w XX wieku*, 173.

30. Gawryszewski, *Ludność Polski w XX wieku*, 84.

31. Gawin, "Planowanie rodziny—hasła i rzeczywistość," 225.

32. Gawin, "Planowanie rodziny—hasła i rzeczywistość," 226.

33. Krystyna Slany, "Legal Regulations of Abortion in Poland in the Interwar Period as a Part of Family Policy," in *Issues through the History of Social Work in Poland and the World*, ed. I. Szczepaniak-Wiecha, A. Małek, and K. Slany (Kraków: Jagiellonian University Press, 2006); Gawin, "Planowanie rodziny—hasła i rzeczywistość," 226.

34. Gawin, "Planowanie rodziny—hasła i rzeczywistość," 227.

35. Marta Gaudyn, "Lata dwudzieste, lata współczesne," in Snochowska-Gonzalez, *A jak hipokryzja*, 117; Kolarzowski, "Polski spór o aborcję," 173–74.

36. Gawin, "Planowanie rodziny—hasła i rzeczywistość," 234–35.

37. Quoted in Gaudyn, "Lata dwudzieste, lata współczesne," 115.

38. Szczuka, *Milczenie owieczek*, 211.

39. Tadeusz Boy-Żeleński, *Piekło kobiet* (Warsaw: Rijafa Roja, 2013), 8–9; and Szczuka, *Milczenie owieczek*, 191.

40. Zofia Galicka, "W sprawie art. 141 i 142," *Bluszcz*, no. 15 (1930): 20.

41. Felicja Kowalewska, "Zanim klamka zapadnie," *Bluszcz*, no. 19 (1930): 19.

42. Czajkowska, "O dopuszczalności przerywania ciąży," 111.

43. Gawin, "Planowanie rodziny—hasła i rzeczywistość," 232–33; Katarzyna Sierakowska, "Macierzyństwo—wizje a rzeczywistość," in Żarnowska and Szwarc, *Równe prawa i nierówne szanse*, 212.

44. Barbara Klich-Kluczewska, "Making Up for the Losses of War: Reproduction Politics in Post-War Poland," in *Women and Men at War: A Gender Perspective on World War II and Its Aftermath in Central and Eastern Europe*, ed. Maren Roger and Ruth Leiserowitz (Osnabruck: Verlag, 2012), 320n37.

45. Gawin, "Planowanie rodziny—hasła i rzeczywistość," 228–30.

46. Gaudyn, "Lata dwudzieste, lata współczesne," 117.

47. Gawin, "Planowanie rodziny—hasła i rzeczywistość," 237.

48. Zielińska, *Przerywanie ciąży*, 49.

49. Czajkowska, "O dopuszczalności przerywania ciąży," 109–10.

50. Reprinted in Gawin, "Planowanie rodziny—hasła i rzeczywistość," 230.

51. Zielińska, *Przerywanie ciąży*, 52–53; Czajkowska, "O dopuszczalności przerywania ciąży," 137.

52. Klich-Kluczewska, "Making Up for the Losses of War," 307.

53. For a more nuanced picture of physicians' attitudes toward law revision, see Kuźma-Markowska, "Transantlantyckie kontakty," 208–10. It is also worth mentioning that the discourse on abortion in postwar Poland can be characterized by a change in the rhetoric used, for example, the term "fetus" was replaced by "unborn child," and that although attempts to tighten Polish abortion law started in 1949 with Stanisław Chrempiński's proposal in a specialist legal journal, proposed amendments never affected the existing law; see Klich-Kluczewska, "Making Up for the Losses," 323–24.

54. Those measures include medals awarded to women (especially from rural areas) with numerous children, financial benefits (maternity, childbirth, family), benefits for nonworking mothers, child facilities for working and single mothers, as well as the introduction of a 1975 law that enabled women to take early retirement. See Klich-Kluczewska, "Making Up for the Losses," 312, 315–18; Jacqueline Heinen and Monika Wator, "Child Care in Poland before, during, and after the Transition: Still a Women's Business," *Social Politics: International Studies in Gender, State and Society* 13, no. 2 (2006): 192–94.

55. Klich-Kluczewska, "Making Up for the Losses," 320; and Agata Ignaciuk, "'Clueless about Contraception': The Introduction and Circulation of the Contraceptive Pill in State-Socialist Poland (1960s-1970s)," *Medicina nei Secoli* 26, no. 2 (2014): 511–12.

56. Klich-Kluczewska, "Making Up for the Losses," 321.

57. Henry P. David and Joanna Skilogianis, eds., *From Abortion to Contraception: A Resource to Public Policies and Reproductive Behavior in Central and Eastern Europe from 1917 to the Present* (Westport, CT: Greenwood Press, 1999), 170.

58. See Agata Ignaciuk, "'Ten szkodliwy zabieg': Dyskursy na temat aborcji w publikacjach Towarzystwa Świadomego Macierzyństwa/Towarzystwa Planowania Rodziny (1956–1980)," *Zeszyty Etnologii Wrocławskiej* 1, no. 20 (2014): 79–80; David and Skilogianis, eds., *From Abortion to Contraception*, 170.

59. Sylwia Kuźma-Markowska, "Aborcja, eugenika, totalitaryzm—czyli czym różniło się przerywanie ciąży 'za Hitlera' i 'za Stalina,'" in Snochowska-Gonzalez, *A jak hipokryzja*, 144.

60. Women worked a "second shift," a term coined by Arlie Russell Hochschild, *The Second Shift: Working Families and the Revolution at Home* (New York: Viking, 1989).

61. Czajkowska, "O dopuszczalności przerywania ciąży," 115–26; Heinen and Wator, "Child Care in Poland," 192.

62. From 1971 to 1979, it was known as the Polish Society for Planned Motherhood, and from 1979 until today as the Polish Society for Family Development. See Ignaciuk, "Ten szkodliwy zabieg," 78.

63. Ignaciuk, "Ten szkodliwy zabieg," 90–95.

64. Czajkowska, "O dopuszczalności przerywania ciąży," 133–35; Małgorzata Fidelis, *Women, Communism, and Industrialization in Postwar Poland* (Cambridge: Cambridge University Press, 2010), 231.

65. Czajkowska, "O dopuszczalności przerywania ciąży," 113, 115, 145–49; Ignaciuk, "Ten szkodliwy zabieg," 81.

66. Czajkowska, "O dopuszczalności przerywania ciąży," 162, 175.

67. Czajkowska, "O dopuszczalności przerywania ciąży," 162–66.

68. Czajkowska, "O dopuszczalności przerywania ciąży," 159–60; Ignaciuk, "'Clueless about Contraception,'" 512.

69. Czajkowska, "O dopuszczalności przerywania ciąży," 164–66; Fidelis, *Women, Communism*, 198–99.

70. Czajkowska, "O dopuszczalności przerywania ciąży," 177.

71. Czajkowska, "O dopuszczalności przerywania ciąży," 177.

72. Reprinted in Czajkowska, "O dopuszczalności przerywania ciąży," 179–80.

73. Czajkowska, "O dopuszczalności przerywania ciąży," 179.

74. Ignaciuk, "'Clueless about Contraception,'" 514; and Czajkowska, "O dopuszczalności przerywania ciąży," 179.

75. Czajkowska, "O dopuszczalności przerywania ciąży," 180.

76. Czajkowska, "O dopuszczalności przerywania ciąży," 179.

77. Kolarzowski, "Polski spór o aborcję," 174.

78. Quoted in Czajkowska, "O dopuszczalności przerywania ciąży," 167.

79. Czerwinski, "Sex, Politics, and Religion," 656; and Chałubiński, "Polityka, kościół, aborcja," 94–95.

80. Jacqueline Heinen and Anna Matuchniak-Krasuska, *Aborcja w Polsce: Kwadratura koła* (Warsaw: Polskie Towarzystwo Religioznawcze, 1995), 93.

81. Kolarzowski, "Polski spór o aborcję," 175; and Heinen and Matuchniak-Krasuska, *Aborcja w Polsce*, 93.

82. Christabelle Sethna and Marion Doull, "Accidental Tourists: Canadian Women, Abortion Tourism, and Travel," *Women's Studies* 41, no. 4 (2012): 470; Lena Lennerhed, "Abortion, Sex-Liberalism and Feminism in Sweden in the 1960s/70s," *Women's History Magazine* 73 (Autumn 2013): 13–18; Elżbieta Korolczuk, "Lekcja szwedzkiego: 'turystyka aborcyjna' a legislacja dotycząca aborcji," in Snochowska-Gonzalez, *A jak hipokryzja*, 83; Per Gunnar Cassel, *Induced Legal Abortion in Sweden during 1939–1974: Change in Practice and Legal Reform*, working paper 2009: 1, 9, http://www.stressforskning.su.se/polopoly_fs/1.18721.1320939636!/WP_2009_1.pdf.

83. See Cassel, *Induced Legal Abortion*, 9–10; and Lennerhed, "Abortion, Sex-Liberalism," 15.

84. Lennerhed, "Abortion, Sex-Liberalism," 13–17.

85. Peter D. Mazur, "Contraception and Abortion in Poland," *Family Planning Perspectives* 13, no. 4 (1981): 196.

86. Heinen and Wator, "Child Care in Poland," 192; Fidelis, *Women, Communism*, 170–71.

87. Fidelis, *Women, Communism*, 245; Zielińska, *Przerywanie ciąży*, 59; Heinen and Wator, "Child Care in Poland," 195.

88. Heinen and Wator, "Child Care in Poland," 195.

89. Ignaciuk, "'Clueless about Contraception,'" 523.

90. Marek Okólski, "Abortion and Contraception in Poland," *Studies in Family Planning* 14, no. 1 (1983): 269. See also Ignaciuk, "'Clueless about Contraception,'" 523–24.

91. Okólski, "Abortion and Contraception in Poland," 265.

92. Kolarzowski, "Polski spór o aborcję," 175.

93. Ewelina Wejbert-Wąsiewicz, *Aborcja między ideologią a doświadczeniem indywidualnym: Monografia zjawiska* (Łódź: Wydawnictwo Uniwersytetu Łódzkiego, 2011), 77.

94. Krystyna Ostrowska, "Psychologiczne problemy kobiet podejmujących decyzję o przerywaniu ciąży," *Studia Philosophiae Christianae* 25, no. 2 (1989): 104. See also Zielińska, *Przerywanie ciąży*, 62.

95. Wejbert-Wąsiewicz, *Aborcja między ideologią*, 77. See also Agata Chełstowska, "Stigmatisation and Commercialization of Abortion Services in Poland: Turning Sin into Gold," *Reproductive Health Matters* 19, no. 37 (2011): 98–106.

96. Zielińska, *Przerywanie ciąży*, 63–64; and Hanna Jankowska, "Abortion, Church and Politics in Poland," *Feminist Review*, no. 39 (Autumn 1991): 176.

97. Zielińska, *Przerywanie ciąży*, 65; Jankowska, "Abortion, Church," 176.

98. Andrzej Piotrowski, 'Tożsamość zbiorowa jako temat dyskursu polityki: Dwa przemówienia parlamentarne—analiza przypadku," in *Rytualny chaos: Studium dyskursu publicznego*, ed. Marek Czyżewski, Sergiusz Kowalski, and Andrzej Piotrowski (Kraków: Aureus, 1997), 197–224.

99. Kramer, "The Polish Parliament," 83.

100. Środa, *Kobiety i władza*, 218–25.

101. Centrum Badania Opinii Społecznej, *Opinia publiczna o prawie do przerywania ciąży* (Warsaw: Centrum Badania Opinii Społecznej, 1992), 7; and Centrum Badania Opinii Społecznej, *Dopuszczalność aborcji w różnych sytuacjach* (Warsaw: Centrum Badania Opinii Społecznej, 2016), 7.

102. Płatek, "Rzecz o bezpieczeństwie kobiet," 664.

103. Okólski, "Abortion and Contraception in Poland," 265–66; Mazur, "Contraception and Abortion in Poland," 195.

104. Irena Kotowska et al., *Kobiety w Polsce* (Warsaw: Główny Urząd Statystyczny, 2007), 88.

105. *Sprawozdanie Rady Ministrów z wykonywania oraz o skutkach stosowania w 2015 r. Ustawy z dnia 7 stycznia 1993 r. O planowaniu rodziny, ochronie płodu ludzkiego i warunkach dopuszczalności przerywania ciąży* (Journal of Laws no. 78, as subsequently amended.) (Warsaw, 2017), 81.

106. Główny Urząd Statystyczny, *Rocznik demograficzny* (Warsaw: Główny Urząd Statystyczny, 2016), 76.

107. "Fikcja legalnej aborcji: To prawo jest martwe," tvn24.pl, October 21, 2016, http://www.tvn24.pl/wiadomosci-z-kraju,3/legalna-aborcja-jest-fikcja-to-prawo-jest-martwe,685673.html; Marcin Kobiałka, "Rzeszów: lekarze Pro-Familii podpisali klauzulę sumienia," Onet.pl, May 11, 2016, https://rzeszow.onet.pl/rzeszow-lekarze-pro-familii-podpisali-klauzule-sumienia/gd6wll; Federation for Women and Family Planning, "Dzień dobry, chcę przerwać ciążę . . ." O procedurach dostępu do legalnej aborcji w polskich szpitalach (Warsaw: Federation for Women and Family Planning, 2016), 12, 17.

108. Paweł Ozdoba, "Kolejny protest działaczy prolife: Antyaborcyjny samochód stanął przed szpitalem w Warszawie," dorzeczy.pl, June 21, 2017, https://dorzeczy.pl/kraj/33145/Kolejny-protest-dzialaczy-prolife-Antyaborcyjny-samochod-stanal-przed-szpitalem-w-Warszawie.html; Paweł Kopeć, "Antyaborcyjny protest przed Szpitalem Uniwersyteckim w Dzień Dziecka," wyborcza.pl (Kraków), June 1, 2017, http://krakow.wyborcza.pl/krakow/7,44425,21898275, antyaborcyjny-protest-przed-szpitalem-uniwersyteckim-w-dzien.html.

109. Federation for Women and Family Planning, 20 *lat*, 69–70; Wanda Nowicka and Agnieszka Walko-Mazurek, *Zawsze po stronie kobiet: 20 lat Federacji na rzecz Kobiet i Planowania Rodziny* (Warsaw: Federation for Women and Family Planning, 2011), 24.

110. Gaudyn, "Lata dwudzieste, lata współczesne," 113; Federation for Women and Family Planning, *Piekło kobiet trwa*, 32; Federation for Women and Family Planning, 20 *lat*, 19–20.

111. Jacqueline Heinen and Stephane Portet, "Reproductive Rights in Poland: When Politicians Fear the Wrath of the Church," *Third World Quarterly* 31, no. 6 (2010): 1008–11, 1015–17.

112. Federation for Women and Family Planning, 20 *lat*, 19.

113. Federation for Women and Family Planning, 20 *lat*, 19.

114. Federation for Women and Family Planning, 20 *lat*, 19.

115. Federation for Women and Family Planning, 20 *lat*, 2.

116. Federation for Women and Family Planning, 20 *lat*, 3–4.

117. Federation for Women and Family Planning, "Skutki ustawy antyaborcyjnej—Raport Federacji 2000," 5 (unpublished report).

118. *Sprawozdanie z realizacji wykonania w roku 1997 zapisów ustawy z dnia 7 stycznia 1993 r. o planowaniu rodziny, ochronie płodu ludzkiego i warunkach dopuszczalności przerywania ciąży*. Form no 592 (Warsaw, 1998), 34–35, 37.

119. Urszula Nowakowska and Maja Korzeniewska, "Prawa kobiet w sferze prokreacji," in *Kobiety w Polsce w latach 90: Raport Centrum Praw Kobiet* (Warsaw: Centrum Praw Kobiet, 2000), 228–29. The current Polish Constitution, Article 18 states: "Marriage, being a union of a man and a woman, as well as the family, motherhood and parenthood, shall be placed under the protection and care of the Republic of Poland." The development of the Polish constitution has its ideological roots in Catholic doctrine. See the statement by Marek Krzaklewski, leader of *Solidarność*, quoted in Aldona Mazur, "Geneza regulacji konstytucyjnych dotyczących ochrony rodziny," *Acta Universitatis Wratislaviensis*, no. 3322 (2011): 196.

120. Nowicka and Walko-Mazurek, *Zawsze po stronie kobiet*, 22–24, 35.

121. "Unijna turystyka aborcyjna," *Gazeta Wyborcza*, July 2, 1997, 10.

122. Nowicka and Walko-Mazurek, *Zawsze po stronie kobiet*, 20; Wanda Nowicka, "Starania o liberalizację ustawy antyaborcyjnej w latach 1993–2005," in *Homofobia, mizoginia i ciemnogród? Burzliwe losy kontrowersyjnych ustaw*, ed. Iza Desperak (Łódź: Omega-Praxis, 2008), 44.

123. Federation for Women and Family Planning, *Prawa reprodukcyjne w Polsce: Skutki ustawy antyaborcyjnej. Raport, September 2007* (Warsaw: Federation for Women and Family Planning, 2007); Federation for Women and

Family Planning, 20 *lat*, 21–22. See also Kalina Błażejowska, "U ginekologa boli bardziej," *Wysokie Obcasy*, July 1, 2017.

124. "Turystyka aborcyjna Polek," *Sejm RP*, August 26, 2010. Online archives of Federation for Women and Family Planning, accessed June 10, 2015, http://www.federa.org.pl/dokumenty_pdf/podrzedne/wysluchaniepodsumowanie .pdf (page no longer available).

125. "Turystyka aborcyjna Polek," 3.

126. See "(Germany) Ciocia Basia," Women Help Women, accessed August 10, 2017, https://womenhelp.org/en/page/405/germany-ciocia-basia; and Claudia Snochowska-Gonzalez, "Pociagiem po aborcję: Ciocia Basia pomoże w zorganizowaniu bezpiecznego zabiegu w Berlinie," *Wysokie Obcasy*, July 23, 2016, http://www.wysokieobcasy.pl/wysokie-obcasy /1,149982,20432960,pociagiem-po-aborcje-kazdy-moze-zadzwonic-do-cioci -basi-i-uzyskac.html.

127. "Dron aborcyjny—pierwszy lot do Polski," Women on Waves, accessed June 30, 2016, http://www.womenonwaves.org/pl/page/5636/abortion-drone— first-flight-to-poland.

128. "Dron aborcyjny przyleciał do Polski," tvn24.pl, June 27, 2015, http://www.tvn24.pl/wiadomosci-z-kraju,3/dron-aborcyjny-przylecial-z -frankfurtu-na-odra-do-slubic,555268.html.

129. "Dron aborcyjny leci nad Polskę," *Niezależna*, June 23, 2015, http:// niezalezna.pl/68286-dron-aborcyjny-leci-nad-polske.

130. Elżbieta Korolczuk, "Explaining Mass Protests against Abortion Ban in Poland: The Power of Connective Action," *Zoon Politikon*, no. 7 (2016): 92, https://www.civitas.edu.pl/collegium/wp-content/uploads/2015/03/Zoon _Politikon_07_2016_091_113.pdf.

131. Chełstowska, "Stigmatization and Commercialisation," 104.

132. Krystyna Kacpura, "Stop This Crackdown on Abortion in Poland," *Guardian*, September 21, 2016, https://www.theguardian.com/commentisfree /2016/sep/21/stop-abortion-law-crackdown-poland-reproductive-rights.

133. Korolczuk, "Explaining Mass Protests," 95.

[12]

Beyond the Borders of Brexit

Traveling for Abortion Access to a Post-EU Britain

NIKLAS BARKE

UNSAFE ABORTIONS performed internationally, and the corresponding maternal mortality rate, are decreasing slowly but remain alarming.[1] The vast majority of unsafe abortions and accompanying maternal deaths occur globally in developing countries.[2] However, the mistaken suggestion that these are *purely* non-European problems serves as an illustration of "us versus them" racialized thinking, or othering, that is becoming more and more characteristic of Europe.[3] The reason for the relatively low number of unsafe abortions and consequent maternal deaths within Europe relates to the greater accessibility of safe and legal abortion services in this region as well as a greater possibility for women to travel in order to access these services.[4]

For women based in countries that have harsh abortion regulations, Britain (England, Scotland, and Wales) has for a long time served as a global destination hub for safe and legal abortion services, as is indicated in several chapters in this volume.[5] Indeed, as Mary Gilmartin and Sinéad Kennedy outline carefully in their own contribution to this volume, travel to Britain is particularly salient in the case of women from the Republic of Ireland (hereafter Ireland),[6] who have suffered under one of the harshest abortion regimes in the region, since Irish law has permitted legal abortion only when the pregnancy is deemed to threaten the life of the pregnant woman.[7]

The 1967 British Abortion Act, as Gayle Davis et al. note in their chapter in this volume, does not apply to Northern Ireland, where the 1861 Offences against the Person Act and the 1945 Criminal Justice Act have prohibited abortions in all situations except when there is a serious and long-term risk to the pregnant woman's mental or physical health. Thus, as recently as 2017, roughly 4,000 abortions were carried out in Britain on women from Northern Ireland and from the latter's geographical neighbor, Ireland.[8] An additional 800 or so abortions were performed on women not residing in either Ireland or Britain.[9] Moreover, it is likely that the number of nonresidents who obtained an abortion in Britain was higher than what the official records tell us, since many women choose to provide a local address for reasons of confidentiality.[10] The lack of accurate data on nonresident women having abortions in Britain is also taken up by Christabelle Sethna in this volume.

The fact that, on average, at least 15 nonresident women have their pregnancies terminated in Britain every day entails an additional observation: Brexit is potentially a dark cloud on the horizon for many women who, in the future, may want to travel to Britain in order to access a safe and legal abortion. However, a referendum held in Ireland on May 25, 2018, that repealed the country's Eighth Amendment may offset, at least in the long term, some of the potential complications Brexit could cause in regard to the cross-border travel of women from Ireland and Northern Ireland.[11]

Brexit is the result of a promise made in 2013 by former British prime minister David Cameron: a referendum on the membership of the United Kingdom (UK), consisting of England, Scotland, Wales, and Northern Ireland, in the European Union (EU).[12] The referendum itself was held on June 23, 2016. With roughly 17.4 million votes (52 percent) cast in favor of leaving the EU, against 16.1 million (48 percent) in favor of remaining, the British electorate voted for an exit from the EU, and the term "Brexit" was coined.[13] Data indicate that Northern Ireland and Scotland were more in favor of remaining within the EU, whereas England and Wales voted in greater numbers to leave. Still, the fairly narrow margin overall between the "Leave" and "Remain" sides demonstrates a clear division regarding how the British have felt toward Europe in recent years, a division reflected also by many British politicians.[14] Cameron had himself championed and promoted the Remain side during referendum campaigning and, as a consequence of the result, decided to resign from office.[15] He was replaced as leader of the Conservative Party by then home secretary Theresa May, who became the new British prime minister.

In March 2017, May invoked Article 50 of the Treaty of Lisbon, which triggered the start of formal negotiations between the UK and the EU to resolve exactly how Brexit would be achieved.[16] In a letter from May to the president of the European Council, Donald Tusk, she raised a number of issues that the UK government believed would require consideration by both sides.[17] Given how decisive the topic was among members of her own parliament, May also called a snap parliamentary election, with the aim of strengthening her position in the Brexit negotiations.[18] The election took place on June 8, 2017, but "backfired spectacularly" for May, who ended up with fewer members of Parliament, lost her party's majority, and was placed in a weaker bargaining position than before.[19]

Negotiations between the UK and EU are ongoing but far from resolved.[20] This is a point in time when little can be said with absolute certainty.[21] However, the aim of this chapter is to consider the possible impact of Brexit on the matter of abortion provision and the freedom of movement across UK borders in a post-EU scenario. While dozens of questions about what Brexit might mean for trade, law and order, investment, and even the price of Scotch whisky[22] have arisen, travel to access abortion services, especially for Northern Irish and Irish women, is isolated on the borders of discussions about Brexit. This chapter examines which direction the Brexit negotiations may take, differentiating between a "soft" and "hard" UK departure from the EU. It investigates the situation in Ireland, an EU member state, both before and after Ireland's recent referendum to repeal the Eighth Amendment and, ultimately, speculates about the implications of both the Brexit and the Irish referendums for Irish and Northern Irish women seeking abortion services.

Abortion Travel to Britain Prior to Brexit

For women living in EU countries where abortions are prohibited, or difficult to obtain, and who are compelled to access abortion services in Britain, three main issues need to be overcome: travel, eligibility, and funding. Funding has been the primary obstacle, as the authors of several chapters in this volume ascertain. While the UK has been a member of the EU, eligibility for and physical accessibility to the procedure has not constituted a major impediment. The UK is bound by one of the EU's cornerstone principles, the Freedom of Movement (FoM) of persons.[23] This means that non-UK EU citizens have the right to travel freely to the UK without having to obtain a visa or otherwise declare the purpose of their visit.[24] Thus for women who normally reside anywhere in the EU, there has been no obstacle per se to entering the UK. In addition, the UK and Ireland have parallel regulatory systems that allow Irish women to enter the UK without even a passport.[25]

British abortion law is in practice quite liberal and termination of pregnancy services accessible. A pregnant woman's personal wish to have an abortion does not constitute sufficient grounds for her to have that abortion: two doctors must agree that the procedure is necessary in order to avert a risk to the pregnant woman's physical or mental health, or to her existing children.[26] However, since the risk of continuing with a pregnancy is generally considered greater than if it were terminated in a safe medical environment, doctors have increasingly felt it appropriate to fulfil the woman's request.[27] In this regard, although it was not the intention of the law, abortion in Britain can arguably be characterized as available "on request." The procedure is legal in Britain up to 24 weeks' gestation, but if there is a substantial risk to the pregnant woman's life, or if the fetus suffers from abnormalities, the time limit is waived.[28] Additionally, there is no requirement that the pregnant woman reside in Britain or be a British citizen. However, British residents are, in theory, eligible for a free abortion funded by the public National Health Service (NHS)—though, as Gayle Davis et al. illustrate, this is not always available in practice—whereas those who are not British citizens have had to pay for the service themselves. While women from Northern Ireland are now entitled to free NHS healthcare, like their mainland counterparts, this situation has not historically extended to abortion provision, which had to be funded by the women themselves. This anomalous position began to change only in mid-2017.[29]

Although carried out by medical professionals, abortions still reside outside the mainstream healthcare system. These procedures are governed effectively by criminal law regulations, quite distinct from other medical measures.[30] If you break your arm or cut yourself, a doctor will alleviate these issues with casts and stitches, no questions asked. Conversely, a pregnant woman will have to fulfil certain requirements to be entitled to obtain a legal abortion; if you get pregnant and do not wish to become a parent, you will need the authorities to approve the necessary medical procedure. The fact that the British government chose to regulate abortion as part of the country's criminal law system might be considered detrimental to maternal health or women's rights.[31] However, within the context of Brexit, this—together with the fact that nonresidents' abortion requests are not covered by public healthcare insurance—is something that could potentially be positive for those traveling to Britain in pursuit of a termination in the future.

Funding is the third and major impediment for women forced to travel in search of abortion services. The lack of affordable transportation and accommodation options can be a very difficult, and sometimes impossible, obstacle to overcome. Whereas Lori A. Brown in this volume has calculated the costs of traveling considerable distances by bus within the state of Texas, the costs of transportation to Britain from the EU can involve buses, cars, trains, and ferries, but the area is most likely accessed by airplane. A return flight to London midweek from Dublin starts at €40, and from Warsaw costs as much as €120. In addition, one requires transportation to and from the airport, as well as overnight accommodation. If the pregnant woman also has to take time off work to make the trip, the issue of lost income can further damage her financial situation. Crucially, one must add to this ledger the cost of the actual procedure, which starts at approximately €500 but can easily total more than €2,000 for abortions between 20 and 24 weeks' gestation, the latest stage at which an abortion can legally be performed in Britain today.[32]

Hence, as things stand before Britain formally leaves the EU, abortion has been readily available and accessible for nonresident women from any EU member state, so long as they can overcome funding hurdles related to their economic status. While more difficult to quantify, further impediments exist in terms of the stigma surrounding abortion in many of the countries from which women travel. The desperation that compels women to travel domestically and internationally for abortion services is driven home keenly throughout this volume; highlighting just two examples, that desperation has led New Zealand women to travel to Australia for abortion services and Australian women to traverse vast distances to a neighboring state within the country for the same purpose, as investigated in this volume by Hayley Brown and Barbara Baird, respectively. It may seem obvious, but should nonetheless be stressed, that women traveling for an abortion typically do so not on account of traveling for fun but out of necessity stemming from the conservative, restrictive, and often aggressively antichoice societies in which they normally reside. Even for women whose financial circumstances are comfortable, where the economic burden of abortion travel is, therefore, less of an issue, the stigma of ending a pregnancy can transcend their social status.[33]

Background to Brexit

Following an expansion of the EU eastward during the early twenty-first century, there was a noticeable movement westward of citizens from Eastern Europe, a region that Anna Bogic and Ewelina Ciaputa examine in their respective chapters in this volume in regard to access to abortion services. Some EU countries responded by imposing restrictions and/or quotas on immigrants, but others—including the UK—did not.[34] Later in the same decade, the "Financial Crisis"[35] affected most of Europe quite severely. This resulted in a political shift toward the Right in many European countries, in which right-wing populist parties began to make significant advances.

The UK, which effectively has a two-party political system with either the Conservative Party or the Labour Party in power, has as of 2018 not seen any such populist party form a national government. However, over the past 10 to 15 years, the UK Independence Party (UKIP)—a populist party based largely on a pro-nationalism, anti-immigration, and "Euroscepticism" agenda—has slowly advanced in popularity. Critics charge that this agenda was fueled variously by racism against immigrants, a backlash against globalization, and the racial and economic discontent of white middle-class and/or working-class voters.[36] Indeed, in the 2014 election to the European Parliament, UKIP became the largest British party, winning more than one-quarter of the votes. However, while becoming the third-largest party in the UK in the 2015 national elections, with 12.6 percent of the vote, UKIP won only one seat in the 649-seat-strong UK parliament.[37] This proportional imbalance is due in part to the fact that the UK consists of four separate countries, and to the fact that these four entities are each guaranteed a certain number of seats in the national parliament. Although having limited institutional political power, UKIP still had the political clout to exert pressure on the government to hold the Brexit referendum, as well as to influence the actual campaign.[38] Following this referendum, and having achieved his party's one main goal—to have the UK leave the EU—Nigel Farage, UKIP's leader, decided to step down. In the subsequent 2017 snap parliamentary election in the UK, UKIP lost its only seat in Parliament.[39]

The two major political parties in the UK—the Labour Party and the Conservative Party—did not present an internally unified approach toward the electorate as to how they should vote in the referendum. While both parties largely opposed leaving the EU, prominent figures in both parties, especially the Conservative Party, favored the idea of leaving. May, who succeeded Cameron as both party leader and prime minister, had maintained a relatively low profile during the fierce referendum debates. During the campaign, she had declared that the UK should not leave the EU but rather quit the European Convention on Human Rights.[40] When forced to champion the concept of Brexit as the new prime minister in honor of the referendum results, she appointed prominent Conservative Party Brexit supporters such as Boris Johnson to her new cabinet.

Throughout the campaign surrounding the referendum, the Leave camp continuously stressed the need for Britain to regain its lost sovereignty, that is, control over its own finances, laws, and borders.[41] It was alleged that too much money, mainly in the form of the membership fee, was being sent to the EU, money that was badly needed domestically.[42] Still, immigration provoked the greatest controversy. As explained previously, FoM—of persons as well as goods, capital, and services—can be considered the four founding principles of the EU.[43] One of the main benefits of being an EU member, which is gaining access to the EU's inner market (the "single market"), entails the requirement to allow for FoM.[44] Although the UK early on decided to opt out of the Schengen Agreement,[45] the FoM principles still apply. Growing rates of immigration to Britain were said to be hampering the economy, because of the burden that immigrants were said to be in terms of welfare and security.[46] Britain's healthcare system, the NHS, was also believed to be under significant financial strain, due in part to the costs associated with providing non-UK citizens with healthcare. Although it was contested just how accurate this calculation was, one of the Leave side's most popular and well-used slogans during the Brexit campaign was "We send the EU £350 million a week, let's fund our NHS instead," painted in tall letters on the side of campaign buses.[47] The shortcomings and underfunding of the NHS was deployed strategically to showcase putative EU meddling with internal British matters and resources.

The fact that the referendum results more or less split the population in half—52 percent Leave, 48 percent Remain—is reflected in the two main paths that British politicians are currently considering, namely, a hard or a soft Brexit. Somewhat simplified here, a soft Brexit refers to an outcome in which the UK is still quite close to the EU, and where the practical differences between being and not being an EU member are not significant. A hard Brexit refers to a solution where all ties to the EU are cut. It might be noted, however, that those who champion the latter often appear to suggest that the UK can continue to enjoy the main benefits of EU membership, conveniently free from all EU requirements and financial commitments. There are a number of alternative scenarios in which the current Article 50 of the Treaty of Lisbon negotiations could result. The most plausible options are reviewed in the next two sections, before I address the question of which direction the UK is likely to take. A description of these alternatives is presented with regard to how relevant they are to the issue of abortion travel and what consequences may be anticipated here.

The Soft Brexit Option

This possible outcome of Article 50 negotiations, where as little as possible is altered in the practical relationship between the UK and the EU, would presumably be favored by most of those who voted to remain in the EU. A key objective for the UK here would be to retain access to the EU single market. A number of European countries are not members of the EU but still have access to the single market. A closer look at some of these reveals various alternative future possibilities for women traveling to Britain to access abortion services.

The "Norwegian model" would, in the case of the UK, mean remaining a member of the European Economic Area (EEA) by rejoining the European Free Trade Association (EFTA), staying within the single market, and allowing FoM of goods, services, capital, and persons.[48] Remaining in the EEA would require the implementation of certain EU legislation connected to the single market but no longer having any substantial say in the decisions made.[49] This model would also require the UK to pay a fee in order to be part of the single market. Norway's financial contribution to the EU budget is currently 15 to 20 percent lower per capita compared to the UK. While this is a substantial difference, the UK government needs to consider whether it is worth the price of losing a seat at the decision-making table. In addition to this cost "saving," the UK would not be bound by the EU's customs union and could hence decide on its own external tariffs. However, EEA exports to the single market would have to conform to EU rules of origin in order to enter the EU duty free.[50] Crucially, for the purposes of this chapter, EEA membership would not directly affect possible travel to Britain. Rather, the EEA requirement to retain the system of FoM of persons would entail upholding the status quo, allowing the same possibility of abortion travel to Britain as existed before Brexit.

A slightly different alternative is what could be called the "Swiss model." Switzerland has bilaterally negotiated a number of treaties with the EU in order to join various programs and benefit from certain EU policies. Switzerland is also a member of the EFTA, but without being part of the EEA. Through the EFTA and other bilateral agreements, Switzerland can engage in free trade with other EFTA members and the EU on all nonagricultural goods. A precondition for these agreements is that the parties also guarantee FoM of persons. This "à la carte" model has practical outcomes similar to the Norwegian EEA model. However, since Switzerland is the only non-EEA EFTA member, there is only one example of what EFTA membership could entail. The practical consequences of a Swiss model for abortion travel would seem to be similar to the Norwegian model, that is, it would be unlikely to alter the current possibilities for nonresident women traveling to Britain. As with the EEA model, any substantial free trade deal with the EU seems to necessitate allowing FoM of persons.

Alternatively, the UK could strike a comprehensive trade deal that differs slightly from those models but is nonetheless similar. Crucially, any substantial free trade deal would be accompanied by a requirement for the FoM of persons. Any favorable trade deal without FoM of persons would be deemed to risk the stability of the EU, since such a system would be too appealing for other member states and would thereby risk additional member state exits. While not a noticeable feature of French president Emmanuel Macron's agenda since his 2017 election win, he did announce before the election that there was a substantial risk of a French EU exit, a "FREXIT," if the EU failed to reform.[51] Thus, in short, any soft Brexit deal would be favorable for the matter of abortion travel. The concept of FoM would continue to be supported by the

British government, which should allow nonresident women to continue to travel to Britain in search of an abortion.

The Hard Brexit Option

This possible outcome of the Article 50 negotiations is generally understood as a solution where the UK cuts all ties with the EU and rejects its policies and regulations henceforth. In such a scenario, what has been labeled "repatriation of its sovereignty"—including regaining control over its borders—is deemed imperative for the UK.[52] However, it is also quite clear that even the most hard-line Brexit proponents tend to favor a comprehensive trade agreement with the EU. The least severe hard Brexit option would suggestively be one where the UK and the EU agree on either a new customs union or a limited tariff-free trade deal. Any deal that would qualify as, and satisfy the supporters of a hard Brexit, would inevitably have to be restricted in what it includes: too inclusive (e.g., trade in goods *and* services) and the EU would demand FoM of persons, something that would contradict the war cry of taking back control over UK borders.

Although subject to increasing opposition,[53] the main idea that has been put forward by May is to cut all existing ties to the EU and then rejoin the sectors that are of particular interest to the UK. Such a model would be tailored to conform to the top two priorities of the Conservative Party: to control EU immigration and to withdraw from the jurisdiction of the European Court of Justice (ECJ).[54] Withdrawing from the ECJ should here be viewed as "regaining sovereignty" and "taking back control over the legal system."[55] Whatever the specificities of a hard Brexit outcome, it could prove highly detrimental to prospective abortion travelers, since the principle of FoM of persons would be relaxed or suspended outright.

In a more moderate Brexit scenario, the UK might secure a trade deal that would allow it to relinquish the FoM of persons system and instead introduce a simplified visa process much like the Electronic System for Travel Authorization (ESTA) in the United States of America (USA), or the Canadian Electronic Travel Authorization (ETA) system. Such a system would typically apply uniformly toward all EU countries, with the possibility of separate treatment of non-Schengen countries such as Romania and Bulgaria. The idea with these types of systems is to have a simple procedure that allows people to travel for the purposes of tourism or short-term visits while being able to observe and control who is actually crossing a nation's borders. In a scenario where an ESTA/ETA-like system is put in place, it would mean an additional obstacle in the way of women wishing to travel to Britain for abortion purposes, although these obstacles should not be too difficult to overcome. However, if it were the case that Romania and Bulgaria, as non-Schengen members, were not included in this system, it should be noted that women from these countries are nonetheless less likely to travel to Britain for an abortion, compared with women located elsewhere in Europe, since abortion is available on request up to 14 weeks' gestation in both Romania and Bulgaria.[56]

Without agreement on the actual terms of the UK's exit from the EU, there can be no negotiations on trade. In such a situation, the UK would automatically fall back on the trade rules of the World Trade Organization (WTO). Trading under these rules would not require the UK to accept any regulations resembling those pertaining to the EU FoM of persons. A formal visa system might be put in place for travel between the UK and EU.[57] Such is the case between China and the EU, with trade based on WTO rules, and EU-China travels require a visa. However, this is not a very likely outcome. The UK economy depends to a great extent on tourism, and introducing complicated visa application systems would risk decreasing the revenues made from the tourism industry. Roughly 10 percent of jobs in the UK, as well as 10 percent of the UK's GDP, comes from the tourism sector.[58] More plausible is a system similar to ESTA and ETA. This way, traveling to the UK would remain a relatively easy option, albeit one now placed under the direct control and regulation of the UK authorities. In this scenario, without any specific trade agreement between the EU and the UK, the EU could not make any demands about EU or Schengen nationals being treated equally. The UK authorities could, therefore, decide on a country-by-country basis how persons from different countries should be allowed to enter the UK, something that could therefore potentially be detrimental to women from those EU countries not favored by the UK. Current complications concerning FoM are reminiscent of those observed decades ago. According to Christabelle Sethna in her contribution to this volume, suggested border controls to manage the flow of nonresident women traveling to Britain for abortion services soon after the passage of the 1967 act were seen as impractical on numerous levels, including the inconvenience such controls would pose to general tourist traffic.

Likely Consequences of Brexit and the Irish Referendum for Abortion Travel

As discussed earlier, immigration and, consequently, the free movement of persons across EU borders have been some of the most contentious issues to dominate the referendum debates and quite possibly led a slim majority of people in Britain to vote in favor of leaving the EU. Only by leaving, it was argued, would the UK regain full control over its borders, acquiring the power to regulate who could enter the UK and under what circumstances.[59] Echoes of this argument can be heard in Lori A. Brown's chapter in this volume. She contextualizes the interstate travel of women from Texas against the backdrop of state and federal deportation policies targeting undocumented migrants. Given that travel for abortion services can heighten the vulnerability of a woman facing an unwanted pregnancy, it is important to consider the extent to which Brexit might affect women traveling to Britain to have their pregnancies terminated.

We have seen that the majority of nonresident women who attempt to obtain an abortion in Britain travel from Ireland and Northern Ireland. For women residing in Northern Ireland, it is possible that Brexit could cause an additional problem, although it would be constitutionally complicated, if not impossible, for any restrictions on travel to be imposed upon them; even though Northern Ireland is separated by water from mainland Britain, it is still part of the UK. As mentioned previously, women living in Northern Ireland do not have the same access to abortion services as do women in the rest of the UK because abortion in Northern Ireland is not governed by the 1967 British Abortion Act. However, recent reform is changing the situation for women from Northern Ireland, who are now considered eligible for NHS-funded abortion services in Britain.[60]

The referendum in Ireland that resulted in a vote to repeal the Eighth Amendment on May 25, 2018, could provide political momentum for changes to the restrictive abortion regulation in Northern Ireland.[61] This amendment is enshrined in article 40.3.3 of the Irish constitution and obliges the state to protect "the right to life of the unborn . . . with due regards to the equal right to life of the mother," effectively prohibiting abortions in all circumstances except when the pregnant woman's life is at risk. The bar for what has been considered a risk to a pregnant woman's life has, however, been set quite high: the death of Savita Halappanavar in 2012 was a tragic, but arguably strong, catalyst for the push to legalize abortions in Ireland.[62] Halappanavar died of sepsis after doctors refused to perform an abortion on her, even though a miscarriage was deemed inevitable.[63] Article 40.3.3 will be replaced by the wording: "Provisions may be made by law for the regulation of termination of pregnancies." While this change should loosen legal restrictions on abortion within Ireland, it is also broadly viewed as a catalyst for similar reform in Northern Ireland.[64] A separate decision from the UK Supreme Court, coincidentally appearing fewer than two weeks after the Irish referendum, has added to the momentum in Northern Ireland. While the case, brought by the Northern Ireland Human Rights Commission, was dismissed on technical grounds, a majority of the justices stated that abortion regulation in Northern Ireland is not compatible with human rights.[65]

The overall picture is further complicated due to the situation that May finds herself in after the failed snap parliamentary election she called.[66] May ended up with a "hung parliament" and became dependent on political support from the Democratic Unionist Party (DUP), a political party from Northern Ireland that is strongly opposed to abortion.[67] Regardless of how May feels about mitigating the abortion regulations in Northern Ireland, or allowing Northern Ireland to hold a referendum on abortion as well, her primary objective is arguably to maintain enough political power to control Brexit developments, and for that purpose, the DUP is essential.[68] Therefore, it is expected that May will withstand the pressure that she has already come under, not only from Northern Irish campaigners for abortion law reform but also from her own party, at least until the Brexit negotiations are concluded.[69]

Border Regulation

In the interim, a new pathway for Northern Irish women seeking abortion services may emerge. The repeal of the Eighth Amendment in Ireland might lead to a situation where Northern Irish women could be eligible for abortion services in nearby Ireland. Taoiseach Leo Varadkar, the prime minister of Ireland, has stated that he cannot see why Northern Irish women, who are already allowed to access healthcare in Ireland, should not also be allowed to access abortion services once they become part of the country's healthcare system.[70] The nature of this special relationship between Ireland and Northern Ireland highlights yet another complication in the context of Brexit: there is a risk that Brexit will create a two-tier UK citizen system. Under the Belfast Agreement, persons born in Northern Ireland are in general entitled not only to British citizenship but also to Irish citizenship and therefore to membership in the EU.[71] In one scenario, it is suggested that any disadvantages to UK citizens that materialize as a result of Brexit will not affect those persons born in Northern Ireland who obtain an Irish passport. Depending on the outcome of Brexit, and legal reforms in Ireland and possibly also in Northern Ireland concerning abortion services, there could be a situation where British women travel to Northern Ireland to give birth in order to entitle their children to an Irish passport, thereby securing their access to the EU, while Northern Irish women could travel to Ireland or Britain for access to abortion services. Consequently, Northern Ireland might end up expanding its reproductive healthcare sector drastically, without necessarily making abortion access facilities part of that expansion.[72]

The situation for women residing in Ireland, which is not part of the UK, may be even less clear. On the one hand, there may be no major changes in the offing for Irish women who must continue to travel to Britain in search of an abortion. Over time, this kind of travel might diminish gradually due to abortion law reform in the wake of the Irish referendum. Parallel to the EU FoM regulations, Ireland and the UK established the Common Travel Area (CTA) before EU FoM rules were applicable to Ireland or the UK. For people wishing to enter the UK from Ireland, as per section 1(3) of the Immigration Act 1971, there is no immigration control. This does not mean that once you have entered Ireland, you have the right to enter the UK. Rather, it means that Irish citizens are allowed to enter the UK without a passport. Under UK law, Ireland is not considered a foreign country,[73] and Irish nationals are not regarded as foreigners.[74] In theory, Irish women traveling to the UK do not need a passport or visa, but in practice it is at the discretion of the air and sea carriers who transport travelers. Staff on all such carriers are required to check travelers' identities, and some regard passports as the only valid identification. At the time of writing, the main option for traveling between Ireland and the UK, the low-cost Irish airline Ryanair, does not require one to show a passport as long as a traveler can produce another valid form of government-issued photo identification. A passport requirement might seem like a small matter to overcome, but for some women who travel for abortion services, the additional cost of a passport would add to their financial and logistical burdens, which might in some cases prove to be an impossible barrier to surmount.[75]

On the other hand, there is a possibility that the land border between Northern Ireland and Ireland, and the sea border between Ireland and mainland Britain, will be subjected to an increased border control mechanism. When the Article 50 negotiations are over and the UK is formally no longer part of the EU, it will still have a land border with Ireland, an EU country, which shares in turn a border with Northern Ireland and a legal arrangement that allows persons traveling from Ireland to enter the UK via Northern Ireland. The concern here is that as long as both Ireland and the UK are EU members, they could mutually guarantee to uphold the EU requirements that apply equally to both of them. But as the UK departs the EU, both sides will have different obligations to fulfill, which might leave the two countries in a situation in which they cannot continue with a business-as-usual approach to the control of their respective borders.[76]

Since Ireland will still be part of the EU after Brexit, its border with the UK will represent an "external border." Depending on the Article 50 negotiations, the EU might very well oblige Ireland to put in place more thorough border controls than it has currently. Likewise, in leaving the EU, if one of the more important things for the UK is to gain control over its borders, the authorities may see Ireland as offering a risky back door into the UK if the borders remain as open as they are today. The easiest way for British authorities to police who enters the UK from Ireland is to impose passport controls in airports and harbors that receive Irish flights and sea vessels. This would require Irish women seeking abortions to acquire a passport in order to enter Britain, although Irish-UK interstate movements are all too prevalent to seem likely. Any requirement for Irish people wishing to visit the UK to obtain a visa also seems unlikely because the two countries have a close historical connection.

As of October 2018, there has arguably been some development on the issue of border control between the UK and Ireland. According to the "December deal," the UK has committed, regarding the Ireland–

Northern Ireland border, to a "full alignment" with internal market rules if a hard border cannot be avoided.[77] While the precise meaning of "full alignment" is yet to be decided,[78] these negotiations have essentially upheld what is otherwise argued in this chapter regarding the future situation between the UK and Ireland: one way or another, trade and border crossing after Brexit will probably be business as usual.[79]

The results of the Irish referendum might eventually slow down the need for Irish women's travel to Britain for abortion services. Still, abortion law reform in Ireland will not happen overnight, and the efforts needed to construct a functioning system of accessible abortion services should not be underestimated. Legislation must materialize. The new wording of the Irish Constitution replacing Article 40.3.3 does not provide effective abortion regulation; it gives only a mandate to the Irish parliament to enact positive legislation concerning termination of pregnancy. Draft legislation provides for free abortion during the first 12 weeks of pregnancy, and abortion without any time limit when the pregnancy is a threat to the woman's life or when the fetus suffers from a fatal condition.[80] Pregnancy as a result of rape was deliberately not included in the draft, since such situations would fall under the general right to abortion on request during the first 12 weeks. Lawmaking is typically a slow process, and the proposed text contains numerous provisions that will lead to contentious and time-consuming deliberations. The Irish prime minister indicated shortly after the referendum that legislation should not be expected before the end of 2018.[81] Even if this draft is passed as proposed, women needing an abortion after the 12th week would have to continue to travel to Britain.

Yet even with new abortion legislation in place, several practical matters also require resolution. More than 1,000 Irish doctors signed a declaration calling for a vote to repeal the Eighth Amendment, but effectuating the practice of abortion will take time.[82] The draft legislation includes provisions for conscientious objection. With the exception of abortions where the pregnant woman's life is at risk, any medical practitioner can refuse to participate in carrying out an abortion. In such a situation, a medical practitioner must arrange for the transfer of care of a pregnant woman requesting an abortion. Rather than risk any delay, some Irish women will continue to travel to Britain for a timely abortion. Additionally, both medical and surgical abortion arguably require the care of experienced medical practitioners. It is not certain that the current Irish healthcare system will be able to accommodate the thousands of Irish women who leave to access abortion services in Britain every year. The Irish referendum result should be viewed as an advancement of reproductive rights in Ireland, with possible positive side effects also for women in Northern Ireland. However, there is a very real chance that women from both these regions will continue to travel to Britain for abortion services for the foreseeable future.

The question of which border regulations will be put in place for the rest of the EU is even more complex. It should be remembered that while the Brexit negotiations are ongoing, no progress made in the talks is deemed valid until a full agreement has been reached. In line with this is the EU condition that there will be no trade talks before all other matters—FoM, the Status of the European Court of Justice, citizens' rights, and so forth—have been resolved. However, it should be pointed out that British abortion providers and organizations working for the advancement of reproductive healthcare, while aware of the ever-present attempts by antichoice organizations to curb abortion rights and access to related services, are confident of the continuous support of such services by the vast majority of the British population. In fact, even though healthcare, and especially healthcare provided to UK nonresidents, was a topic to which significant attention was devoted during Brexit discussions, abortion services were never used as an argument for or against Brexit and have been on the sidelines of the Brexit discussions altogether.[83]

A final word may be said about the related concept of "human rights." May received a significant degree of criticism for her idea that the UK should not leave the EU but rather the Convention on Human Rights. She has not dropped this idea. Rather, May is promoting it as a foundation for her platform for reelection in 2020.[84] The Convention is a supranational legal instrument separate from the EU. Its 47 signatories must award certain fundamental rights to people within their jurisdictions. While protecting important values, May claims, the Convention is also impeding the UK government from attending to matters of national importance, such as deporting Islamic fundamentalists and other perceived threats to the UK's national security.[85]

The Convention is fairly complicated where the subject of abortion is concerned.[86] While there is typically a reluctance from the Convention's governing judicial body, the European Court of Human Rights, to express any clear principles, the Convention offers a minimum level of rights that permits pregnant women to choose to have an abortion to safeguard their well-being.[87] Since Britain already has a fairly liberal abortion system, the Court is unlikely to have reason to reprimand it. However, states can deviate from this right so long as they fulfil certain requirements, in the case of abortion typically relating to the protection of "morals." Morals are included in the handful of legitimate grounds on which a state can base its deviations from certain rights under the Convention to ensure a state's right to sovereignty or self-determination when there is no consensus on the matter in Europe. The Convention does currently provide an additional safety net for abortion rights in Britain; they cannot be altered in a more restrictive direction without the demonstration of a clear democratic foundation for any such changes. However, were the UK to reject the Convention, it could possibly open up a number of opportunities to restrict access to abortion services.

Any substantial changes in British abortion law are not particularly likely at this point. However, the political shift in a more conservative direction that has been observed throughout the UK and Europe over the past decade should not be dismissed lightly in regard to women's rights in general, and reproductive rights more specifically. Ewelina Ciaputa's contribution to the present volume is especially pertinent because it reveals the steady rollback of reproductive rights in Poland, an EU member since 2004. Furthermore, a glance at the USA shows how quickly threats to certain hard-won reproductive rights victories can be mobilized.[88] At the moment, the Convention serves as a reassuring defense against such a possibility, but its rejection could leave abortion services in Britain in a much more vulnerable position, both for resident and nonresident women alike.

Conclusion

Three main items that could negatively affect travel to Britain for abortion services were steadfastly on the agenda of the Brexit campaigners: controlling entry to the UK, creating more restrictive criteria for nonresidents attempting to access healthcare in the UK, and reducing general expenditures for nonresidents in the UK. While each of these items might complicate the lives of nonresidents wishing to travel to or live in the UK, they do not necessarily pose an insurmountable obstacle for women who come to Britain to obtain an abortion. Women traveling to the UK for abortion services, even in a worst-case scenario, could simply do so as visiting tourists, and at most might require a simplified visa system. Furthermore, since abortion services are generally not subsidized under the NHS for nonresidents, there are few indications, if any, leading to a scenario where issues of access and funding will become more onerous.

While we are as yet uncertain of what the actual results of the Brexit negotiations will be, several matters, including the prospect of a second UK referendum,[89] point toward the possibility for EU residents to enter the UK much as before. State revenues from trade and tourism are in all likelihood too important for UK politicians to risk, so complete isolation from the EU would not appear to be a practical option, a matter that has gained credibility as Brexit negotiations have advanced.[90] Irish women might face the additional burden of being required to hold a valid passport, but if this is part of the final agreement between the UK and EU, it is most likely that this requirement will be phased in over a period of time. Additionally, due to upcoming abortion law reform in Ireland, Irish women will probably become less dependent on travel to Britain to access abortion services and so too may Northern Irish women in the future.

In general, since there is strong support among the British public for women's reproductive rights, support seemingly shared by the authorities,[91] there would appear to be no political points to be won by imposing further restrictions on access to abortion services. Yet in a world where the contemporary trend is a strong shift toward populism and nationalist agendas, in Europe and elsewhere, there are no certainties anymore, if there ever were. Countries that previously enjoyed a strong reputation for their views on human rights, such as Sweden, have adopted remarkably restrictive immigration discourses and laws. Few commentators really believed that the UK would vote to leave the EU, or that the American electorate would choose Donald Trump as their president. The past number of years have seen violent attacks of different magnitudes and with various consequences from political and religious fanatics all over Europe. Contemporary global politics points in a direction where nothing should be taken for granted, and there is always a risk of greater restrictions and further regulation over time. However, in this chapter I have concluded that the most likely outcome of the Brexit process is one where women can continue to travel to Britain in order to gain access to a procedure that they are denied or find difficult to access in their home country, without any new major impediments being placed in their path.

Toward the close of 2018, the seemingly inextricable catch-22 that is the border issue between Ireland and Northern Ireland remained unresolved. Its resolution will be decisive for the Brexit outcome and has substantial consequences for Irish women's accessibility to abortion services: a continued soft border would mean Northern Irish women could potentially benefit from any easing up of Ireland's abortion legislation; a hard border could make matters more difficult. Although an increasing volume of voices sounds the alarm about a "no-deal" Brexit, a rapprochement between the UK and the EU is still probable. Regardless, if the official date for the UK's exit from the EU (March 29, 2019) is prolonged or if there is a no-deal divorce between the UK and the EU, the argument remains: the UK cannot afford to isolate itself from the EU to the extent that traveling in general to the UK will be anything but easily achievable, and hence, abortion travel to Britain will also be possible in the future for those who can afford the journey.[92]

Notes

1. World Health Organization, *Unsafe Abortion: Global and Regional Estimates of the Incidence of Unsafe Abortion and Associated Mortality in 2008*, 6th ed. (Geneva: World Health Organization, 2011), http://apps.who.int/iris/bitstream/10665/44529/1/9789241501118_eng.pdf.

2. Elisabeth Åhman and Iqbal H. Shah, "New Estimates and Trends Regarding Unsafe Abortion Mortality," *International Journal of Gynecology and Obstetrics* 115, no. 2 (2011): 124.

3. Gabriella Lazaridis, Giovanna Campani, and Annie Benveniste, *The Rise of the Far Right in Europe: Populist Shifts and "Othering"* (Basingstoke: Palgrave Macmillan, 2016).

4. Caitlin Gerdts et al., "Experiences of Women Who Travel to England for Abortions: An Explanatory Pilot Study," *European Journal of Contraception and Reproductive Health Care* 21, no. 5 (2016): 401–2; Lisa Kelly and Nicole Tuszynski, "Introduction: Banishing Women: The Law and Politics of Abortion Travel," *Columbia Journal of Gender and Law* 33, no. 1 (2016): 27.

5. "Britain" and the "UK" will be used throughout the text to signify slightly different things. Britain is used to mean England, Wales, and Scotland, whereas the UK includes Northern Ireland. This is a necessary distinction since it is the UK as a whole that is a member of, and plans to leave, the EU, while it is to Britain (and mainly England) that women travel to have an abortion performed. The main difference lies in the separate and much more restrictive abortion laws in force in Northern Ireland, where abortion is only permitted when the pregnant woman's life is at risk.

6. Ann Rossiter, *Ireland's Hidden Diaspora: The Abortion Trail and the Making of a London-Irish Underground, 1980–2000* (London: IASC Publications, 2009); Alyssa Best, "Abortion Rights along the Irish-English Border and

the Liminality of Women's Experiences," *Dialectical Anthropology* 29, nos. 3–4 (September 2005): 424.

7. Article 40.3.3 of the Irish Constitution and the Protection of Life during Pregnancy Act (2013).

8. Department of Health [UK], *Abortion Statistics, England and Wales: 2017, Summary Information from the Abortion Notification Forms Returned to the Chief Medical Officers of England and Wales* (London: Crown, 2018), https://assets.publishing.service.gov.uk/government/uploads/system/uploads /attachment_data/file/714183/2017_Abortion_Statistics_Commentary.pdf.

9. Department of Health [UK], *Abortion Statistics, England and Wales*, 4.

10. Best, "Abortion Rights along the Irish-English Border," 431.

11. "The Irish Times View on the Referendum: This Belongs to the Women of Ireland," *Irish Times*, May 29, 2018, https://www.irishtimes.com/news /politics/abortion-referendum/the-irish-times-view-on-the-referendum-this -belongs-to-the-women-of-ireland-1.3510518.

12. Nicholas Watt, "EU Referendum: In-Out Choice by End of 2017, Cameron Promises," *Guardian*, January 23, 2013, https://www.theguardian.com /politics/2013/jan/22/eu-referendum-2017-david-cameron.

13. "EU Referendum Results," BBC News, accessed February 15, 2018, http://www.bbc.com/news/politics/eu_referendum/results.

14. John Charlton, "Brexit Schmexit," *Information Today* 33, no. 7 (2016): 1–3.

15. Heather Stewart, Rowena Mason, and Rajeev Syal, "David Cameron Resigns after UK Votes to Leave European Union," *Guardian*, June 24, 2016, https://www.theguardian.com/politics/2016/jun/24/david-cameron-resigns-after -uk-votes-to-leave-european-union.

16. George Parker and Kate Allen, "Brexit Begins as Theresa May Triggers Article 50," *Financial Times*, March 30, 2017, https://www.ft.com/content /22c0d426-1466-11e7-b0c1-37e417ee6c76.

17. "Prime Minister's Letter to Donald Tusk, Triggering Article 50," March 29, 2017, https://www.gov.uk/government/publications/prime-ministers -letter-to-donald-tusk-triggering-article-50.

18. Joe Watts, "Theresa May Calls for a Snap UK General Election Saying Brexit Process Needs a Strong Government," *Independent*, April 18, 2017, https://www.independent.co.uk/news/uk/politics/general-election-theresa-may -snap-uk-2017-what-date-tory-labour-jeremy-corbyn-conservative-a7688396 .html.

19. Niall McCarthy, "Theresa May's Snap Election Gamble Has Backfired Spectacularly," *Forbes*, June 9, 2017, https://www.forbes.com/sites/niallmccarthy /2017/06/09/theresa-mays-snap-election-gamble-has-backfired-spectacularly -infographic/#14ba4fb473c3.

20. Daniel Boffey, "EU Leaders Agree Brexit Talks Can Move on to Phase Two," *Guardian*, December 15, 2017, https://www.theguardian.com/politics /2017/dec/15/brexit-talks-eu-next-phase-brussels-theresa-may; James Rothwell, "Brexit, Phase Two: What Happens Next," *Telegraph*, December 15, 2017, https://www.telegraph.co.uk/news/2017/12/15/happens-next-brexit-talks/.

21. James Galbraith, "Europe and the World after Brexit," *Globalizations* 14, no. 1 (2017): 164.

22. Mark Leftly et al., "42 Questions about Brexit That Need Answering," *Time*, March 29, 2017, http://time.com/4699743/brexit-theresa-may-questions-unanswered/.

23. Treaty of the Functioning of the European Union (TFEU), Articles 4(2)(a), 26. For more information about abortion rights at the EU level, see Christina Zampas, "Legal and Political Discourses on Women's Right to Abortion," in *A Fragmented Landscape: Abortion Governance and Protest Logics in Europe*, ed. Silvia De Zordo, Joanna Mishtal, and Lorena Anton (New York: Berghahn Books, 2017), 23–45.

24. TFEU, Article 21; Charter of Fundamental Rights of the European Union (2000/C 364/01), Article 45.

25. Terry McGuinness and Melanie Gower, "The Common Travel Area, and the Special Status of Irish Nationals in UK Law," *House of Commons Library* 7661 (2017): 4–5.

26. Abortion Act 1967, c. 87, October 27, 1967.

27. Jennie Bristow, *Britain's Abortion Law: What It Says, and Why* (Stratford-upon-Avon: British Pregnancy Advisory Service, May 2013), 4, http://www.reproductivereview.org/images/uploads/Britains_abortion_law.pdf.

28. Abortion Act 1967, Article 1(1)(a)-(d).

29. Jessica Elgot and Henry McDonald, "Northern Irish Women Win Access to Free Abortions as May Averts Rebellion," *Guardian*, June 29, 2017, https://www.theguardian.com/world/2017/jun/29/rebel-tories-could-back-northern-ireland-abortion-amendment.

30. Gavin Colthart, "Abortion Law," *House of Commons Library*, SN/SES/4309 (2009): 2.

31. Meda Chesney-Lind and Syeda Tonima Hadi, "Patriarchy, Abortion, and the Criminal System: Policing Female Bodies," *Women and Criminal Justice* 27, no. 1 (2017): 74.

32. "Private Abortion Fees," Marie Stopes UK, accessed February 15, 2018, https://www.mariestopes.org.uk/abortion-services/fees/.

33. Joanna N. Erdman, "The Law of Stigma, Travel, and the Abortion-Free Island," *Columbia Journal of Law and Gender* 33, no. 1 (2016): 29–37.

34. Jonathan Portes, "Immigration, Free Movement and the EU Referendum," *National Institute Economic Review* 236, no. 5 (2016): 16.

35. The "Financial Crisis" refers to the global financial crisis that originated in the subprime mortgage market in the USA then spread to the banking sector, first in the USA and later in Europe.

36. Gurminder K. Bhambra, "Brexit, Trump, and 'Methodological Whiteness': On the Misrecognition of Race and Class," *British Journal of Sociology* 68, no. S1 (November 2017): 214–32.

37. "Current State of the Parties," UK Parliament, accessed February 15, 2018, http://www.parliament.uk/mps-lords-and-offices/mps/current-state-of-the-parties/.

38. Eiko Thielemann and Daniel Schade, "Buying into Myths: Free Movement of People and Immigration," *Political Quarterly* 87, no. 2 (2016): 139.

39. Ben Kentish, "Election Results: Ukip Leader Paul Nuttall Loses by Wide Margin as Party Collapses Nationwide," *Independent*, June 9, 2017, https://www.independent.co.uk/News/uk/politics/election-results-latest-ukip-seats-vote-share-paul-nuttall-a7780406.html.

40. Gavin Stamp, "Who Is Theresa May: A Profile of UK's New Prime Minister," *BBC News*, July 25, 2016, http://www.bbc.com/news/uk-politics -36660372.

41. Ben Riley-Smith, "Leave or Remain in the EU? The Arguments for and against Brexit," *Telegraph*, June 20, 2016, https://www.telegraph.co.uk/politics /2016/06/16/leave-or-remain-in-the-eu-the-arguments-for-and-against-brexit/.

42. Macer Hall, "Taxpayers to Fork Out £370m A WEEK if Britain Does Not Leave the EU," *Express*, March 16, 2016, https://www.express.co.uk/news /politics/652817/British-taxpayer-EU-bill-pay-out-Brussels-hundreds-millions-if -not-leave-Brexit-referendum.

43. Mariusz Maciejewski and Louis Dancourt, "The Internal Market: General Principles," European Union Parliament, November 2017, http://www .europarl.europa.eu/atyourservice/en/displayFtu.html?ftuId=FTU_2.1.1.html.

44. Joe Watts, "Angela Merkel Vows to Block Full Single Market Access without Free Movement after Theresa May Interview," *Independent*, January 9, 2017, https://www.independent.co.uk/news/uk/politics/brexit-latest-angela -merkel-single-market-free-movement-theresa-may-a7517951.html; Chris Campbell, "Single Market Access NOT POSSIBLE without Full Freedom of Movement, Says Macron Aide," *Express*, April 22, 2017, https://www.express .co.uk/news/uk/795082/No-single-market-access-without-freedom-movement -Emmanuel-Macron-French-presidential-EU.

45. The Schengen Agreement is an agreement between 22 of the EU member states to abolish internal border controls, meaning mainly that once someone is within this area, they can move freely between the different countries that constitute the Schengen Area.

46. Sofia Vasilopoulou, "UK Euroscepticism and the Brexit Referendum," *Political Quarterly* 87, no. 2 (2016): 219–20.

47. Ben Chu, "EU Referendum: Statistics Regulator Loses Patience with Leave Campaign over '£350m a Week' EU Cost Figure," *Independent*, May 27, 2016, https://www.independent.co.uk/news/business/news/eu-referendum -statistics-regulator-loses-patience-with-leave-campaign-over-350m-a-week-eu -cost-a7051756.html.

48. "The European Free Trade Association," European Free Trade Association, accessed February 15, 2018, http://www.efta.int/about-efta/european-free -trade-association.

49. Swati Dhingra and Thomas Sampson, *Life after BREXIT: What Are the UK's Options Outside the European Union?* (London: Centre for Economic Performance, London School of Economics and Political Science, 2016), 5.

50. Dhingra and Sampson, *Life after BREXIT*, 5.

51. Henry Samuel, "The EU Must Reform or Face a Frexit, Says Emmanuel Macron," *Telegraph*, May 1, 2017, https://www.telegraph.co.uk/news/2017/05 /01/eu-must-reform-face-frexit-says-macron/.

52. Adrian O'Dowd, "Hunt Wants 'New Relationship' with Europe on Health after Brexit," *British Medical Journal* 356, no. j447 (2017): 1.

53. Rob Merrick, "Theresa May Lacks Power to Force Hard Brexit through Parliament, Warns George Osborne," *Independent*, February 1, 2018, https:// www.independent.co.uk/news/uk/politics/theresa-may-hard-brexit-george -osborne-parliament-support-tory-conservatives-eu-a8188751.html.

54. Jon Henley, "Key Points from May's Brexit Speech: What Have We Learned?," *Guardian*, January 17, 2017, https://www.theguardian.com/politics/2017/jan/17/key-points-from-mays-what-have-we-learned.

55. On the development of UK-ECJ issues, see Laura Hughes, Steven Swinford, and Gordon Rayner, "Brexit Deal: Britain Must Accept European Court of Justice Rulings Until 2021, EU Says," *Telegraph*, December 15, 2017, https://www.telegraph.co.uk/news/2017/12/15/theresa-may-applauded-eu-leaders-made-big-effort-jean-claude/; Daniel Boffey, "Brexit: UK Fails to Retain Voice in European Court of Justice," *Guardian*, December 7, 2017, https://www.theguardian.com/politics/2017/dec/07/brexit-uk-fails-to-retain-voice-in-european-court-of-justice.

56. Romanian Penal Code, Law no. 140, November 5, 1996, Article 185; Bulgarian Decree no. 2, February 1, 1990, on the conditions and procedures for the artificial termination of pregnancy, Articles 1–19.

57. "Proper visa system" loosely refers to a system where an individual would have to apply for a visa, including filling out personal information forms, possibly presenting medical certificates or insurance papers, and so forth, in order to visit another country.

58. Deloitte and Oxford Economics, *Tourism: Jobs and Growth. The Economic Contribution of the Tourism Economy in the UK* (London: Deloitte MCS, 2013), https://www.visitbritain.org/sites/default/files/vb-corporate/Documents-Library/documents/Tourism_Jobs_and_Growth_2013.pdf.

59. Matthew Goodwin and Caitlin Milazzo, "Taking Back Control? Investigating the Role of Immigration in the 2016 Vote for Brexit," *British Journal of Politics and International Relations* 19, no. 3 (2017): 450–64.

60. Elgot and McDonald, "Northern Irish Women."

61. Jon Henley, "Irish Abortion Referendum: Yes Wins with 66.4%—as it Happened," *Guardian*, May 26, 2018, https://www.theguardian.com/world/live/2018/may/26/irish-abortion-referendum-result-count-begins-live.

62. Megan Specia, "How Savita Halappanavar's Death Spurred Ireland's Abortion Rights Campaign," *New York Times*, May 27, 2018, https://www.nytimes.com/2018/05/27/world/europe/savita-halappanavar-ireland-abortion.html.

63. Robin de Peyer, "Ireland Abortion Vote: How the Death of Savita Halappanavar Helped Bring about Referendum," *Evening Standard*, May 25, 2018, https://www.standard.co.uk/news/world/savita-halappanavar-how-an-indian-dentists-death-helped-bring-about-the-referendum-on-abortion-in-a3848356.html.

64. Melissa Davey, "'North Is Next': Fresh Fight for Grassroot Power the Beat Ireland Abortion Ban," *Guardian*, June 1, 2018, https://www.theguardian.com/world/2018/jun/02/north-is-next-fresh-fight-for-grassroots-power-that-beat-ireland-abortion-ban.

65. Owen Bowcott, "Northern Ireland Abortion Law Clashes with Human Rights, Judges Say," *Guardian*, June 7, 2018, https://www.theguardian.com/world/2018/jun/07/supreme-court-dismisses-bid-to-overturn-northern-ireland-abortion-laws.

66. Watts, "Theresa May Calls for a Snap UK General Election Saying Brexit Process Needs a Strong Government"; McCarthy, "Theresa May's Snap Election Gamble Has Backfired Spectacularly."

67. Elizabeth Nelson, "We Are the Invisible Victims of the DUP's Anti-Abortion Hardliners," *Guardian*, June 19, 2017, https://www.theguardian.com/commentisfree/2017/jun/19/invisible-victims-dup-anti-abortion-womens-rights-northern-ireland.

68. Jessica Elgott, "Abortion Rights in NI 'Blocked by Deal with DUP' Says Sinn Fèin," *Guardian*, June 7, 2018, https://www.theguardian.com/world/2018/jun/07/abortion-rights-in-ni-blocked-by-deal-with-dup-says-sinn-fein.

69. Jessica Elgot, "May Resists Tory Calls to Act on Northern Ireland Abortion," *Guardian*, June 4, 2018, https://www.theguardian.com/uk-news/2018/jun/04/theresa-may-resists-tory-calls-to-act-on-northern-ireland-abortion; Peter Walker, "No Plans to Intervene on Northern Ireland Abortion Laws, Says No 10," *Guardian*, May 29, 2018, https://www.theguardian.com/politics/2018/may/29/no-plans-to-intervene-on-northern-ireland-abortion-law-says-no-10.

70. Kevin Rawlinson, "Varadkar: Northern Irish Women May be Able to Have Abortion in the Republic," *Guardian*, May 29, 2018, https://www.theguardian.com/world/2018/may/29/varadkar-northern-irish-women-have-abortions-republic-ireland.

71. "The Belfast Agreement (The Good Friday Agreement; Northern Ireland Peace Agreement)," Belfast, 1998, Annex A, Article 1(vi) and Annex 2, https://www.dfa.ie/media/dfa/alldfawebsitemedia/ourrolesandpolicies/northernireland/good-friday-agreement.pdf.

72. Tristan Cork, "Abortions, Births and the Belfast Child Question: Will the Brexit Deal Make Bristolians Second Class Citizens in Bristol?," *Bristol Post*, December 10, 2017, https://www.bristolpost.co.uk/news/bristol-news/abortions-births-belfast-child-question-901136.

73. Ireland Act 1949, Section 2.

74. British Nationality Act 1981, Section 50(1).

75. The fee for obtaining a passport is €80, as of May 23, 2018. See "Passport Fees," Department of Foreign Affairs and Trade [Ireland], accessed May 23, 2018, https://www.dfa.ie/passports-citizenship/top-passport-questions/passport-fees/.

76. Alexandra Porumbescu, "Freedom of Movement within the European Union vs. Border Security," *Annals of the "Constantin Brâncuşi" University of Târgu Jiu, Letter and Social Science Series* 4 (2015): 90–99.

77. Joint report TF50 (2017) 19—Commission to EU 27:§§ 43, 49.

78. John Campbell, "Brexit: Michel Barnier Says Part of Border Deal Not Fully Agreed," BBC News, February 1, 2018, http://www.bbc.com/news/uk-northern-ireland-politics-42895358.

79. Commission to EU 27, *Joint Report from the Negotiators of the European Union and the United Kingdom Government on Progress during Phase 1 of the Negotiations under Article 50 TEU on the United Kingdom's Orderly Withdrawal from the European Union*, TF50 (2017) 19, December 8, 2017, especially §§ 42, 49–50, accessed February 22, 2018, https://ec.europa.eu/commission/sites/beta-political/files/joint_report.pdf.

80. "General Scheme of a Bill to Regulate Termination of Pregnancy," Department of Health, Dublin, 2018, https://health.gov.ie/wp-content/uploads/2018/03/General-Scheme-for-Publication.pdf.

81. Harriet Agerholm, "Ireland to Enact New Abortion Law 'by End of this Year,' PM Leo Varadkar Says," *Independent*, May 26, 2018, https://www .independent.co.uk/news/world/europe/ireland-abortion-law-new-end-year -varadkar-referendum-result-latest-a8370506.html.

82. Sorcha Pollak, "Abortion: Over 1,000 Doctors Call for Yes Vote in Referendum," *Irish Times*, May 12, 2018, https://www.irishtimes.com/news/social -affairs/abortion-over-1-000-doctors-call-for-yes-vote-in-referendum-1.3493355.

83. Regarding the absence of abortion as a rationale for voters, see Harold D. Clarke, Matthew Goodwin, and Paul Whiteley, "Why Britain Voted for Brexit: An Individual-Level Analysis of the 2016 Referendum Vote," *Parliamentary Affairs* 70, no. 3 (2017): 439–64; Sasha O. Becker, Thiemo Fetzer, and Dennis Novy, "Who Voted for Brexit? A Comprehensive District-Level Analysis," *Economic Policy* 32, no. 92 (October 2017): 601–51.

84. Christopher Hope, "Theresa May to Fight 2020 Election on Plans to Take Britain out of European Convention on Human Rights after Brexit is Completed," *Telegraph*, December 28, 2016, https://www.telegraph.co.uk/news /2016/12/28/theresa-may-fight-2020-election-plans-take-britain-european/.

85. Charlie Cooper, "Theresa May Says UK Should Leave European Human Rights Convention," *Independent*, April 25, 2016, https://www.independent.co .uk/news/uk/politics/european-convention-human-rights-eu-referendum-brexit -theresa-may-a6999701.html. The fact that the UK was instrumental in the creation of the convention appears to be an irony lost on the prime minister. See Patrick Stewart, "What Has the ECHR Ever Done for Us?," *Guardian*, April 25, 2016, https://www.theguardian.com/culture/video/2016/apr/25/patrick-stewart -sketch-what-has-the-echr-ever-done-for-us-video.

86. Joanna N. Erdman, "The Procedural Turn: Abortion at the European Court of Human Rights," in *Abortion Law in Transnational Perspective: Cases and Controversies*, ed. Rebecca Cook, Joanna Erdman, and Bernard Dickens (Philadelphia: University of Pennsylvania Press, 2014), 121–42.

87. A, B, and C v. Ireland, December 16, 2010, ECHR-2010:§214.

88. "Trump's 'Mexico City Policy' or 'Global Gag Rule,'" Questions and Answers, Human Rights Watch, last modified February 8, 2018, https://www .hrw.org/news/2018/02/14/trumps-mexico-city-policy-or-global-gag-rule; Emily Bazelon, "Trump's Abortion Policy," *New York Times*, March 10, 2017, https://www.nytimes.com/2017/03/10/opinion/trumps-abortion-strategy.html.

89. David Schrieberg, "Brits Overwhelmingly Favor a Second Brexit Referendum, New Poll Shows," *Forbes*, January 26, 2018, https://www.forbes.com/sites /davidschrieberg1/2018/01/26/brits-overwhelmingly-favor-a-second-brexit -referendum-new-poll-shows/#686b902424e0; Rowena Mason, "Farage's Call for Second Brexit Vote Greeted with Glee by Remainers," *Guardian*, January 12, 2018, https://www.theguardian.com/politics/2018/jan/11/nigel-farage-backs -fresh-brexit-referendum-to-kill-off-issue. However, see also C.W., "Why the British Economy Has Done Better Than Expected since the Brexit Vote," *Economist*, January 15, 2018, https://www.economist.com/the-economist -explains/2018/01/15/why-the-british-economy-has-done-better-than-expected -since-the-brexit-vote, which explores the reasons why Brits might not be motivated to push for a second referendum.

90. Dan Roberts, "Leaked Brexit Impact Report: Key Questions Answered," *Guardian*, January 30, 2018, https://www.theguardian.com/politics/2018/jan/30/key-questions-latest-leaked-brexit-forecasts.

91. Home Office and the RT Hon Amber Rudd MP, "Review into Harassment and Intimidation near Abortion Clinics," GOV.UK, November 26, 2017, https://www.gov.uk/government/news/review-into-harassment-and-intimidation-near-abortion-clinics.

92. John Crace, "Why Brexit and the Northern Irish Border Issue Remains Centre Stage," *GQ*, October 15, 2018, https://www.gq-magazine.co.uk/article/brexit-northern-ireland-border-issue; Elizabeth Piper and Gabriela Baczynska, "Despite 'Big Gaps,' UK and EU Talk Up Brexit Prospects," Reuters, October 18, 2018, https://www.reuters.com/article/uk-britain-eu-summit/despite-big-gaps-uk-and-eu-talk-up-brexit-prospects-idUSKCN1MS0X2; and Abigail Aiken et al., "The Impact of Northern Ireland's Abortion Laws on Women's Abortion Decision-Making and Experiences," *BMJ Sexual and Reproductive Health* (2018), https://srh.bmj.com/content/early/2018/10/19/bmjsrh-2018-200198.

Christabelle Sethna is a historian and professor at the Institute of Feminist and Gender Studies, University of Ottawa. She researches and publishes in the areas of sex education, contraception, and abortion. As principal investigator, she has been funded by the Social Sciences and Humanities Research Council of Canada. Her research includes a first-time study on the domestic travel of Canadian women to abortion clinics and a current study on the international travel of women for abortion services. Her most recent book, coauthored with Steve Hewitt, is *Just Watch Us: RCMP Surveillance of the Women's Liberation Movement in Cold War Canada* (2018).

Gayle Davis is senior lecturer in the history of medicine at the University of Edinburgh. She has published widely on reproductive health, clinical practice, and policy-making in post–World War II Britain. Recent publications include (with Tracey Loughran) *The Palgrave Handbook of Infertility in History: Approaches, Contexts and Perspectives* (2017) and (with Roger Davidson) *The Sexual State: Sexuality and Scottish Governance, 1950–80* (2012).

Barbara Baird works in women's studies at Flinders University in Adelaide, South Australia, a university built on the unceded land of the Kaurna people (the Indigenous traditional owners). Her research focuses on the history and cultural politics of sexuality and reproduction, and the mutually constitutive nature of the politics of sexuality, gender, race, and nation. Her recent work on abortion has been published in *Australian Feminist Studies*, *Australian Historical Studies*, *Reproductive Health Matters*, and *Health and Human Rights Journal*.

Niklas Barke is a doctoral candidate at Åbo Akademi University in Finland and a visiting fellow at Sciences Po in Paris. His research focuses on how anti-abortion groups use human rights language and so-called legal arguments to try to influence cases before the European Court of Human Rights. Other areas of interest include legal methodology and discourse analysis, structural aspects of law, and the relationship between laws and people's behavior.

Anna Bogic holds a PhD in women's studies and an MA in translation studies from the University of Ottawa, Canada. Her doctoral dissertation examined the

Serbian translation of the American feminist health classic *Our Bodies, Ourselves* (1971), while her master's thesis focused on the first English translation of Simone de Beauvoir's *The Second Sex* (1949). Her areas of research include feminist translation studies, women's reproductive rights, and feminism in postcommunist Eastern Europe. She is also a freelance translator and teaches courses in women's studies and translation studies.

Hayley Brown is a research fellow at the Centre for History in Public Health, London School of Hygiene and Tropical Medicine. She was previously an honorary research fellow in history at Birkbeck, University of London, from 2012 to 2014. Her research interests cover the fields of the histories of New Zealand, Britain, and Australia in the nineteenth and twentieth centuries. She is interested in the histories of sexuality, reproduction, and gender; the social history of families; legal history; and the history of public health. She is currently working on a history of health system reform in Britain and New Zealand, focusing on the years 1948–1993.

Lori A. Brown is professor of architecture at Syracuse University and a licensed architect in New York, USA. Her creative practice examines relationships between architecture and social justice. She is the author of *Contested Spaces: Abortion Clinics, Women's Shelters and Hospitals* (2016) and *Feminist Practices: Interdisciplinary Approaches to Women in Architecture* (2013). Her current projects include "Birthing Centers, Borders and Bodies" and the *Bloomsbury Global Encyclopedia of Women in Architecture* with Dr. Karen Burns. She is the cofounder of and leads ArchiteXX in New York City.

Cathrine Chambers is a feminist trauma therapist in private practice as well as president of the Kamala Institute: Centre for the Integrated Treatment of Trauma and Anxiety in Antigonish, Nova Scotia, Canada. She was the research assistant for the study "Understanding for a Change: Interrogating the Effects of 20 Years of Denying Women Access to an Abortion in PEI" under the direction of Dr. Colleen MacQuarrie, Department of Psychology, University of Prince Edward Island, Canada. Furthermore, she is a member of the PEI Abortion Rights Network and is passionate about reproductive justice, feminist approaches to healing, and advocating for the rights of women and girls in Atlantic Canada.

Ewelina Ciaputa is a feminist, sociologist, and researcher at the Institute of Sociology, Jagiellonian University in Kraków, Poland. Her interests include gender studies, reproductive health and rights, and citizenship and identity studies. Her latest publications include "Reproductive Rights and Gender Equality in Poland after 1989," in *Gender Equality and Quality of Life: Perspectives from Poland and Norway*, edited by Marta Warat, Ewa Krzaklewska, Anna Ratecka, and Krystyna Slany (2016), and "Motherhood of Women with Physical, Visual and Hearing

Disabilities" (coauthored with Aleksandra Migalska, Agnieszka Król, and Marta Warat), *Studia Socjologiczne* 2 (2014): 203–24.

Mary Gilmartin is a professor in the Department of Geography at Maynooth University, Ireland. She writes about contemporary migration and mobility in Ireland, and is the author of *Ireland and Migration in the Twenty-First Century* (2015).

Agata Ignaciuk holds a doctorate in women's and gender studies from the University of Granada, Spain. She is a fellow at the Institute of Ethnology and Cultural Anthropology, University of Warsaw, Poland, and a collaborator in both the Department of the History of Science, University of Granada, and the Institute of Feminist and Gender Studies, University of Ottawa. Her research interests include the transnational history of reproductive health, contraception, and abortion, as well as the history of women and gender in Spain and Poland.

Sinéad Kennedy teaches in the Department of English at Maynooth University, Ireland. She is a coeditor of *The Abortion Papers Ireland: Volume 2* (2015) as well as a longtime abortion rights activist in Ireland and national secretary of the Coalition to Repeal the Eighth Amendment.

Lena Lennerhed is professor of the history of ideas. Her research focus is sexuality and gender in twentieth-century Sweden, including the Swedish sex-liberalism movement of the early 1960s and the formation and development of Swedish sex reform organization Riksförbundet för sexuell upplysning (RFSU). Her publications include books on illegal abortion, *Historier om ett brott* (2008), and legal abortion, *Kvinnotrubbel: Abort i Sverige 1938–1974* (2017).

Jo-Ann MacDonald is an associate professor in the Faculty of Nursing at the University of Prince Edward Island, Canada. She joined the university in 2002 after completing 20 years of work experience in local and provincial health programs.

Colleen MacQuarrie is a professor in the Department of Psychology at the University of Prince Edward Island, Canada. Active in feminist organizations for more than 20 years, she is an academic activist and developmental health researcher whose program of research is directed to understand better the multifaceted nature of health and wellness across the life span and within diverse community settings. She teaches a range of courses from foundational through to upper level, including classes in adulthood, aging, qualitative methodologies, as well as in social justice in psychology.

Jane O'Neill obtained her Economic and Social Research Council–funded PhD from the University of Edinburgh, where she is now a research associate on the

Arts and Humanities Research Council–funded project "The Abortion Act (1967): A Biography" with principal investigator Sally Sheldon. Her research interests include twentieth-century histories of gender, sexuality, courtship, and youth. Recent publications include "'Education not Fornication'? Sexual Morality among Students in Scotland, 1955–1975," in *Students in Twentieth-Century Britain and Ireland*, edited by Jodi Burkett (2018).

Clare Parker obtained her PhD from the University of Adelaide and is now a research associate on the Arts and Humanities Research Council–funded project "The Abortion Act (1967): A Biography" (with principal investigator Sally Sheldon). Her publications include "From Immorality to Public Health: Thalidomide and the Debate for Legal Abortion in Australia," *Social History of Medicine* 25, no. 4 (2012): 863–80; "A Parliament's Right to Choose: Abortion Law Reform in South Australia," *History Australia* 11, no. 2 (2014): 60–79; and *Sex and the State: Abortion, Homosexuality and the Sexual Revolution in South Australia* (forthcoming).

Sally Sheldon is professor of law at the University of Kent, where she researches in the area of healthcare ethics and law. Her extensive list of publications includes "British Abortion Law: Speaking from the Past to Govern the Future," *Modern Law Review* 79, no. 2 (2016): 283–316; "The Decriminalisation of Abortion: An Argument for Modernisation," *Oxford Journal of Legal Studies* 36, no. 2 (2015): 1–32; and *Beyond Control: Medical Power and Abortion Law* (1997). She is a trustee of the British Pregnancy Advisory Service, a founding member of Lawyers for Choice, and an editor of the journal *Social and Legal Studies*.

New Zealand Contraception, Sterilisation and Abortion Act (1978), 75, 80, 82

New Zealand Royal Commission on Contraception, Sterilisation and Abortion, 76–77

nonresident women, 46–48, 50–55, 59, 61–64, 66, 69n38, 117, 248n44

North America, 2, 186. *See also* Canada; United States of America

Northern Ireland, 9–10, 133, 142n39, 310–311, 321–329

Northern Ireland Human Rights Commission, 322

Norway, 317–318; "Norwegian model," 317

nurses, 54, 82, 242, 250n64, 251n76, 295

Obama, Barack, 175; administration of, 175, 179

"Obamacare," 179

"obstacle race," 116

obstetricians, 80, 104, 109, 113. *See also* American Congress of Obstetricians and Gynecologists; Royal Australian and New Zealand College of Obstetricians and Gynaecologists; Royal College of Obstetricians and Gynaecologists

Ofstad, Harald, 34–35

Our Bodies, Ourselves (OBOS), 15, 252–257, 266–267, 270–271. See also *Naša tela, mi*

outpatients, 182, 241, 289, 291

Pacific Island women, 78

Partido Popular, 231

passports, 61, 78, 83, 241, 260, 313, 323, 324, 328, 334n75

Patient Assisted Travel Scheme (Australia), 152–153

patients, 4, 5–6, 8, 26–27, 52, 53, 60, 62, 64, 73, 77, 201; American, 173, 177, 179, 183–184, 185, 186, 187, 188, 256; Australian, 73, 79, 90; British, 102, 105, 106, 107, 109, 111, 113, 114, 115, 116, 142–143n48; Canadian, 9, 208, 219; experience of abortion, 207–210, 212, 214–221; foreign, 59, 240, 242; New Zealand,

77, 79, 82, 85, 87, 90, 91; Polish, 283; private, 60, 107; Spanish, 240, 242. *See also* outpatients

Perry, Rick, 178–179, 180

persecution, 207–208, 211

pharmacists, 9, 148, 207, 300–301

physicians. *See* doctors

plane travel, 4, 29, 156, 158, 205, 300, 314. *See also* airports

Planned Parenthood, 181

Poland, 16, 260–261, 278–283; abortion law reform, 284–285; constitution, 296, 308n119; Constitutional Tribunal, 296; government, 288–289, 299–300; legislation, 281–285, 288–289, 293–294, 303n53; Penal Code, 282, 286–287; "Poland Affair," 41–42; Second Republic of, 281–282; Third Republic of, 292–293

Polish Society for Conscious Motherhood, 288, 305n62

politicians, 66, 103, 137, 203–205, 279–282, 298, 311, 317, 328; antichoice, 54, 80–81, 205, 270, 287; pro-choice, 49; right-wing, 300

politics. *See* communism; conservatism; democracy; fascism; feminism; liberalism; radicalism; socialism

postabortion healthcare, 10, 30, 242, 243

postabortion insight, 58

Potts, Malcolm, 48

pregnancy, carrying to term, 1, 115, 128–129, 215, 220, 269–270

Pregnancy Advisory Centre (Australia), 151

"pregnant from Ireland" (PFI), 126

Preterm Clinic (Sydney), 91

Prince Edward Island, 15, 201–210, 221–222

Prince Edward Island Abortion Rights Network, 206

Prince Edward Island Reproductive Rights Organization (PRRO), 205–206

prison, 34, 133, 143n51, 178, 243, 248n28, 263, 282, 285–286, 295, 296. *See also* incarceration

private sector: Australia, 147, 153, 155–157; Britain, 46–47, 49–50, 53–55, 60, 106-7, 110, 111–112, 147; "profiteering," 108–109; Spain, 237

pro-choice activism, 5, 73, 81, 142n45, 203–204, 221, 245, 265–266, 298
pro-choice discourse, 147–148, 252
pro-gun regime, 178, 192–193
pro-life activism, 300–301
pro-life lobby, 10
pro-life organizations, 82, 180, 204, 224n17, 292–293, 299
pro-life regimes, 15, 178, 205, 321–322
pro-life sentiment, 9, 294, 300–301
pronatalism, 15–16, 262, 265, 280–281, 292, 299
psychiatrists, 112, 115–116

race, 7, 8, 12, 26, 60, 65, 194n19, 201, 210, 234. *See also* blacks, non-Hispanic; whites
racism, 160, 315
radicalism, 80, 133, 257,
Reagan, Ronald, 2, 191
referral agencies, 46, 47, 50, 53, 56, 62, 64–65, 66n2, 89–90, 97n86, 131, 186, 240–241, 242, 295, 296
Regius Chair of Midwifery, 103, 104
Regulation of Information Act (Ireland), 135
religion: Baptist, 180; Christian, 27, 40, 78, 180; church as political actor, 280; Episcopal, 104, 284; fanatics, 328; Islamic, 326; Methodist, 180; Muslim, 180; organizations, 125, 138, 208, 224n17, 273n24; Protestant, 202, 204; religious education, 294–295; traditionalism, 203–204, 209–210. *See also* Catholicism
Report on the Working of the Abortion Act, 63
reproductive activism, 131–137
reproductive healthcare, 1–2, 164–165, 172–173, 181, 184–186, 189, 191–193, 299–301, 323, 326
"reproductive mobility," 123–126, 137–138; restriction of, 127–129; reclaiming of, 130–136. *See also* mobility
Republican Party (USA), 179–180
Rex v. Bourne (1938), 108. *See also* Bourne Decision
"right to life," 127, 128, 130, 180, 204, 321–322

Right to Life Association, 204
Roe v. Wade, 1, 3–4, 146, 173, 186–187, 189, 245, 255–257, 259, 261, 271n4
Royal Australian and New Zealand College of Obstetricians and Gynaecologists, 154
Royal College of Midwives (Britain), 117
Royal College of Obstetricians and Gynaecologists (RCOG), Britain, 53, 110, 111–112, 117
rubella, 29, 37–38, 41, 44n50, 49, 258
Ruiz Gallardón, Alberto, 231
Russia, 3, 282
R v. Davidson, 75
R v. Morgentaler, 186–187, 204

Sanford, Wendy, 254
Schengen Agreement, 297, 316, 332n45; non-Schengen countries, 319–320
Scotland, 46, 61, 102–109, 114, 118, 119n8, 310, 311; Aberdeen, 103–106, 110, 114, 116; Dundee, 105; Edinburgh, 105–107; Glasgow, 103, 104–106, 110, 112–114, 119n9; Highlands and Islands, 107
Scottish abortion law, 102–104
Scottish Episcopal Church, 104
Sección Femenina (female branch of La Falange, fascist party), 241
Second Spanish Republic, 233–234
self-induced abortion, 36–37, 217–219, 258, 279, 283
Serbia, 15–16, 252, 265–268, 270–271; abortion bill, 268–269; government of, 268–269; Orthodox Church, 269
Sex and Society Conference (Stockholm, 1964), 291–292
sex education, 25, 32, 172
Simms, Madeleine, 48–49, 67–68n14
Sisters Overseas Service (SOS), 80, 82–83; Christchurch branch, 86–87; Nelson branch, 87
skill, 52, 61, 172, 236, 244–245
Smart, George, 77, 78, 94n23
Smith, Thomas, 103
Smyth, Ailbhe, 1
Social Democratic Party (Sweden), 25; Women's Federation, 38
socialism, 15, 241, 253

Unborn Child Protection Bill (Poland), 293

United Kingdom (UK), 1, 10, 311, 315–320, 323–328, 329n5; parliament, 315–316

United States of America (USA), 1, 3–4, 9, 25, 31, 172–173, 257–261, 270–271, 271n4; Arizona, 28, 31; Louisiana, 187; New Mexico, 187–188; New York, 259–260; Oklahoma, 187–188; Texas, 2, 15, 172–185, 187–192, 197n49

United States v. Texas, 177

vacuum aspiration, 48, 243

Valencia group (abortion provider "Los Naranjos," Spain), 243–244

Vandeput, Suzanne, 34–36, 49

Varadkar, Taoiseach Leo, 126, 137

viability, of a pregnancy, 107, 190; financial, 157–158

Vindicacción Feminista, 233

visas, 29, 78, 128, 313, 319, 320, 323, 324, 328, 333n57

Wales, 46, 61, 102, 108–110, 133–134, 310, 311, 329n5

Weddington, Sarah, 255–256

Western Europe, 2, 13, 59, 253, 283

West Germany, 26–27, 59, 264

"white coat abortion," 241

whites, 2, 7, 160, 178; non-Hispanic, 174; settler societies, 72; voters, 315; women, 28, 33, 40, 49, 51, 53, 297

Whole Woman's Health v. Hellerstedt, 190–191

Women on Waves (WOW), 135, 297–299

Women on Web, 135

Women's Abortion Action Campaign (WAAC), Australia, 73; Adelaide branch, 87

Women's Coalition Group (Ireland), 133–134

Women's Health Foundation (Hobart, Australia), 157

Women's Legal Education and Action Fund (LEAF, Canada), 206

Women's National Abortion Action Campaign (WONAAC), 73

Women's Wellness Program (Canada), 206–207

Women to Blame (exhibition, Ireland), 131, 141n30

World Health Organization, 148

World Trade Organization, 320

Yugoslavia, 252–253, 260–261, 264, 270–271; abortion law, 262–263; feminism, 253, 261, 276n85; language of, 276n90; socialist government of, 262–264